SIXTH EDITION

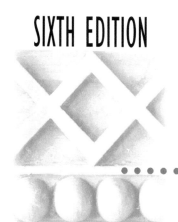

NURSE-CLIENT INTERACTION

Implementing the Nursing Process

Sandra J. Sundeen, RN, MS, CNAA

Chief Psychiatric Nurse,
Mental Hygiene Administration,
Maryland Department of Health and Mental Hygiene;
Adjunct Assistant Professor,
School of Nursing,
University of Maryland,
Baltimore, Maryland

Gail W. Stuart, PhD, RN, CS, FAAN

Center for Health Care Research,
Professor, Colleges of Nursing and Medicine,
Department of Psychiatry & Behavioral Sciences,
Medical University of South Carolina,
Charleston, South Carolina

Elizabeth Anne DeSalvo Rankin, PhD, RN, CMH

Professor,
Department of Nursing,
Salisbury State University,
Salisbury, Maryland

Sylvia Ann Cohen, RN, PhD

School Psychologist,
Scottsdale School System,
Scottsdale, Arizona

with 58 illustrations

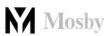 Mosby

St. Louis Baltimore Boston Carlsbad Chicago Minneapolis New York Philadelphia Portland
London Milan Sydney Tokyo Toronto

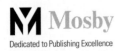

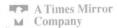

PUBLISHER *Sally Schrefer*
EDITOR *Jeff Burnham*
DEVELOPMENTAL EDITOR *Linda Caldwell*
ASSOCIATE DEVELOPMENTAL EDITOR *Jeff Downing*
PROJECT MANAGER *Dana Peick*
SENIOR PRODUCTION EDITOR *Dottie Martin*
DESIGNER *Amy Buxton*
MANUFACTURING SUPERVISOR *Karen Boehme*

SIXTH EDITION
Copyright © 1998 by Mosby, Inc.

Previous editions copyrighted 1976, 1981, 1985, 1989, 1994

Printed in the United States of America
Composition by Accu-color, Inc.
Printing/binding by R. R. Donnelley & Sons Company

Mosby-Year Book, Inc.
11830 Westline Industrial Drive
St. Louis, Missouri 63146

Library of Congress Cataloging-in-Publication Data
Nurse-client interactions - implementing the nursing process / Sandra Sundeen...[et al.].—6th ed.
    p. cm.
  Includes bibliographical reference and index.
    ISBN 0-8151-2605-0
    1. Nurse and patient.   2. Nursing—Psychological aspects.
  I. Sundeen, Sandra J., 1940–
    [DNLM: 1. Nurse-Patient Relations.   2. Nursing Process. WY 87 N974 1998]
RT86.3.N85 1998
610.73'06'99—dc21
DNLM/DLC
for Library of Congress
                                                         97-42735
                                                           CIP

97 98 99 00 01 / 9 8 7 6 5 4 3 2 1

NURSE-CLIENT
INTERACTION

· ·

Implementing the Nursing Process

PREFACE

The education of professional nurses must meet quality standards. To accomplish this, it is necessary to balance clinical skills and theoretical information. In searching the literature, we have found that a variety of fields, such as psychology, anthropology, cybernetics, humanities, and sociology, contribute to the theoretical basis for the behavioral component of nursing education. However, other than in reference to psychiatric settings, this information does not apply explicitly to the nursing process. In addition, the models used to present theoretical information vary greatly among disciplines and among theorists within a discipline. Other sources provide fragments of the necessary theoretical materials. Therefore the student must independently absorb a wealth of information from a variety of sources, select salient aspects of the theories, and appropriately apply them to the nursing process. We believe that it is advantageous to have one text as a compilation of basic resources with the incorporation of recent research.

This sixth edition will continue to be helpful to students as they grapple with the new challenges of professional interpersonal relationships. Faculty will appreciate the updated and annotated reference materials. The content of the book has been completely reviewed and revised to include any additional pertinent theory that has evolved since the last edition was published. In particular, the section on nursing diagnosis includes the most recent list of NANDA diagnoses. The format of the book has also been revised to add more tables and figures when appropriate, and pages were broken up with additional headings whenever possible.

When the communication process in a human-to-human relationship is viewed as the vehicle through which nursing is accomplished, it becomes necessary to incorporate psychodynamic and socio-logical information into the nursing process. This trend toward integration requires psychiatric nursing, or the therapeutic use of self, to move into the total and varied dimensions of nursing education and practice.

This book is an integrated compilation of psychodynamic principles presented as a single source, synthesizing nursing content based on a broad background of information from primary theorists and research. Since nursing education, to a great extent, builds upon an integration of basic concepts, this text provides a resource for nursing programs and the practicing nurse clinician.

Understanding the behavioral aspects of the nursing process requires an analysis of self, communication, and interpersonal relationships. Chapter 1 of the text presents a brief overview of the phases of the nursing process. Chapters 2 and 3 present theory relative to the development of a self-concept and the growth of self-awareness. Chapters 4, 5, 6, and 7 examine the concepts and phases of the nurse-client relationship, as well as the behavioral manifestations of those concepts and phases—communication. All of the preceding aspects of the nursing process deal with the nurse's ability to help clients move toward their maximum potential.

Chapter 8 focuses on interaction in groups, including introductory information on group dynamics and process. The emphasis is on assisting the student to understand and contribute to the groups that are commonly encountered in the work setting. Chapter 9 presents theory that enables the nurse to analyze the stress states of self and client, as well as the coping and adaptation mechanisms used by each to deal with the stress of daily existence. Chapters 10 and 11 focus on application of the basic concepts of interpersonal relationships in specific client situations involving health promotion and crisis intervention. Changes in the health care system are increasing the need for all nurses to be skilled at providing nursing care before the development of an illness or early in the course of an illness. Chapter 12 is essentially a summary and practical application of the theory presented throughout the book. It should help the reader understand the reciprocal nature of the concepts presented and discussed.

The ideas within the book arose from combined thinking and mutual planning. All of us collaborated in the review and revision of each other's work in an attempt to interrelate the ideas and content of the text. We also created a structure for the book that is designed to facilitate learning. Each chapter begins with learning objectives. An annotated list of additional readings encourages students to explore further concepts that are new to them or difficult to understand. To assist instructors and students in the application of the theory that is presented, each chapter concludes with suggested discussion questions and learning activities.

In recognition of the diversity of the clients that are served by nurses and the diversity of the nurses themselves, we have added a new feature, "Cultural Considerations" boxes, which highlight an aspect of the content that is affected by the cultural background of the client. It is our hope that these cultural inserts will help the student recognize the need to consider the individual differences of clients and incorporate recognition of diversity into nursing practice. In this edition we have also added critical thinking questions throughout each chapter. These are intended to assist students in examining and exploring for themselves challenging aspects of the theoretical material.

Throughout the text an attempt has been made to avoid pronouns that express bias and to give recognition and support to the commitment of both men and women to the nursing profession. However, this has not always been possible. Therefore, for expediency and clarity, the nurse is often referred to in the third person, feminine gender, and the client in the third person, masculine gender. It should also be noted that Ms. is used instead of Miss or Mrs. based on our personal preferences. Finally, because the focus of the book is on wellness, growth, and health, the term *client* is used to describe the individual, family, or group interacting with the nurse throughout the health-illness continuum.

We would like to express our gratitude to all of our family and friends who contributed to the success of this endeavor by sharing their thoughts, ideas, and support. Special thanks to Ms. Elizabeth Faraci DeSalvo for her patience and assistance in typing the original manuscript. Grateful acknowledgments are due to Ms. Dianne Franklin Bald for her artistic contributions. We are particularly appreciative of the many helpful comments we have received from those for whom we wrote this book—the students and faculty of schools of nursing.

CONTENTS *in Brief*

1   *The Nursing Process,* 1

2   *The Emergence of the Self,* 33

3   *The Dynamics of Self-Growth,* 55

4   *The Communication Process,* 81

5   *Therapeutic Communication,* 107

6   *The Nurse-Client Relationship: Theoretic Concepts,* 147

7   *The Course of the Helping Relationship,* 173

8   *Small Groups and Group Process Dynamics: An Overview,* 199

9   *Stress and Adaptation,* 217

10   *Health Promotion Strategies,* 243

11   *Crisis Intervention,* 285

12   *Comprehensive Case Study,* 301

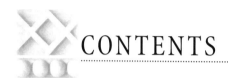

CONTENTS

1 The Nursing Process, 1
Learning Objectives, 1
Philosophical Beliefs, 1
  The Person, 1
  Nursing, 2
Nursing Functions and Levels of
Prevention, 3
  Primary Prevention, 3
  Secondary Prevention, 4
  Tertiary Prevention, 5
Nursing Process, 6
  Assessment, 7
  Nursing Diagnosis, 10
  Outcome Identification, 14
  Planning, 16
  Implementation, 18
  Evaluation, 22
Summary, 24

2 The Emergence of the Self, 33
Learning Objectives, 33
Infancy: Birth to 1 1/2 Years, 36
Toddler Years: 1 1/2 to 3 1/2 Years, 39
Early Childhood: 3 1/2 to 7 Years, 41
Middle Childhood: 7 to 12 Years, 43
Adolescence: 12 to 19 Years, 45
Adulthood, 47
Middle Age, 48
Old Age, 49

3 The Dynamics of Self-Growth, 55
Learning Objectives, 55
Variables of the Self, 56

Body Image, 57
  Developmental Changes, 57
  Effect on Self-Conceptions, 59
  Nursing Assessment, 60
  Related Problems, 61
Self-Ideal, 63
Self-Concept, 64
  Developmental Changes, 64
  Nursing Assessment, 66
Self-Esteem, 66
  Developmental Changes, 67
  Nursing Assessment, 69
Influences on the Self, 69
  Family and Social Relations, 71
The Healthy Personality, 73
  Maslow's Hierarchy, 73
  Dynamics of the Self, 75
Nursing and Self-Awareness, 76

4 The Communication Process, 81
Learning Objectives, 81
Communication Defined, 82
Levels of Communication, 83
  Verbal Level, 83
  Nonverbal Level, 86
Metacommunication, 92
Congruent Communication, 93
Examination of the Communication
Process, 94
Functional Components of the
Communication Process, 95
Additional Processes Necessary for
Communication, 96
  Perception, 96
  Evaluation, 97
  Transmission, 97

Patterns of Communication, 97
  Relating Pattern, 97
  Defensive Communication Patterns, 98
  Games as Communication Patterns, 99
  Interactional Patterns, 100
Factors affecting the Communication Process, 101
  Pattern Organization, 101
  Relationship, 101
  Purpose, 101
  Content, 102
  Time, 102
Summary, 102

5 *Therapeutic Communication, 107*
Learning Objectives, 107
Therapeutic Communication Techniques, 107
  Listening, 107
  Silence, 108
  Establishing Guidelines, 109
  Giving the Client Broad Openings, 109
  Reducing Distance, 109
  Acknowledgment, 110
  Restating, 110
  Reflecting, 110
  Clarification, 111
  Consensual Validation, 111
  Focusing, 111
  Summarizing and Planning, 112
Nontherapeutic Communication Techniques, 112
  Nontherapeutic Techniques of Omission, 112
  Nontherapeutic Techniques of Commission, 115
Barriers to Communication, 116
Special Communication Problems, 120
  Lack of Common Language, 120
  The Aphasic Client, 121

The Sensory-Impaired Client, 121
The Noncommunicative Client, 122
The Child, 123
Structured Communication, 125
  Health Education, 125
  Oral Reports, 126
  Written Reports, 128
Organizational Communication, 129
  Administrative Communication, 129
  Horizontal Communication, 131
  Staff Communication, 131
  Government, 132
  Medical Organizations, 133
  Community Groups, 133
  Media and Public Opinion, 133
  Assessment of Organizational Communication, 134
Acquisition of Communication Skills, 135
  Understanding the Communication Process, 135
  Self-Assessment, 136
  Methods of Skill Acquisition, 136
  Student-Teacher Relationship, 136
  Factors that Handicap Skill Acquisition, 137
Evaluation of Nurse-Client Communication, 138
  Who are the Participants?, 138
  What are They Saying?, 138
  Is Their Purpose being Accomplished?, 138
Summary, 141

6 *The Nurse-Client Relationship: Theoretic Concepts, 147*
Learning Objectives, 147
The Helping Relationship, 147
  The Nurse-Client Relationship, 148
  Characteristics of the Helping Relationship, 148
  Values Clarification, 149

Concept of Trust, 151
  Trust in the Nurse-Client
  Relationship, 151
  Characteristics of the Trusting
  Person, 152
  Building a Trusting Relationship,
  152
Concept of Empathy, 152
  Empathy Research, 153
  Empathy in Everyday Life, 153
  Sympathy, 154
  Development of Empathy, 154
  The Empathy Process, 155
  Nonverbal Behaviors that
  Communicate Empathy, 156
  Self-Assessment of Level of Empathy,
  156
Concept of Caring or Love, 157
  Definitions of Caring, 157
  Development of the Ability to Care,
  158
  Development of the Caring
  Relationship, 158
  The Use of Touch, 159
Concept of Hope, 160
  Definitions of Hope, 160
  Faith and Hope, 160
  Components of Hope, 161
  Dimensions of Hope, 161
  Nursing Interventions, 161
  Nursing Strategies related to Hope,
  161
Concepts of Autonomy and Mutuality,
162
  Sick Role Behaviors, 162
  Definitions of Autonomy and
  Mutuality, 163
  Autonomy, 163
  Mutuality, 166
Summary, 166

7 *The Course of the Helping
Relationship, 173*
  Learning Objectives, 173
  Preinteraction Phase, 174
  Introductory or Orientation Phase, 174
    Introductions, 175
    The Contract, 175
    Roles of the Nurse and Client, 176
    Location, Frequency, and Length of
    Meetings, 176
    Overall Purpose of the Relationship,
    176
    Duration of the Relationship and
    Indications for Termination, 177
    Way in which Confidential Material
    will be Handled, 177
    Summarizing the Contract, 177
    Beginning Client Assessment, 178
  Maintenance or Working Phase, 178
    Patterns of Growth and Resistance,
    178
    Facilitating Expression of Feelings,
    179
    Responding to the Client's Feelings,
    182
  Termination Phase, 189
    Termination and Interpersonal
    Growth, 190
    Behavioral Responses to
    Termination, 190
  Summary, 192

8 *Small Groups and Group
Process Dynamics: An
Overview, 199*
  Learning Objectives, 199
  Types of Groups, 199
    Task Groups, 199
    Therapeutic Groups, 203
    Other Groups, 204

The Dynamic Processes and Development Phases of a Group, 205
  Group Set, 205
  Group Process, 206
  Group Phases, 208
Implication for Nurses, 210
Summary, 211

9 Stress and Adaptation, 217
Learning Objectives, 217
Definitions Relative to Stress, 217
  The Stress State, 219
The Stress Response, 221
  Appraisal, 221
  Frustration, 221
  Threat, 221
  Conflict, 222
  Anxiety, 222
Psychophysiology of the Stress Response, 224
Adaptation, 228
  Behavior Adaptation, 229
  Defense Mechanisms, 231
  Physical Reactions, 234
Stress, Adaptation, and Nursing, 234
Summary, 236

10 Health Promotion Strategies, 243
Learning Objectives, 243
Health Education, 244
  Definitions, 245
  Goals, 246
  Theoretic Basis, 248
Establishing Health Education Programs, 252
  Assessment, 252
  Planning, 253
  Planning Goals, 255
  Instructional Activities, 255
  Implementation, 258
  Obstacles to Health Education, 261
Crisis Intervention, 262

Advocacy, 263
  Definitions of Advocacy, 263
  Models of Advocacy, 263
  Advocacy and Tertiary Prevention, 264
  Self-Help Groups, 264
  Definition, 265
  The Advocacy Role of the Nurse, 269
Holistic Health, 273
  Home Health/Community Services, 275
  Values in Health Promotion, 276
  Health Promotion and Stages of Development, 276
  Spirituality, 277
Summary, 277

11 Crisis Intervention, 285
Learning Objectives, 285
  The Concept of Crisis Intervention Explored, 286
  Theoretic Basis of Crisis Intervention, 288
  Techniques of Crisis Intervention, 290
  Families in Crisis, 293
  Application of Crisis Intervention Techniques, 295
  Situational Crises, 295
  Maturational Crises, 298
Summary, 298

12 Comprehensive Case Study, 301
Learning Objectives, 301
Process Recording, 302
Nursing Care Plan, 304
Supervision, 306
Case Study, 307
  First Meeting, 308
  Second Meeting, 317
  Third Meeting, 326
  Fourth Meeting, 327
  Fifth Meeting, 338
  Sixth Meeting, 339
  Seventh Meeting, 341

NURSE-CLIENT
INTERACTION
Implementing the Nursing Process

The Nursing Process

....

What is the thing called health? Simply a state in which the individual happens transiently to be perfectly adapted to his environment. Obviously, such states cannot be common, for the environment is in constant flux.

H. L. Mencken
American Mercury

LEARNING OBJECTIVES

After studying this chapter, the student should be able to:

- Describe one's beliefs about the nature of the individual and the profession of nursing.
- Identify nursing functions related to primary, secondary, and tertiary prevention.
- Discuss the process and content of a nursing assessment.
- Define *nursing diagnosis* and differentiate between it and *medical diagnosis*.
- Formulate long-term and contributory short-term expected outcomes using behavioral terms.
- Assign priorities to expected outcomes and discuss the rationale for priority assignment.
- Identify the need to base nursing actions on sound nursing theory.
- Describe the need to identify alternative approaches to meeting the nursing care needs of clients.
- Use a structured format for the documentation of client care.
- Describe criteria for the evaluation of nursing care.
- Use peer review and faculty supervision to evaluate professional growth.

PHILOSOPHICAL BELIEFS

One's view of the individual will influence one's perception of the nature of nursing, as well as of the nurse's role and function. A discussion of nursing and the nursing process, therefore, should begin with a statement of beliefs regarding the nature of the person and the profession of nursing.

The Person

In this text the person is believed to be an integrated whole with biologic, psychologic, sociocultural, philosophic, and intellectual components. Innately, individuals are neither good nor bad; their values and characteristics arise from their interactions with the social and physical world. These interactions occur within themselves, with significant others, and with the environment. Thus the person exists in a world of changing experiences of which he or she is the center, and interaction with the world is based on personal dynamics. In addition, as the person grows to a fuller realization of her or his potential, each of these changing experiences and perceptions combine in such a way that they have meaning beyond the moment.

Every individual faces a variety of situations and stimuli each day that arise from the environment and from within oneself. These produce a dynamic, evolving life situation to which the person reacts and responds in an attempt to meet the ever-present challenges of existence, growth, and development. In modern society, such stimuli might include term paper deadlines, conflicts with co-workers, commuting to school or work through traffic, or generalized pressures related to one's role responsibilities.

Whenever a person experiences an event, whether real or imagined, initial cognitive appraisal of the event plays an important role in the way an individual responds. A situation that is viewed as biologically or psychologically threatening is more likely to produce a strong response than is a situation perceived as relatively harmless. Similarly, the same situation may evoke very different responses from different individuals. When the situation is seen as being the least bit uncertain or stressful, several phenomena occur at the same time. There is arousal of emotional responses such as fear, anger, or anxiety, and the expression of physiologic responses such as an increase in blood pressure, a more rapid respiratory rate, and enhanced muscle tone. This integrated psychophysiologic response has evolved to allow human beings to deal with life situations in a manner that promotes survival. Thus the behaviors that one demonstrates are attempts to cope with the demands of life. Facing the stresses of day-to-day life promotes the dynamic nature of the individual as the person struggles with change, adaptation, and development.

Within a nurturing environment the goal of the person is one of growth, autonomy, and self-actualization. In an environment of respect and acceptance individuals direct their energies toward self-definition, constructive relationships with others, and positive control over their lives and destinies. In this movement the person reacts as a whole being to the environment, combining the biopsychosocial components of behaviors. These behaviors arise from personal needs and goals and can be understood only from the individual's own frame of reference. Also basic to this philosophy is the belief that individuals are autonomous, free to make decisions regarding their own goals, and responsible for the consequences of their own actions. Exploring the nature of the individual and stating some basic assumptions help formulate a definition of nursing and a description of nursing functions.

Nursing

Nursing is a service profession that effects changes in the client's biopsychosocial environment to promote health, learning, and growth. The nurse is supportive and therapeutic, interacting with the client to explore his needs, feelings, and goals. The nurse facilitates the client's positive adaptation as a unique individual to the stress he is experiencing. Nursing

care can be given in any setting, and the goal of this care is to maximize the person's positive interactions with his environment, level of wellness, and degree of self-actualization.

The ANA in their 1980 publication entitled *Nursing: a Social Policy Statement* defined nursing as "the *diagnosis and treatment of human* responses to actual or potential health problems."[4] Since 1980, nursing philosophy and practice have been influenced by a greater elaboration of the science of caring and its integration with the traditional knowledge base for diagnosis and treatment of human responses to health and illness. As such, definitions of nursing more frequently acknowledge the following four essential features of contemporary nursing practice:[5]

- Attention to the full range of human experiences and responses to health and illness without restriction to a problem-focused orientation
- Integration of objective data with knowledge gained from an understanding of the patient's or group's subjective experience
- Application of scientific knowledge to the processes of diagnosis and treatment
- Provision of a caring relationship that facilitates health and healing

Nursing is a profession that has both dependent and independent functions. As a nurse, one is involved with all of the components of a person in dynamic interaction. The focus of nursing is the diagnosis and treatment of nursing problems. These are areas in which the client's health may be promoted or in which the client needs help with biopsychosocial adaptation to stress. The helping relationship is the vehicle through which the nurse interacts with the client and promotes his health. The nurse engages the client as a partner in health care, using an assessment based on his total life structure. She does not separate and treat the biologic or psychosocial components in isolation but focuses on their interplay and their effect on the client's total life process. The nurse evokes the client's perceptions of his experiences, and together they attempt to find solutions to his health problems. Nursing actions are directed toward finding meaning in the client's coping responses, maximizing strengths, and maintaining integrity.

In the implementation of these actions, other aspects of nursing emerge. One of these concerns the intensity of the nurse-client relationship over time. The nurse in an inpatient setting is the health professional who has the most contact with the client throughout the day, as well as over a period of time. Another aspect concerns the continuity of care that can be provided by the nurse as the primary caregiver. She may be the professional most accessible and open to the client regardless of the setting or time of day. These aspects describe the uniqueness of the nurse as a health team member sharing and coordinating the health care and growth of clients with other members of the health care team.

This description of nursing demonstrates the nurse's need for self-awareness, observational skills, facilitative communication, and interpersonal competence. The nurse must continuously clarify with the client the meaning of his behavior and the nature of his present needs and goals. The actions implemented and the nursing role assumed depend in part on the time, place, and people involved. However, professional nursing actions, whether dependent or independent, are ultimately decided by the nurse, based on her diagnosis of the client and her appraisal of her own potential.

The nature of nursing, then, requires that the nurse be assertive in giving care to the client. The nurse must actively define nursing functions and be prepared to challenge the existing practice, structure, and power relationships. The purpose is quality nursing care of the client, and the nurse is responsible to the client for providing this care. This is reflected in the Code for Nurses (see box), which summarizes the nurse's responsibility.

The range of nursing functions may be further described and analyzed. The concepts of primary prevention, secondary prevention, and tertiary prevention provide a framework for discussing nursing activities throughout the health-illness continuum.

CRITICAL THINKING *Question* ....

The medical model and overall health care system are often described as "paternalistic." Discuss what this means and how it relates to the philosophy of the nature of the person and the profession of nursing as presented in this chapter.

Code for Nurses

1. The nurse provides services with respect for human dignity and the uniqueness of the client unrestricted by considerations of social or economic status, personal attributes, or the nature of health problems.
2. The nurse safeguards the client's right to privacy by judiciously protecting information of a confidential nature.
3. The nurse acts to safeguard the client and the public when health care and safety are affected by the incompetent, unethical, or illegal practice of any person.
4. The nurse assumes responsibility and accountability for individual nursing judgments and actions.
5. The nurse maintains competence in nursing.
6. The nurse exercises informed judgment and uses individual competence and qualification as criteria in seeking consultation, accepting responsibilities, and delegating nursing activities to others.
7. The nurse participates in activities that contribute to the ongoing development of the profession's body of knowledge.
8. The nurse participates in the profession's efforts to implement and improve standards of nursing.
9. The nurse participates in the profession's efforts to establish and maintain conditions of employment conducive to high-quality nursing care.
10. The nurse participates in the profession's effort to protect the public from misinformation and misrepresentation and to maintain the integrity of nursing.
11. The nurse collaborates with members of the health professions and other citizens in promoting community and national efforts to meet public health needs.

From American Nurses' Association: *Code for nurses with interpretive statements,* Kansas City, Mo, 1976, American Nurses' Association.

NURSING FUNCTIONS AND LEVELS OF PREVENTION
Primary prevention

Primary prevention is a community concept that involves lowering the incidence of illness in a community by counteracting the causative factors before they have had a chance to do harm. It is a concept that precedes disease and is applied to a generally healthy population. It includes health promotion, illness prevention, and protection against disease. Within this area lie many of nursing's independent functions that have as their goal decreasing the vulnerability of the individual to illness.

Health promotion and illness prevention include those nursing activities that encourage and strengthen the person's capacity to withstand stressors. Examples of such a nursing function include a nurse in an industrial setting who encourages the employees to engage in regular exercise or who teaches good nutrition by emphasizing the basic four food groups, limiting salt intake, and adequate hydration. A school nurse might promote health by establishing classes in sex education and personal hygiene for high school students. Specific provisions against disease are evidenced when the nurse promotes immunizing children or encourages the parent to "childproof" the house to prevent accidental illness such as poisoning or lead ingestion. The purpose of these interventions is to safeguard persons from a disease or stressor by removing or reducing the risk factors.

Consumer education is another nursing function in this area and is demonstrated by the nurse who warns clients about the dangers of unprotected sexual activity. In still another example an alert nurse working in a nursing home might notice that the temperature in a refrigerator used to keep high-protein snacks has risen to 40° F (4.44° C). This is a good environment for the growth of bacteria. Providing for the disposal of the food and the repair of the refrigerator are nursing actions that will prevent future problems.

Primary prevention by the nurse also includes consultation with community caregivers. An example of this function is the nurse who is a consultant to elementary schools. At a school the nurse spends time talking with the teachers and administrators, reviewing the principles of promoting health and exploring the problems or questions they might have regarding student behavior, classroom programs, staff relationships, or curriculum policies. This nurse might also function in a counseling role by meeting with the parents of some of the schoolchildren and reviewing with them growth and developmental milestones, family developmental tasks, or child management techniques. Finally, the area of political involvement is also a concern of primary prevention nursing intervention, whether the nurse is lobbying for reimbursement of nurses rendering care to the chronically ill or lobbying for federal funding of community day care centers for working parents.

Secondary prevention

Secondary prevention involves the reduction of actual illness by lowering the prevalence of the problem in the community. This can be accomplished in two ways: by lowering the factors that led to the illness, or by shortening the duration of existing problems by early diagnosis and effective treatment. Secondary prevention begins when pathology is involved, and it includes symptom identification, as well as prompt intervention.

Independent nursing functions in this area might include screening an adult population for high blood pressure or school-age children for vision impairments. Screening procedures such as breast self-examination and the use of the Denver Developmental Screening Test are types of secondary prevention. Another example is a nurse working in a clinic who notices the increasing incidence of venereal disease. Evaluating the community statistics might lead to the creation of an educational program concerned with venereal disease that could be incorporated into the high school curriculum and that would encourage ways to prevent venereal disease, as well as early diagnosis and treatment. This example shows the overlap between secondary prevention and primary prevention nursing functions.

An additional activity of the nurse relative to secondary prevention is the coordination of the care that the ill client receives. A dependent function would be to administer medical treatments and medications. An independent function would be to engage the client as a partner in his health care treatment and formulate a nursing diagnosis regarding his experience of illness. The nurse would identify nursing problems, develop a treatment plan, and be responsible for its implementation and evaluation. The nurse would also facilitate the client's relationships with family or significant others, including them in the nursing care plan and goals. In the area of secondary prevention the nurse would also help the terminally ill client die with dignity and support the family during the mourning process.

Tertiary prevention

Tertiary prevention involves reducing the residual impairment resulting from illness, such as the lowered capacity to contribute to the occupational and social life of the community. Once again, primary, secondary, and tertiary prevention nursing functions overlap. Tertiary prevention activities focus specifically on the client's habilitation or rehabilitation. Habilitation involves helping the client attain a new level of functioning that is a higher level than previously had. An example is the help given to a withdrawn, suspicious, teenage boy who dropped out of high school because of feelings of inadequacy. The community nurse working with his family spent time talking with the boy and exploring his feelings. Her intervention motivated him to pass his high school equivalency examination and later attend college. Rehabilitation involves helping the client achieve a level of functioning less than or equal to his previous level. This is evident in the nurse's rehabilitative efforts to maximize the functioning of a client who has experienced a stroke.

In habilitation or rehabilitation the nursing care plan is subject to continued evaluation and modification based on changing biopsychosocial problems and the formulation of new goals. In rehabilitation activities the nurse also strives to prevent recurrence of the problem. For instance, the nurse might help plan and reinforce an appropriate exercise program for the client who has had a heart attack.

The Clinical Example box shows how nursing actions can be described using the primary preven-

CLINICAL EXAMPLE

Ms. L. is a nurse working in the pediatric clinic of a community hospital. As part of her health teaching she reviews normal developmental behavior of children with the parents she sees in the clinic. She stresses to them the importance of proper nutrition, adequate rest, and social peer relationships for growing children. She might also initiate parent effectiveness training groups within the clinic or community setting. These are some of the nursing activities that describe her role in primary prevention.

In her work in the pediatric clinic she has identified that a number of children are referred to the clinic because of problems in school. Most of these children are sent by the county schools because of their disruptive behavior and inability to learn. Ms. L. recognizes that prepubescent children who are behavior problems in the classroom often have learning disabilities. From her epidemiologic case finding she realizes the need for health teaching of parents and consultation to the county schools. Ms. L. visits the schools and discusses the diagnosis and treatment of children with learning disabilities with the teachers and the school nurse. She finds that the schools do not have sufficient funds for special education classes and that there is only one resource teacher within the three schools to provide the individual attention needed for these children. Ms. L. becomes politically involved, campaigning for additional educational funds

and the reallocation of existing funds to form special education classes. She meets with parent groups to teach them about behaviors that are characteristic of learning disabilities, and she also works with the one available special education teacher to establish an ongoing workshop for teachers to increase their skills in teaching the child with a learning disability. Ms. L. also supervises the administration of drugs to children diagnosed as having a learning disability. She works with the school nurse to set up a parents' group for the families of children with learning disabilities so that they can share their experiences, help each other solve problems, and identify agencies within the community that may help alleviate the problem. In addition, she refers children who are having adjustment problems because of their inability to learn to the mental health department. These nursing actions describe her roles in secondary prevention.

Her functions in tertiary prevention revolve around working with the families and teachers of children with learning disabilities to maximize the children's potential and to decrease possible adverse psychologic effects from their poor interpersonal relationships and slow learning. Her goal is not only to help these children reach a higher level of functioning (habilitation) but also to assist those who have already lost interest in school to return to their former level of social development (rehabilitation).

tion, secondary prevention, and tertiary prevention model.

All of these nursing functions are actions for which the nurse is directly responsible. They are carried out whether or not the client is under medical care and in any setting agreed on by the nurse and the client. Use of the nursing process aids in analyzing the nursing problem, planning the appropriate actions, organizing their implementation, and evaluating the nursing care.

CRITICAL THINKING *Question* ················

Which level of prevention do you believe is the priority of the current health care system? Defend your answer based on the type of health care reimbursed by third-party payers and the allocation of federal research funding in health care.

··

NURSING PROCESS

Many nursing scholars have formulated conceptual models for nursing. These models are outlines or frameworks designed for use in nursing education, practice, and research. From these models are developed nursing theories of principles for practice. In presenting the content of this book, no attempt is made to endorse or further develop one particular model of nursing. Rather, the focus is on the implementation of the nursing process and its behavioral manifestations.

The nursing process is an interactive, problem-solving process used by the nurse as a systematic and individualized way to fulfill the goal of nursing care. It is a deliberate and organized approach requiring thought, knowledge, and experience. The nursing process acknowledges the autonomy of the individual and his freedom to make decisions regarding his own goals and to be involved in his own care. Together, the nurse and client emerge as partners in a relationship built on trust and directed toward maximizing the client's strengths and maintaining his integrity.

The problem-solving process is a scientific way of thinking and dealing with problems, and its principles are included in the nursing process (Table 1-1).

Many disciplines incorporate aspects of the problem-solving process. The nursing process, however, is distinguished from the problem-solving process in its purpose and method. The purpose of the problem-solving process is the development of new knowledge. The purpose of the nursing process is to maximize a client's positive interactions with his environment, his level of wellness, and his degree of self-actualization. The methods also differ. With the scientific process one can problem solve in isolation, manipulating objects and ideas without interacting with other people. The nursing process, however, is founded on the helping, interpersonal relationship; the nurse interacts with the client to analyze and meet his biopsychosocial needs.

One uses the nursing process with an individual client, as well as with a family or group, at any point on the health-illness continuum. The setting and the client's needs will determine whether this process is directed toward primary, secondary, or tertiary prevention. The nursing process is the basic framework for nursing, and it is used to provide quality, professional care. It requires that the nurse have a sound knowledge base, be able to communicate effectively and think logically, be technically efficient, and be

TABLE I-I   Comparison of steps in problem solving with phases of the nursing process

STEPS IN PROBLEM SOLVING	PHASES OF NURSING PROCESS
Observation and recognition of the problem	Data collection
Definition of the problem	Formulation of the nursing diagnosis
Formulation of hypotheses or possible solutions	Planning of nursing care
Implementation of the hypotheses or possible solutions	Implementation of nursing actions
Formulations of conclusions	Evaluation of nursing assessment, care plan, and actions

receptive to internal and external evaluation. Because it is a disciplined approach to care of the client, the nurse must be able to demonstrate flexibility, openness, creativity, and leadership in directing change.

The phases of the nursing process—assessment, diagnosis, outcome identification, planning, implementation, and evaluation—are reflected in the ANA's *Standards of Nursing Practice.* The standards strive to improve the practice of nursing, which occurs in a variety of settings. The standards for the nursing profession are defined as follows:

Standard I. Assessment—The nurse collects client health data.

Standard II. Diagnosis—The nurse analyses the assessment data in determining diagnoses.

Standard III. Outcome identification—The nurse identifies expected outcomes individualized to the client.

Standard IV. Planning—The nurse develops a plan of care that prescribes interventions to attain expected outcomes.

Standard V. Implementation—The nurse implements the interventions identified in the plan of care.

Standard VI. Evaluation—The nurse evaluates the client's progress toward attainment of objectives.[6]

The nursing process, however, does not consist of separate, discrete phases followed in strict sequence. Rather, they are continuous and interdependent. All phases may overlap or occur simultaneously. For example, when collecting data from an elderly woman who has recently suffered a stroke, the nurse diagnoses the problem of impaired mobility and implements a regimen of muscle exercises to increase joint mobility and muscle strength. Each day, while assisting the client with exercises, the nurse also evaluates the client's progress and identifies new goals and actions. Thus the nursing process is dynamic and dependent on ongoing validation and evaluation.

For the purpose of studying the process, however, it is helpful to temporarily separate the phases and examine each one. This provides for increased understanding of the elements of each phase and the relationship of each phase to the others.

 CULTURAL CONSIDERATIONS

Current U.S. data suggest that the following sociocultural trends will influence the health care system and the way health care is provided:

- The population will increase by 60% to almost 400 million by the year 2050.
- Growth will be concentrated at the two ends of the age spectrum. By 2050 the population aged 65 and over will more than double, and the population aged 85 and older will be the fastest growing age group.
- The U.S. population is becoming more diverse by race and ethnicity. Hispanics will be the largest ethnic group, making up one quarter of the population.
- The United States has become a predominantly urban nation with the population occupying only 2.5% of the land mass.

Discuss the impact these changes will have on the health care delivery system and the roles and career opportunities for nurses.

Assessment

The first phase of the nursing process marks the beginning of the nurse-client relationship and consists of the collection of data about the client. Many factors can influence this important phase. The nursing conditions and nursing behaviors related to assessment are depicted in Fig. 1-1. As in any communication process, the perception, transmission, and evaluation of the data are subject to the personal interpretation of both the nurse and the client. Specifically, the nurse and client are influenced by their respective:

- Physical, mental, and emotional states and needs
- Cultural, social, and philosophical backgrounds
- Number and functional ability of senses
- Past experiences with the present situation
- Perceptions of the meaning of the event
- Interests, preoccupations, preconceptions, and motivational levels
- Knowledge or familiarity with the situation
- Environmental conditions and distractions
- Presence, attitudes, and reactions of others

To accomplish the tasks of this phase successfully, the nurse needs certain knowledge and skills. Basic to these is the need for self-awareness. The nurse needs to know herself and feel comfortable with her-

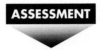

NURSING CONDITIONS	NURSING BEHAVIORS
Self-awareness	Establish nursing contract
Accurate observations	Obtain information from client and family
Therapeutic communication	Validate data with client
Responsive dimensions of care	Organize data

Fig. 1-1 Nursing conditions and behaviors related to assessment.

self before she will be able to reach out to the client and actively listen to his verbal and nonverbal communication. The nurse must be able to separate her own feelings from those of the client and identify her own needs and personal and professional goals. It is also necessary for the nurse to objectively analyze how she affects the client. Clients should not be stereotyped but should be respected as individuals. If this is done, the client's communication can be viewed as his perception of the situation, and the client's behavior can be seen as his coping response.

The nurse also needs accurate observation and communication skills to draw out the client verbally and be keenly aware of his nonverbal behaviors. This includes knowledge of the components of the nurse-client helping relationship. Because this is the basis for implementing care, the nurse should understand the dynamics of the relationship and her participation in it. Finally, the nurse needs knowledge of the biologic, physical, and behavioral sciences to provide herself with a theoretic base for collecting data.

The nurse must first establish a nursing contract that defines explicit mutual expectations for the interaction of nurse and client. The specific elements of a contract are discussed in detail in Chapter 7. Once this has been established, the nurse can obtain information about the client's past history, present situation, and health care expectations. The client is always the first and primary source of data, but the nurse may also obtain information from family members or friends, other health team members, medical and social records, and laboratory or testing results.

On some occasions the client may not be able to enter into a contract and give the nurse the necessary information. This may occur with a small child, an unconscious adult, or a person who is so anxious and emotional that he cannot respond to outside questions. In these instances the nurse may obtain the necessary information from other family members or friends accompanying the client. However, as soon as the client is able to interact with others, the nurse should establish a contract and validate or confirm the data with him and complete the nursing assessment (Fig. 1-2).

CRITICAL THINKING *Question* ....

Obtaining data about the client from family members and others is important to the nursing assessment. What problems does it potentially create, however, in relation to confidentiality and the client's right to privacy?
....

Omission of this step can seriously impair the quality of the nursing care. For example, a nurse was caring for a client who was brought in unconscious after an automobile accident. The family reported that they knew of no existing health problems or allergies pertaining to the client. When the client gained consciousness, however, and the nurse began to validate her information, the client said that he once had a serious reaction to penicillin but saw no need to tell his family about it. If the nurse had not validated her data, the client's health might have been seriously jeopardized.

The focus of the nurse is on gaining a total view of the client's biopsychosocial components. The nurse reviews the biologic aspects of the client,

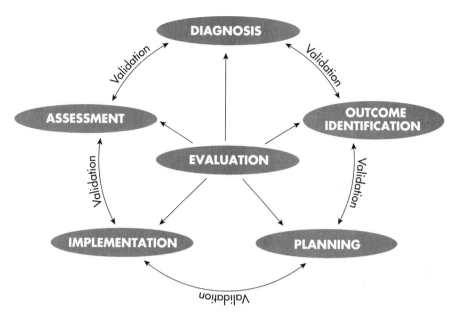

Fig. 1-2 The nursing process.

including anatomy, physiology, chemistry, and genetic background. She examines the psychologic component of the client, assessing growth and development, behavior, motivation, feelings, and coping responses. Socially, the client's family relationships, involvement in groups, culture, religion, and occupation are additional areas of information.

These are particularly important factors to include in every nursing assessment. They exert a powerful influence on the success of the nursing process, because sociocultural factors contribute to a client's belief system regarding health and illness. Any one of these factors, including religion, sex, race, cultural background, family ties, economic status, or social support systems, may play a dominant role in the person's life. Therefore any attempt to promote the well-being of a client must be based on an understanding of him as a unique individual who lives in a larger social, cultural, and religious community. The nurse strives to obtain as complete a picture as possible of the client's life situation.

The quality of the nursing assessment will be enhanced by the use of a standard format to organize the data. Use of a standardized assessment tool or nursing history form will improve the quality of the

nursing process, reduce the client's repetition of his history, and provide a source of information available to all health team members. Various nursing programs and health care institutions have developed their own tools or forms. The nurse might use one of these forms or develop an original form based on a particular setting, client population, or nursing role.

In collecting the data, the nurse should select a private place, free from noise and distractions, to interview the client. Observing, interviewing, and examining are the basic methods for gathering information. During the data collection process, the nurse uses all five senses. With hearing she responds to the client's statements, inflections, and verbal communication, as well as to the sounds of the client's heart, lungs, and bowels. With sight the nurse can observe nonverbal communication, body integrity, skin color, and physical growth patterns or abnormalities. The senses of taste and smell help the nurse note distinctive or unusual odors. Finally, the sense of touch is greatly used when the nurse palpates, percusses, and presses while using the various physical assessment skills.

In the process of collecting data, the nurse uses interpersonal and physical assessment skills to understand the client's life situation. Throughout the interview the nurse clarifies and validates all information with the client to be sure that the data are accurate. Accurate data collection reflects only what the client actually said and the behaviors observed by the nurse. It is essential that the nurse differentiate between reporting specific, observable client behaviors and inferences or interpretations of the client's behavior based on the nurse's own assumptions, value judgments, or generalizations. If the data collection is precise, standardized, and organized, the nurse will be able to identify the particular problems and needs of the client. None of them will be overlooked or misinterpreted. Thus thorough data collection facilitates the nurse's analysis and formulation of the nursing diagnosis.

Nursing diagnosis

On completion of the data collection, the nurse compares the information with documented norms of health and wellness, making proper allowance for the client's individual variations. Based on this comparison the nurse formulates inferences regarding the client's responses to actual or potential health problems. In this analysis or formulation of inferences, the nurse engages in decision making. Many decisions are made throughout the nursing process, from the decision concerning what data one should collect to the decision or evaluation of how successful the nursing care was for the client. Some decisions require only a few seconds of thought, whereas much time is needed for others. The nursing conditions and nursing behaviors related to nursing diagnosis are depicted in Fig. 1-3.

Nursing decisions may be logical or illogical. Examples of illogical decision making include intuition, tradition, prejudice, and trial and error. In illogical decision making the nurse does not attempt to objectively examine data to derive inferences. Instead, the nursing judgment is based on guessing or little thought, as in intuition; rules, regulations, or previous results, as in tradition; biased beliefs, as in prejudice; or lack of goal direction, as in trial and error. Logical decision making implies knowledge and thought that may be either inductive or deductive. Inductive thinking is reasoning from the specifics to the generalization; deductive thinking is reasoning from the generalization to the specifics. Both types of thought are useful to the nurse in analyzing data, as can be seen in the Clinical Example box.

CLINICAL EXAMPLE

The nurse notes that the calf of Ms. P.'s right leg is swollen, reddened, warm, and painful when touched. Inductive thinking allows the nurse to infer from these specifics that the client may have thrombophlebitis or a clot in her vein. When the doctor prescribes complete bed rest for the client, however, the nurse anticipates additional problems. From her general knowledge of immobility and Ms. P.'s lifestyle, the nurse deduces the following, more specific, potential problems: constipation, muscle weakness, boredom, anxiety regarding the care of her children, and guilt feelings because of the increased burden she feels she is placing on her husband.

NURSING DIAGNOSIS

NURSING CONDITIONS	NURSING BEHAVIORS
Logical decision making	Identify patterns in data
Knowledge of normal parameters	Compare data with norms
Inductive and deductive reasoning	Analyze and synthesize data
Sociocultural sensitivity	Problems/strengths identified
	Validate problems with client
	Formulate nursing diagnosis
	Set priorities of problems

Fig. 1-3 Nursing conditions and behaviors related to nursing diagnosis.

In this phase the nurse uses logical decision making to analyze the collected data and derive a nursing diagnosis. The analysis and synthesis of the data can also assume a logical progression consisting of the following:

- Categorizing all data
- Identifying data gaps and incongruencies
- Determining patterns
- Applying theories, models, frameworks, norms, and standards
- Identifying health concerns and strengths
- Establishing causal relationships

The outcome of this careful evaluation of client data is a summary statement or nursing diagnosis.

A *nursing diagnosis* is the independent judgment of a nurse that identifies the nursing problems of the client. These nursing problems concern aspects of the client's health that may need to be promoted or with which the client needs help in his biopsychosocial adaptation to stress. The subject of nursing diagnoses, therefore, is the client's behavioral response to stress. This response may lie anywhere on the coping continuum, from adaptive and healthy to maladaptive and ill.

Nursing diagnoses are to be distinguished from medical diagnoses. Although they may be complementary to each other, one is not a component of the other, nor contingent on the other. A *medical diagnosis* identifies a pathologic disease, and the focus of medical treatment is to cure the disease process. A nursing diagnosis identifies a person's response to an actual or potential health problem, and the focus of nursing treatment is to promote health and prevent illness.

Thus a client with one specific medical diagnosis may have a number of complementary nursing diagnoses related to his range of health responses. On the other hand, a client may have a specific nursing diagnosis without any identified medical diagnoses. The Clinical Example box helps clarify the difference between a medical and a nursing diagnosis.

In this case the medical diagnosis was specific to the disease process, and the treatment plan involved the use of medication. The nursing diagnosis, however, identified a factor interfering with the medical management of the disease, a stressor in the family relationships, and a problem evident in the child's environment. Obviously, in maximizing the health of the client, medicine and nursing are interrelated

and interdependent. Each profession serves as a resource to the other as physicians and nurses collaborate for the improved health of the client.

The nursing diagnosis states the identified nursing problems, which may be overt, covert, existing, or potential. The nursing diagnosis also may include promoting adaptive human responses. The statement of the nursing diagnosis should be as clear and precise as possible. It should reflect the client's health-related response and not be a restatement of the medical diagnosis, treatment plan, or nursing limitation.

According to the North American Nursing Diagnosis Association (NANDA), a nursing diagnostic statement ideally consists of three parts:

1. Health problem
2. Etiologic or contributing factors
3. Defining characteristics

The first, the health problem, identifies the behavioral disruption or threatened disruption that can be improved through nursing intervention. The second, the etiologic factors, identifies stressors that contribute to the problem. The third, the defining characteristics, describes the signs and symptoms that relate to the identified health problem. All three components are important in formulating a nursing diagnosis. The defining characteristics are particularly helpful, because they reflect the objective and subjec-

 CLINICAL EXAMPLE

An 8-year-old boy is brought by his mother to the hospital emergency room; he is wheezing and having difficulty breathing. After examining the boy, the physician makes a medical diagnosis of acute asthmatic attack and prescribes medication and inhalation therapy. The clinic nurse working with this family completes a thorough nursing history. Based on her analysis and validation with the mother and son, the nurse's diagnosis identifies the following nursing problems:

1. *Knowledge deficit of medication used to control asthmatic attacks*
2. *Alteration in family process because of sibling rivalry with 9-year-old brother*
3. *Ineffective individual coping evidenced in poor school performance*

tive behaviors that are the target of nursing intervention. They also provide specific indicators for evaluating the outcomes of nursing interventions or whether the expected goals of the nursing care were met. Some examples of possible nursing diagnoses are

- Body-image disturbance related to cerebrovascular accident, evidenced by lack of acceptance of body limitations
- Altered thought processes related to Alzheimer's disease, evidenced by inaccurate interpretation of environment, deficit in recent memory, and impaired ability to reason

- Altered sexuality patterns related to embarrassment about one's body after a mastectomy, evidenced by lack of desire for sex

The classification of nursing diagnoses is evolving. Since 1973, a national task force of nursing professionals has been working on a taxonomy of nursing diagnoses. In 1994 NANDA identified the diagnoses listed in the accompanying box. As nurses agree on nursing diagnoses, they will be better able to define the science of nursing to other health professionals and the public. This will result in improved communication among nurses, greater

NANDA Diagnoses

Activity intolerance
Activity intolerance, risk for
Adaptive capacity, decreased: intracranial
Adjustment, impaired
Airway clearance, ineffective
Anxiety
Aspiration, risk for
Body-image disturbance
Body temperature, altered, risk for
Bowel incontinence
Breastfeeding, effective
Breastfeeding, ineffective
Breastfeeding, interrupted
Breathing pattern, ineffective
Cardiac output, decreased
Caregiver role strain
Caregiver role strain, risk for
Communication, impaired verbal
Community coping, ineffective
Community coping, potential for enhanced
Confusion, acute
Confusion, chronic
Constipation
Constipation, colonic
Constipation, perceived
Coping, defensive
Coping, family: potential for growth
Coping, ineffective family: compromised
Coping, ineffective family: disabling
Coping, ineffective individual
Decisional conflict (specify)
Denial, ineffective
Diarrhea

Disuse syndrome, risk for
Diversional activity deficit
Dysreflexia
Energy field disturbance
Environmental interpretation syndrome, impaired
Family processes, altered: alcoholism
Family processes, altered
Fatigue
Fear
Fluid volume deficit
Fluid volume deficit, risk for
Fluid volume, excess
Gas exchange, impaired
Grieving, anticipatory
Grieving, dysfunctional
Growth and development, altered
Health maintenance, altered
Health-seeking behaviors (specify)
Home maintenance management, impaired
Hopelessness
Hyperthermia
Hypothermia
Incontinence, functional
Incontinence, reflex
Incontinence, stress
Incontinence, total
Incontinence, urge
Infant behavior, disorganized
Infant behavior, disorganized: risk for
Infant behavior, organized: potential for enhanced
Infant feeding pattern, ineffective
Infection, risk for
Injury, perioperative positioning: risk for

From *NANDA Nursing Diagnosis Definitions and Classification 1995-1996*, Philadelphia, 1994, North American Nursing Diagnosis Association.

continuity of care for the client, improved quality of nurse-client interactions, and stimulation of research related to the scientific body of nursing knowledge.

Again, after the nursing diagnosis has been formulated, the nurse validates the identified problems with the client and ranks them in their priority or order of importance. Having collected the necessary data and identified the nursing problems, the nurse has now completed the diagnostic process and begins to plan for the nursing care.

CRITICAL THINKING *Question* ....

The nursing diagnosis of "noncompliance" has been subjected to criticism because it implies that the client is not meeting the expectations of the nurse with regard to implementing the treatment plan. Another view of this issue is that client "noncompliance" is really a failure of the nurse to adequately engage the client as a true partner in the treatment process. Discuss the pros and cons of this issue from your perspective as a nurse and the perspective of the client.

NANDA Diagnoses—cont'd

Injury, risk for
Knowledge deficit (specify)
Loneliness, risk for
Management of therapeutic regimen, community: ineffective
Management of therapeutic regimen, families: ineffective
Management of therapeutic regimen, individuals: effective
Management of therapeutic regimen, individuals: ineffective
Memory, impaired
Mobility, impaired physical
Noncompliance (specify)
Nutrition, altered: less than body requirements
Nutrition, altered: more than body requirements
Nutrition, altered: potential for more than body requirements
Oral mucous membrane, altered
Pain
Pain, chronic
Parent/infant/child attachment, risk for altered
Parental role conflict
Parenting, altered
Parenting, risk for altered
Peripheral neurovascular dysfunction, risk for
Personal identity disturbance
Poisoning, risk for
Posttrauma response
Powerlessness
Protection, altered
Rape-trauma syndrome
Rape-trauma syndrome: compound reaction
Rape-trauma syndrome: silent reaction
Relocation stress syndrome
Role performance, altered

Self-care deficit, bathing/hygiene
Self-care deficit, dressing/grooming
Self-care deficit, feeding
Self-care deficit, toileting
Self-esteem disturbance
Self-esteem, chronic low
Self-esteem, situational low
Self-mutilation, risk for
Sensory/perceptual alterations (specify) (visual, auditory, kinesthetic, gustatory, tactile, olfactory)
Sexual dysfunction
Sexuality patterns, altered
Skin integrity, impaired
Skin integrity, impaired, risk for
Sleep pattern disturbance
Social interaction, impaired
Social isolation
Spiritual distress (distress of the human spirit)
Spiritual well-being, potential for enhanced
Suffocation, risk for
Swallowing, impaired
Thermoregulation, ineffective
Thought processes, altered
Tissue integrity, impaired
Tissue perfusion, altered (specify type) (renal, cerebral, cardiopulmonary, gastrointestinal, peripheral)
Trauma, risk for
Unilateral neglect
Urinary elimination, altered
Urinary retention
Ventilation, inability to sustain spontaneous
Ventilatory weaning process, dysfunctional
Violence, risk for: self-directed or directed at others

Outcome Identification

Outcome identification builds on the assessment and nursing diagnosis phases of the nursing process and increases the probability of successful planning, implementation, and evaluation. The development of clearly stated objectives, expected outcomes, and goals for nursing care is built on educational theory. The work of Mager[8] is highly recommended as a resource on this topic. The nursing conditions and nursing behaviors related to outcome identification are depicted in Fig. 1-4.

A primary concern in the development of expected outcomes for nursing care is that it will be possible to evaluate the degree to which they were accomplished. It is, therefore, necessary that they be written in behavioral terms. This means that the *verb* used in the

TABLE I-2   Comparison of terms with many and few interpretations

TERMS WITH MANY INTERPRETATIONS	TERMS WITH FEW INTERPRETATIONS
To know (recall, relate, understand, identify?)	To identify
To understand (know, relate, identify?)	To list
To be familiar with (know, understand, recognize?)	To compare and contrast
To realize (discover, appreciate, comprehend?)	To predict
To appreciate (realize, know, understand?)	To interpret
To believe (realize, hope, trust?)	To recall
To have faith in (believe, hope, trust?)	To label
To be interested in (be aware of, to like?)	To choose
To enjoy (relish, love, be pleased with?)	To select
To value (appreciate, hold in high esteem?)	To volunteer
To feel (receive an impression, be impressed with, respond?)	To translate
	To apply
To think critically (evaluate, apply, synthesize?)	To recognize
To think (understand, conceive, imagine, reflect, infer, judge?)	To state
	To classify
To really understand	To differentiate
To fully appreciate	To construct
	To order
	To describe
	To demonstrate

From Redman B: *The process of patient education,* St Louis, 1993, Mosby.

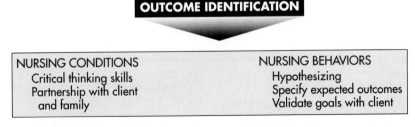

Fig. 1-4 Nursing conditions and behaviors related to outcome identification.

statement should represent a behavior that may be observed. Examples of verbs representing observable behaviors include the following: to state, to write, to demonstrate, to perform, to list, to describe, and to identify. There are, of course, many more. Table 1-2 presents an extensive list developed by Redman.[10] There are a number of other verbs that do not represent observable behaviors but are tempting to use in goal writing. A few examples are to know, to understand, to accept, to realize, to think, and to feel. None of these behaviors can be seen; each requires resorting to another means of validation and would probably be better described by one of the terms in the first list.

Which of the following expected outcomes would be a behavioral description of the activity of the client in Fig. 1-5?

1. The client will hold her baby in a safe and secure manner.
2. The client will be aware of safety principles when holding her baby.
3. The client will provide her baby with a sense of security.

The first describes the behavior that the client is to demonstrate. Her ability to accomplish the goal may be determined by observing her while she cares for her baby. Nursing intervention can be based on these observations. The second assumes that the mother knows the reason for her behavior and would be able to identify safety principles. If the nurse wants to validate the client's knowledge of safety principles, the objective must be reworded as follows:

The client will state the safety principles that are involved in holding her baby.

This information may be validated by interviewing the client. The third outcome assumes a response on the part of the baby, which at this stage of psychosocial development may be inferred but not validated. It would be better to identify a maternal behavior such as that described in the first outcome, which can then be validated by direct observation.

The more specifically an outcome can be stated, the more useful it is in planning nursing care. Conditions may be added to an outcome to better delineate the context in which the expected behavior should occur. The first expected outcome related to

Fig. 1-5 might be modified to include a condition for performance such as:

Having seen a demonstration of how to hold an infant, the client will hold her baby in a safe and secure manner.

Similarly, an outcome for teaching an obese client a weight reduction diet might state:

Given a sample menu plan, the client will plan well-balanced meals within the allowed caloric allotment.

Both of these specify conditions that must be met to maximize the probability of successful goal achievement.

Even when goals are stated behaviorally and include conditions, it is still possible to make them

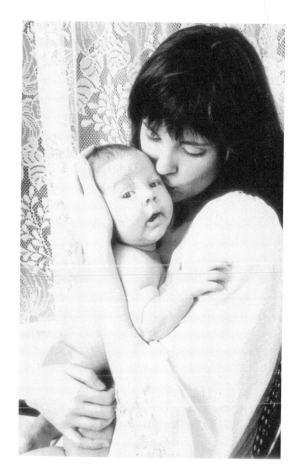

Fig. I-5 Client demonstrates her accomplishment of the goal to hold her baby safely and securely.

more specific. This is done by the addition of criteria for successful goal accomplishment. The outcome for teaching the obese client could be made more precise by adding criteria as follows:

Given a sample menu plan, the client will plan and eat three well-balanced meals. The total caloric value is not to exceed 1200 calories per day.

The goal now states that the client will eat three meals and specifies the upper limit of calories that the client is allowed to consume. Another goal for the same client might state:

Adhering to a diet of 1200 calories per day, the client will lose 10 lb in 6 weeks.

Again, the goal states specifically the amount of weight the client should lose and over what period of time the loss should take place.

Commonly, it is difficult for beginners to write specific, behaviorally stated goals. This is particularly true when the focus of nursing intervention is on the psychosocial aspect of the client's behavior. Attitudinal or emotional changes are somewhat more intangible than the behaviors described in the foregoing examples. However, nursing care is enhanced by specific planning, whether the focus is on the client's physical, psychologic, or attitudinal behavior. For instance, the low-calorie diet for the obese client will probably result in a transient weight loss unless the client experiences a basic attitudinal change concerning dietary habits and patterns. A nursing goal that focuses on that need would state:

The client will verbalize the need to permanently alter his eating habits to maintain his desired weight of 185 lb.

Basic attitudes, values, and habits are the most difficult behaviors for people to change. Therefore the nurse can expect that such change will take place slowly after a great deal of consistent encouragement and reinforcement.

To keep expectations realistic, it is advisable to plan nursing care in terms of a series of short-term goals that lead to a long-term, terminal goal. This is accomplished by identifying the ultimate outcome that the client is to achieve. Then, the component behaviors that must occur before that outcome is reached should be determined.

For example, long-term terminal and short-term contributory goals related to the nursing diagnosis of altered nutrition, more than body requirements, might be organized as follows:

Long-term goal: The client will lose 30 lb in 4 months by adhering to a 1500-calorie diet and a prescribed exercise program.

Short-term goal:
1. The client will lose an average of 2 lb per week to be calculated at each monthly clinic visit.
2. The client will plan menus of 1500 calories per day based on nutritionally sound basic diet guidelines.
3. The client will participate in an exercise stress test before the next clinic visit.
4. If not contraindicated by the stress test, the client will engage in an aerobic form of exercise for at least 1 hour three times weekly.
5. At each clinic visit the client will discuss with the nurse feelings about the reactions to changed dietary and activity patterns.

If care is planned in this manner, both nurse and client can periodically experience a feeling of success even if they are working toward a complex final outcome. This helps prevent discouragement and abandonment of a goal because it seems to be too difficult or unrealistic.

Planning

The nursing care plan is based on application of theory from nursing and related physical and behavioral sciences to the unique needs of the individual client. This presupposes that as the nurse identifies areas of client need, appropriate theoretical resources will again be consulted. Failure to approach nursing care in this scientific manner is likely to result in illogical decision making and a plan based on tradition, intuition, or trial and error. Although use of any of these decision-making methods may result in a valid plan, consistency of depth and accuracy over time will probably suffer, as will the overall care of the client. The nursing conditions and nursing behaviors related to planning are depicted in Fig. 1-6.

Successful care planning is facilitated by active involvement of the client. This enhances the nurse-client relationship by conveying respect for the client and his preferences. Client involvement is essential for individualized nursing care to occur. If the nurse collects the data and returns to the nurses' station, consults the textbooks, and then writes up a plan of care, an important step has been missed. Once the nurse has formulated a tentative care plan, it must be validated with the client. This saves time and effort for both nurse and client as they continue to work together. The client can very quickly tell the nurse that a proposed plan is unrealistic regarding financial status, lifestyle, value system, or perhaps even personal preference. There are usually several possible approaches to a given client problem. Using the one that is most acceptable to the client enhances the likelihood of goal accomplishment. The Clinical Example box illustrates the value of client involvement in care planning.

Priority setting Most clients exhibit a number of nursing problems, each of which must be incorporated into the plan of care. Several goals may need to be written related to each identified problem. As the nurse and client work together to meet client needs, new ones often arise. For this reason it is necessary to make decisions concerning the importance or priority of meeting the various nurse-client goals. Otherwise, care would become haphazard and fragmented, with the focus first on one goal and then on the next, based only on what happened to come up at the time. Important and immediate needs could get lost.

Highest priority is usually given to goals related to problems that threaten the life of the individual. Hence, teaching a 3-year-old who lives on a busy

 CLINICAL EXAMPLE

Billy J. was a 6-year-old child who was placed in a foster home. The pediatrician requested a community-health nursing visit after the foster mother reported that Billy ate very little and was losing weight. The nurse was initially concerned that Billy might be having difficulty with emotional adjustment to his new home and to separation from his parents. However, the foster mother stated that Billy seemed happy and played well with other neighborhood children. She agreed to try to get Billy to talk about his feelings. When she did so, Billy said he liked his new home and hoped he would never leave, because his new parents didn't beat him. The nurse then decided to talk with Billy about his eating problem. He stated readily that he did not like the foods offered in his foster home. The foster parents were of Greek origin and served many ethnic dishes that were strange to Billy. Billy shared his preference for

chicken, hamburgers, and peanut butter–and–jelly sandwiches. With this additional information the nurse and foster mother planned some menus with Billy, who promptly began to eat and gain weight. In this instance the nurse initially devised a plan of care based on knowledge from the behavioral sciences that children who are separated from their parents become depressed. She also knew that appetite loss is a sign of depression. However, because she ignored the information that Billy seemed happy, and primarily because she initially failed to interview Billy, time and energy were lost in determining an appropriate plan of care. When Billy was involved in mutual planning with the nurse and his foster mother, the correct nursing diagnosis was made, an objective was agreed on, and successful goal accomplishments quickly ensued.

NURSING CONDITIONS	NURSING BEHAVIORS
Application of theory	Prioritize goals
Respect for client and family	Identify nursing activities
	Validate plan with client

Fig. I-6 Nursing conditions and behaviors related to planning.

street to play in the yard would take priority over teaching hand washing. Next priority is usually given to those problems that are likely to cause destructive changes in the client. Helping a pregnant woman who has had some bleeding get to her physician would take priority over teaching her prenatal exercises. Lowest priority is assigned to problems related to normal developmental experiences.

Establishing priorities helps organize nursing care and contributes to efficient management of time and energy. A client who is frightened that the lump in her breast may be malignant will have a difficult time concentrating on a discussion of sex education for her preadolescent daughter. If the nurse were to persist in pursuing the latter topic, neither of the client's needs would be met, and the client would rate her health care experience as unhelpful.

Because the nursing care plan is dynamic and should ensure responsiveness to the client's problems throughout the client's contact with the health care system, priorities are constantly changing. For instance, if the client in the aforementioned example learned that her breast biopsy was negative and had a chance to share her feelings, she may then ask the nurse for sex education information for her daughter. This problem would then be given higher priority, and the nurse and client would develop objectives related to it. If the focus is always kept on client problems, priorities can be set and modified as the client changes. Nursing care is then personalized, and the client cooperates in its implementation.

Implementation

After expected outcomes for nursing care have been mutually determined and priorities assigned, the nurse must decide on nursing actions that will lead to goal achievement. Implementation refers to the actual delivery of nursing care to the client and the client's response to the care that is given. Good planning maximizes the probability of successful implementation. Such factors as available people, equipment, resources, time, and money must be considered as nursing actions are planned. The nursing conditions and nursing behaviors related to implementation are depicted in Fig. 1-7.

Well-planned nursing care also takes into account the personalities and experiences of the nurse and the client. Sometimes the nurse's past experience will suggest possible approaches to meeting an objective. For instance, a nurse in a pediatric clinic may have noted that many cases of diaper rash clear up when the mother switches from detergent to soap for her baby laundry. This experience would suggest to the nurse that the mother of a baby with diaper rash should use soap rather than detergent. The pediatric nurse should also become curious about the reason for this. She would then ask an authority, such as a pharmacist, or explore scientific literature to uncover the reason for her observation. As a result, future nursing interventions would be based on sound theory.

The most valid basis for nursing action is that which has been investigated by nursing researchers who have applied the scientific method to nursing practice. As nursing has matured as a profession, the quantity and quality of clinical research conducted by nurses has increased dramatically. This is a positive development that has significantly improved the theory resources available to the practicing nurse. However, if relevant nursing research is unavailable or the nurse wants to explore other points of view, it is also acceptable to judiciously use nursing literature

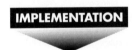

NURSING CONDITIONS	NURSING BEHAVIORS
Past clinical experiences	Consider available resources
Knowledge of research	Implement nursing activities
Responsive and action	Generate alternatives
dimensions of care	Coordinate with other team members

Fig. 1-7 Nursing conditions and behaviors related to implementation.

and theory from the physical and behavioral sciences to provide a rationale for nursing interventions.

Every nursing action should be supported by a rationale. A nurse who is unable to give a reason for nursing actions is practicing irresponsibly. Having a rationale for nursing actions also implies a continuing process whereby the nurse keeps up with new developments and modifies nursing actions in keeping with current, acceptable standards of practice.

Nursing intervention classification McCloskey and Bulechek[9] published a nursing intervention classification (NIC) system. The included interventions are supported by references from the nursing literature and describe what nurses *do* as they provide care to their patients. The authors identify eight reasons that this classification is important:

1. To standardize nomenclature
2. To expand nursing knowledge
3. To develop information systems
4. To teach decision making
5. To cost out nursing
6. To allocate nursing resources
7. To communicate nursing to non-nurses
8. To link nursing content

McCloskey and Bulechek[9] define a nursing intervention as "any direct care treatment that a nurse performs on behalf of a client." They include treatments initiated by nurses or by physicians. Nursing interventions are carried out by a series of nursing activities or actions, and nursing activities are the behaviors that nurses do to assist clients to attain their desired health goals. The box below presents the nursing intervention of "health screening" and related nursing activities. As with the NANDA taxonomy of nursing diagnoses, it is likely that revisions of the NIC will occur as nurses have an opportunity to work with it and nursing research provides better definitions for practice.

In most nurse-client situations there is more than one possible approach to accomplishing the stated outcomes. It is helpful when planning care to identify alternative nursing activities that are appropriate to the goal. If this is done, the nurse is not left floundering should the only identified activity fail. For instance, the community-health nurse who brings pamphlets to explain a low-sodium diet to her hypertensive client could be unsuccessful if the client cannot read. If, however, she also brought pictures

Health Screening

Definition

Detecting health risks or problems by means of history, examination, and other procedures

Activities

- Provide for privacy
- Measure blood pressure, height, weight, percent body fat, cholesterol, blood sugar as appropriate
- Perform pap smear, mammography, prostate check, electrocardiogram, testicular examination, and vision check as appropriate
- Obtain health history as appropriate
- Perform physical assessment as appropriate
- Complete appropriate Department of Health or other records for monitoring abnormal results such as high blood pressure
- Instruct on rationale and purpose of health screenings and self-monitoring
- Provide results of health screenings
- Counsel patient appropriately with alternatives for abnormal findings
- Inform patient of limitations and margin of error of specific screening tests
- Provide appropriate self-monitoring information during screening
- Refer patient to other health care providers as necessary
- Provide follow-up contact for patient with abnormal findings

From McCloskey JC, Bulechek GM: *Nursing interventions classification (NIC)*, ed 2, St Louis, 1997, Mosby.

 CULTURAL CONSIDERATIONS

Decisions about nursing interventions must also be based on an understanding of the client's cultural background. What factors would you consider when planning to teach the following clients about infant feeding?

- A first-generation Mexican American family with both parents in the household and employed in low-paying jobs.
- An upper-middle-class African American family with both parents present and only the father working.
- An unmarried Caucasian teenager who lives with her mother and grandmother. The family is middle class and has been in the United States for several generations.

How would differences in socioeconomic status or family situation affect nursing interventions?

of high- and low-sodium foods to reinforce verbal health teaching, the nurse and the client would be able to continue to progress toward their goal. Consideration of several alternative nursing activities lends a great deal of flexibility to the implementation phase of the nursing process.

Clinical practice guidelines In 1989 the federal Agency for Health Care Policy and Research was established. This agency was given the responsibility for developing clinical practice guidelines related to specific health care problems. Sets of guidelines have been published for a number of conditions, including acute pain management, urinary incontinence in adults, pressure ulcers in adults, and depression.[1-3] These guidelines were developed by multidisciplinary teams of experts. Nurses were included in each panel convened to develop guidelines. Publications such as these provide a valuable resource for practicing nurses as they consider alternative nursing actions. Nurses can obtain information about new guidelines as well as revisions of the existing ones by reading professional journals and newsletters.

Clinical pathways As more health care is provided in managed care systems, there has been an effort to identify and describe the typical course of treatment for various health problems. Clinical pathways, based on a medical or nursing diagnosis, identify usual interventions and expected client behaviors at time-oriented stages of recovery. The progress of treatment can be measured based on a comparison of an individual's progress with the clinical pathway. "Outliers," clients who do not demonstrate the expected behavior, are examined carefully to try to identify the reason for the variation. For instance, if a client who has had hip replacement surgery is expected to ambulate with assistance in physical therapy by the second postoperative day and is unable to stand up after 4 days, the treatment team would focus on identifying the reason for the problem. Causes could be physical, such as a wound infection, or psychosocial, such as fear of burdening other family members after discharge. Interventions would be planned to help the client overcome the problem.

Team relationships Implementation of nursing care must not take place in isolation from the client's other experiences with the health care team and the health care system. The nurse has a responsibility to be sure that the nursing care plan is congruent with the plans of other health care professionals who are involved with the client. Some degree of conflict can be avoided by personal contact with other professionals to discover how they define their roles and responsibilities. Knowledge of the distribution of responsibility within the health team enables the nurse to consult colleagues appropriately as indicated by the needs of the client, as in the following example:

The nurse in the medical clinic assessed that a client ate a diet that was excessively high in starchy foods. The nurse was concerned because the client was slightly obese and had a family history of hypertension and diabetes. The client stated that she ate starchy foods because she could not afford meats, fruits, and vegetables. She had never had any instruction about nutrition. She had heard about food stamps but had no idea whether she was eligible. The nurse decided that this client's needs could best be met by referring her to the nutritionist for information about a balanced, low-cost diet and to the social worker for information about food stamps.

Although the nurse may have information about these areas, it is a much more efficient and appropriate use of time and energy to refer the client to team members who specialize in dealing with the client's needs. Table 1-3 lists some other health professionals and their usual areas of expertise who may receive referrals from nurses. Referral should be accompanied by adequate background information so that the assessment process is not duplicated.

Documentation Written communication is essential to the successful planning and implementation of nursing care. One such means of communication is the written nursing care plan. Most clinical agencies and schools of nursing have devised a format for the nursing care plan, and one such plan is presented in the last chapter of this book. Although there may be differences in format, the care plan is almost always based on the nursing process. Therefore a nurse who is familiar with the nursing process should have little difficulty adapting to various nursing care plan formats. There are a number of advantages to formulating a written record of the nursing care plan as it evolves. The nurse who initiates and writes the plan must think through the whole nursing process in a logical and structured manner. The likelihood of basing nursing care on sound rationale is greater,

TABLE 1-3   Other health care professionals and their areas of expertise

TITLE	AREA OF EXPERTISE
Nutritionist/dietitian	Assessing dietary status, planning nutritional intake; planning prescribed therapeutic diets; diet teaching; budgeting; purchasing and preparing food
Occupational therapist	Assessment of self-care abilities; teaching activities of daily living; rehabilitation; teaching leisure time skills
Physical therapist	Assessment of gross motor function; restoration of motor functioning; use of special therapeutic approaches such as diathermy and whirlpool baths
Physician	Assessment and diagnosis of medical illness; interpretation of diagnostic studies; prescription of treatment approaches, including medication; prescription and supervision of long-term illness care; performance of invasive interventions such as surgery
Play therapist	Assisting children to express feelings and thoughts through the use of age-appropriate play; social skills development; motor skills development
Psychologist	Assessment of mental and emotional functioning; psychotherapy; application of specialized therapeutic techniques such as behavior modification; group psychotherapy; family psychotherapy
Social worker	Social systems assessment and intervention at family, small group, and community levels; social skills training; referral to appropriate community resources; family assessment and support; group therapy; family therapy
Speech therapist	Assessment of speech disruptions; language skills training; speech training or retraining; training in alternative modes of communication
Teacher	Assessment of educational level and learning ability; tutoring; specialized education for the learning disabled; general education for children and adults

because nursing care plans are generally scrutinized by others and the reasons for specific components of the plan may be questioned. Self-evaluation by the nurse is also facilitated. A working care plan that is kept up-to-date requires that application of the nursing process be consistently reviewed and revised. Many agencies are becoming aware that well-written nursing care plans reflect the course of the client's contact with nursing personnel. It is generally a practice to include the nursing care plan in the client's permanent agency record. This can greatly enhance the quality of nursing care if the client contacts the agency again in the future. Much data from the original assessment need not be collected again, thereby freeing the energy of both client and nurse to work on current concerns.

To provide clarity and prevent duplication, most agencies maintain chronologic client records. This means that all health care providers record their observations of the client's progress in one section of the chart as they occur rather than in a separate section reserved for physicians, nurses, or others. Many also organize documentation according to a "problem list" that includes the health care problems and needs that have been identified by the client in conjunction with the team. Each problem is assigned a number that serves as a reference point in the progress note.

Many agencies organize nurses' progress notes according to the nursing process. In this case the note usually begins with an assessment of the client's behavior, including both the client's description of his response to care and the nurse's observations. Next, there is a reference to the nursing care goal or expected client outcome that was addressed. Any nursing interventions that were provided are described. Finally, the nurse records an evaluation of the effectiveness of the intervention and recommendations for modification if indicated. If a problem list is used, the note should also be coded according to the problems that were addressed. The use of a nursing-process format for documentation facilitates feedback for modification of the nursing care plan.

il document. It is
itries be factual and
y to record specific
ehavior and include
nunication whenever
cise and avoid repeti-
included. The focus
person's condition or
onclusions about the
meaning of the .... vior should be avoided.
Greve[7] wrote that "the chart tells the patient's story,"
and he advises using descriptive terminology for
interventions and cautions nurses not to omit documentation of client teaching.

CRITICAL THINKING Question.................

It has been said in relationship to nursing actions, "If it
is not recorded, it was not done." Do you agree or disagree with this statement? What are the implications
for nursing documentation?

Recently attention has been focused on using
standardized formats for client record keeping. Flow
sheets may be used to document routine observations. Documentation forms may be developed
related to nursing or medical diagnoses, including
the aspects of care that are usually involved for
clients with a particular health care problem. If standardized forms are used, it is important to ensure
that they provide for individualization of the client's
care; the risk in this approach is that all clients may
be treated the same without regard to their specific
needs. The problems related to such assumptions
were addressed earlier in this chapter.

Some agencies have instituted computerized documentation systems. Expense has slowed the pace of
this change, but it seems likely that the trend will
continue. As with standardized written forms, it is
important to allow for recognition of the client's
individuality. The advantage of automated record
systems is increased efficiency. In hospital settings,
this is especially true when the computer terminal is
located at the bedside.

The specific format used may vary, but the important issue is that information about the plan of care
be disseminated so that there can be consistency and
continuity in the approach to the client. Fragmented
care can only be detrimental. In addition, written
planning for care requires that the planner have a
logical, well-organized rationale. This avoids a hit-
or-miss or intuitive approach to the client that may
or may not be beneficial. Implementation of care has
the greatest potential for success when it is based on
a sound plan.

Evaluation

Nursing care is incomplete unless it is systematically
evaluated. Evaluation includes an element of
reassessment. Once care has been implemented, the
client's response must be analyzed. This analysis
must be based on the client's response to the intervention and includes both the client's verbal description of the results of the care and nonverbal reactions. For instance, if a client is given eyedrops for
an inflammation of the eye, it is necessary to ask if
the discomfort has been alleviated. The nurse also
needs to observe the eye to see if the redness and
swelling have subsided. Both of these data sources
are then combined to determine the effectiveness of
the nursing intervention.

When evaluating nursing care, one should review
the other steps of the nursing process. The success
or failure of nursing intervention may reflect the
adequacy of the assessment. If important data are
not assessed, there is greater likelihood of inadequate
intervention. Even if the assessment is sufficient, the
analysis of the data must be accurate. Therefore it is
necessary to reconsider the nursing diagnosis and
the client's nursing needs. The right plan for the
wrong need will not help the client.

The plan for nursing intervention must be evaluated next. If expected outcomes of care have been
written behaviorally and mutually validated with the
client, they may serve as a guide for evaluating
nursing care. However, even if goal attainment has
been achieved, the nurse should review the total
nursing process to thoroughly evaluate the nursing
care that the client has received. There are usually a
number of alternative approaches to a client's
problem. Commonly, the first action chosen is not
the most effective in meeting the client's needs. Consideration must also be given to whether the action
was efficient in use of time and energy by both the

nurse and client. An inefficient approach, even though effective, should be modified.

The manner of implementation of the plan should also be reviewed. The goals and nursing actions may be entirely appropriate, but if the nurse does not carry them out adequately, the desired results will not be achieved. For instance, if the nurse assesses that the client needs to learn about prevention of hypertension but then presents the information in complicated medical terminology, the manner of implementation needs modification. The nurse must be flexible when applying the nursing process. The process is dynamic, and it is necessary to respond to the client in terms of the situation at the time of the nursing contact. A total plan may become irrelevant if the client's situation has changed since the last contact. The need to modify a care plan does not connote failure of nursing care. Failure occurs if the plan of care is not relevant to the client's needs and is not revised as the needs change or are clarified.

Clinical supervision It is often difficult for the nurse to evaluate nursing care alone. Supervision by a peer, a group of peers, or a more experienced person is an important part of professional development. Most nurses use a combination of these approaches to supervision. Peer evaluation often goes on informally when the nurse validates the success or failure of nursing approaches with colleagues who are also familiar with the client. Formal supervisory sessions are of utmost importance. Nurses who work in isolation tend to become stale and develop habitual approaches to clients that may not always be the most effective means to accomplish

stated goals; examination of nursing care plans with a supervisor or a supervised group helps prevent this staleness. It also stimulates the nurse to try new approaches, thus encouraging innovation. When the nurse feels frustrated because several approaches to a client have been unsuccessful, supervision can be supportive, provide encouragement, and suggest new ideas. Supervisory sessions are enhanced when they are planned in advance and the nurse presents the written plan of care for the client who is being discussed. It is then possible to review the application of the nursing process in terms of its adequacy, appropriateness, effectiveness, efficiency, acceptability, comprehensiveness, and flexibility. The nurse's thought processes in planning care become apparent and can be examined, facilitating learning. The nursing conditions and nursing behaviors related to evaluation are depicted in Fig. 1-8.

Quality improvement Evaluation of the nursing process is an ongoing activity that is the professional responsibility of every nurse. In addition, health care agencies conduct periodic surveys of the nursing care that is provided within that agency. Organizational evaluation such as this is referred to as the *quality improvement* function of the agency. The emphasis on continuous quality improvement is reflected in the standards of the Joint Commission on Accreditation of Healthcare Organizations (JCAHO). JCAHO accreditation is requested by health care agencies to document that their services have been evaluated by objective, professional surveyors.

Nurses should be directly involved in any quality improvement activity that evaluates nursing care. Sometimes nursing care will be reviewed separately.

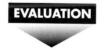

NURSING CONDITIONS	NURSING BEHAVIORS
Supervision	Compare client's response and expected outcome
Self-analysis	
Peer review	Review nursing process
Client and family participation	Modify nursing process as needed
	Participate in quality improvement activities

Fig. 1-8 The nursing conditions and behaviors related to evaluation.

At other times, it is included as part of a review of interdisciplinary client health care.

An important aspect of quality improvement is the *monitoring and evaluation* of client care. One approach to monitoring and evaluation is the *client care audit.* An audit that focuses on the caregiver is sometimes referred to as a *process audit.* Data may be collected by observing the nurse providing care to the client, reviewing nursing care plans and nurses notes, interviewing clients, or a combination of these sources. The data collected are compared with a preset standard of nursing care. This could be a set of behaviors determined by nursing experts; the nursing staff of the agency; or the professional organization, such as the ANA *Standards of Nursing Practice* mentioned earlier. The standard to be used is selected based on the information that is being sought. For instance, standards set by nurses in an agency could pinpoint behavior specific to the care expected by nurses in that setting.

Another type of audit is the *outcome audit.* The outcome audit focuses on the behavior of the client in response to the care that has been provided. It is compatible with the nursing process because it essentially parallels the evaluation phase. Standards of behaviors are written for a group of clients with a common health care problem or need. These standards usually reflect behaviors expected at the end of a health care episode, although it is possible to conduct an audit at an intermediate point in the caregiving process. Proponents of this method point out that the process itself has meaning only in terms of the effect on the client. Data are usually collected from client records, although they can be obtained by direct client observation and interview. Managed care organizations review client outcomes and compare them with established standards to decide whether to authorize continued reimbursement for health care services.

Both process and outcome audits have advantages depending on the information desired. Many agencies do both types of review. Commonly, outcome audits reveal possible problems in the caregiving process that can be validated by initiating a process audit. Nursing research relative to evaluation of care is critically needed. At the present time, it is generally difficult to connect the client outcome to a specific caregiving process because of the lack of valid research in this area.

No matter what approach is taken to client care evaluation, the last step in the process is the most important one. This step is the action that is taken to address the opportunities for improvement that the audit reveals. Sometimes administrative changes in policies or procedures are required. An in-service education program directed toward the area of need is generally sufficient to produce the recommended changes. Audit is viewed by some nurses as a threat, but it is really an opportunity to improve the quality of the care that clients receive. Even the best system can usually find room for improvement. Evaluation of care and monitoring of quality are integral parts of the professional accountability of nurses to clients.

SUMMARY

The nursing process is an interactive, problem-solving process used by the nurse to give organized and individualized care. The goal of nursing care is to maximize a person's level of wellness, degree of self-actualization, and positive interactions with the environment. Through the nursing process the nurse facilitates the client's positive adaptation as a unique individual to the stress he or she may be experiencing. There are five continuous and overlapping phases of this process, and the nursing conditions and behaviors associated with each are summarized in Fig. 1-9.

Data collection is the first phase and marks the establishment of the nursing contract and the beginning of the nurse-client relationship. The focus of the nurse during this phase is to gain a total view of the client's interacting biopsychosocial components. If the data collection is validated, precise, standardized, and organized, the nurse will be prepared to move into the second phase of the nursing process.

The next phase involves formulation of the nursing diagnosis. In this phase logical decision making is used to analyze the collected data and derive a nursing diagnosis through which the nursing problems of the client are identified. Nursing problems are areas in which the client's health may be promoted or areas in which the client needs help adapting to stress. Nurses diagnose a wide range of health-related responses observed in sick and well persons. These responses can be reactions

ASSESSMENT

NURSING CONDITIONS	NURSING BEHAVIORS
Self-awareness Accurate observations Therapeutic communication Responsive dimensions of care	Establish nursing contract Obtain information from client and family Validate data with client Organize data

NURSING DIAGNOSIS

NURSING CONDITIONS	NURSING BEHAVIORS
Logical decision making Knowledge of normal parameters Inductive and deductive reasoning Sociocultural sensitivity	Identify patterns in data Compare data with norms Analyze and synthesize data Problems/strengths identified Validate problems with client Formulate nursing diagnosis Set priorities of problems

OUTCOME IDENTIFICATION

NURSING CONDITIONS	NURSING BEHAVIORS
Critical thinking skills Partnership with client and family	Hypothesizing Specify expected outcomes Validate goals with client

PLANNING

NURSING CONDITIONS	NURSING BEHAVIORS
Application of theory Respect for client and family	Prioritize goals Identify nursing activities Validate plan with client

IMPLEMENTATION

NURSING CONDITIONS	NURSING BEHAVIORS
Past clinical experiences Knowledge of research Responsive and action dimensions of care	Consider available resources Implement nursing activities Generate alternatives Coordinate with other team members

EVALUATION

NURSING CONDITIONS	NURSING BEHAVIORS
Supervision Self-analysis Peer review Client and family participation	Compare client's response and expected outcome Review nursing process Modify nursing process as needed Participate in quality improvement activities

Fig. 1-9 The nursing process.

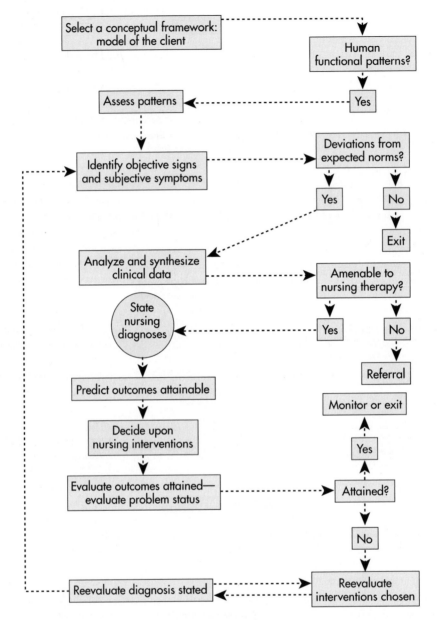

Fig. I-10 Flowchart of nursing process. (From Gordon M: The concept of nursing diagnosis, *Nurs Clin North Am* 14:492, 1979.)

to an actual problem, such as disease, or they can anticipate a potential health problem.

When appropriate nursing problems have been identified and validated, the nurse enters the planning phase of the nursing process. Included in this phase are the setting of priorities, identification of expected outcomes, and determination of nursing interventions and activities.

Implementation is the fourth phase of the nursing process and refers to the actual delivery of nursing care to the client and the client's response to the care that is given. Written communication is essential to the successful planning and implementation of nursing care. The written nursing care plan is a means of communication that is based on the phases of the nursing process. Written planning for care requires the use of a sound rationale and provides for consistency and continuity in the approach to the client.

Evaluation is the fifth phase of the nursing process and includes reassessment of the client based on verbal and nonverbal responses to nursing intervention. When evaluating nursing care the nurse should review each preceding phase of the nursing process. Through supervision and peer evaluation the nurse can review the application of the nursing process and critically examine the care that the client received.

These five phases of the nursing process commonly overlap or occur simultaneously. Each phase builds on the previous one, and all depend on validation with the client to ensure the mutuality of the nursing care. Thus the nursing process is dynamic, interpersonal, and the basic framework used to provide quality, professional nursing care (Fig. 1-10).

This chapter on the nursing process is meant to provide a structural framework for the rest of the text. For this process to be carried out successfully the nurse and client must interact with each other on a human-to-human level. There are several aspects of interpersonal theory that provide the nurse with knowledge necessary to establish the nursing process on an interpersonal level and carry it out successfully. Theory is presented relative to the development of a self-concept and the growth of self-awareness, basic communications, the therapeutic nurse-client relationship, and the application of these concepts to stress and adaptation. Basic concepts are presented relative to the role of the nurse in small groups. The application of the nursing process is studied relative to the three levels of prevention. The final chapter demonstrates the application of the theoretic concepts to the nursing process through the presentation of a hypothetic nursing assessment and nursing care plan. This should help the reader understand the reciprocal nature of the concepts that are presented and discussed.

DISCUSSION QUESTIONS

1. Write your own definition of nursing. Is this the way you would have defined nursing 2 years ago? If not, how is it different?

2. Critique the image of nurses and nursing presented in some recent novels, movies, television shows, and commercials. Discuss ways you and your fellow nurses can improve the image of nursing in the media. Implement at least one of your own suggestions.

3. It has been said that tertiary prevention nursing functions include those of primary and secondary prevention. Why is this true? Give an example to support your explanation.

4. Go to the library and read the ANA *Standards of Nursing Practice* in their entirety. What purpose do they serve? How are they valuable to the profession? How are they helpful to you at this point in your nursing career?

5. What data do you find most difficult to elicit from clients? Why? How can you overcome this discomfort?

6. Think of a nursing decision you made recently in caring for a client. Evaluate whether it was logical, illogical, inductive, or deductive.

7. A nursing student friend is discussing the difficulty she's having identifying the nursing diagnoses for her client. A medical student who overhears the conversation says, "Nurses don't have or need their own diagnoses. Why waste your time? Just carry out the doctor's orders." How would you respond?

8. Identify a personal goal that you would like to achieve a month from now. Write a measurable behavioral expected outcome with short-term contributory goals. On a regular basis, evaluate your progress toward goal attainment.

9. You walk into your neighbor's house and observe the following scene:

   The mother is asleep on the sofa; the 9-month-old is vomiting in his playpen; the 2-year-old is trying to place an electrical plug into a socket; and a pot is boiling over on the stove.

   Describe and give priority to the actions that you would take. State your rationale for both the actions and the priorities.

10. Select a nursing topic that is of interest to you. Survey the literature to identify nursing research

that has been conducted relative to this topic. Can you find additional research studies that have been carried out by scientists from other disciplines? How do the various studies complement or contradict each other?

11. Go to the library and find the professional journal of another health care discipline. Review several issues and identify the client care and other professional concerns of members of that discipline. Compare and contrast with nursing concerns.

12. Briefly interview a friend or relative about how they are feeling. Write a progress note to document your conversation.

13. Using the criteria of adequacy, appropriateness, effectiveness, efficiency, acceptability, comprehensiveness, and flexibility, evaluate your method of study for your last examination.

14. Select an activity that you enjoy. This could be a hobby, sport, or game. Identify three expectations for your performance *during* the activity (process standards) and at least one expectation to be met at the completion of the activity (outcome standard). For example, a game of golf might have process standards of (1) to make par or less on at least nine holes, (2) to hit into no more than two sand traps, and (3) to hit no balls into the water. The outcome standard would be to score 90 or less for 18 holes. Evaluate your performance based on your standards.

EXPERIENTIAL & SIMULATED LEARNING EXERCISES

1. Beliefs about man, health, and illness

PURPOSE: To sensitize the students to the influence a person's belief system can have on his or her perception of health and illness.

PROCEDURE: Assign a different religion or philosophic belief system to each student. Ask each person to study the premises of the religion, its beliefs about the nature of man, and its perspective on health and illness.

DISCUSSION: In a discussion group have the students compare and contrast the various beliefs. How do they correspond with present medical science? What

implications might arise in giving nursing care to someone with these beliefs? What conflicts may arise and how should they best be handled? What would happen if a nurse's belief system was different from that of the institution in which she worked? What alternatives would she have?

2. Perceptions of nursing

PURPOSE: To survey the perceptions people in general have about nursing and good nursing care.

PROCEDURE: Have each student take an informal survey among friends, acquaintances, and relatives, asking the following three questions: (1) What is nursing? (2) What do nurses do? (3) What do you ideally expect from a nurse?

DISCUSSION: Share the results of the survey with a large group. What stereotyped views of nursing emerge? Categorize the nursing functions identified into physical care, psychologic care, and meeting social needs. Which category dominates? Analyze whether dependent or independent nursing functions were most often mentioned. How do the views of the people surveyed compare with the nursing group's views? How might the nursing group go about changing the views of the general public?

3. Identifying behavior

PURPOSE: To differentiate statements describing behavior from those communicating an idea, inference, value judgment, or other nonbehavioral observation.

PROCEDURE: At the start of the exercise, quietly ask one student to perform a certain task within the room (such as to find the latest issue of the *American Journal of Nursing* or to line up three chairs in a row) and nod his or her head to you in response. Then begin the exercise. The first point to make is that in communicating, people do not express themselves clearly enough, so you're going to discuss "identifying behavior" with them. Most often, instead of describing another person's behavior, we discuss his attitudes, motivations, emotions, or personality traits. Often our statements are more expressive of the way we feel about the other person's actions than they are informing about his behavior. We often tend to "read into" other people's actions. What we would like to do is describe behavior that means reporting specific, observable actions of others without placing a value judgment on them as right or wrong, good or bad, and without generalizing about the person's attitude, motives, or personality traits. Ask the students if they have had any difficulty identifying behavior. Tell them you have some statements and you're going to ask each one to say whether one particular statement describes behavior or not.

SAMPLE STATEMENTS:

1. "Sue, you're being stubborn today."
2. "Sue, you cut in before I was finished."
3. Sue resented Joe's question.
4. Sue has a cold.
5. Sue's voice got louder when she said, "Cut that out."
6. Sue was cooperative.
7. Sue walked out of class 10 minutes before it was over.
8. Sue wanted to have her way and dominate the group.
9. Sue answered all the questions asked of her.
10. Sue feels good about herself.
11. "Sue, you want to be the center of attention."
12. Sue looked away from me every time I asked about her father.
13. Sue was upset and worried.
14. Sue interrupted me every time I began a sentence.
15. "Sue, you eat good meals."
16. "Sue, you make me feel uncomfortable."
17. "Sue, you're staring at me and that makes me feel uncomfortable."

DISCUSSION: When you've finished, ask the students if they recall that at the beginning of the exercise, one of them did something different. From memory ask them to describe the student's behavior. Watch out for statements describing her motivation, intent, or goal, which would all be inferences. Then, based on the group's response, either ask the student to repeat his or her actions or tell them what you asked the student to do. Finally, ask them if they feel more comfortable identifying behavior and if they have any additional questions.

4. Collecting data

PURPOSE: To practice the skills involved in gathering information of a clinical nature.

PROCEDURE: Break the students into groups of two. Have one student assume the role of the client and

the other student be the nurse. Ask them to complete a full assessment of their "client" using your institution's data collection tool.

DISCUSSION: The students should share their experiences with data collection in a small group. How long did the assessments take to complete? How did the client feel about the way the interview was conducted? Specifically, what made the client nervous, relaxed, defensive, or embarrassed? Was all of the required data collected? If not, what was omitted or overlooked? What aspect of the data collection was most difficult for the nurse? What would have improved the assessment in both process and content? Ask the students to repeat the exercise reversing their roles.

5. Observable behavior

PURPOSE: To distinguish statements reflecting observable behavior from those reflecting assumed behavior.

PROCEDURE: Assign each student a verb and ask them to write a client-centered goal using that verb. Ask the group to identify whether the behavior described is observable. If it is not observable, ask the student to rephrase the goal using a new verb that will describe observable behavior.

SAMPLE VERBS: Describes, applies, writes, states, believes, thinks, identifies, sees, understands, performs, feels, takes, accepts, learns, assists.

6. Peer review

PURPOSE: To apply standards of nursing practice by giving and receiving feedback on nursing care provided.

PROCEDURE: Each student should become familiar with the ANA *Standards of Nursing Practice*. Assign students in pairs to two clients. Each student should be the primary caregiver for one client, while the other observes and assists if necessary. Following the clinical practice time, they should review the *Standards* and give each other feedback on the nursing care that was observed.

DISCUSSION: The entire group should then discuss the experience of peer review, including the application of predetermined standards to their practice and feelings (positive and negative) about being critiqued by a classmate rather than by a teacher.

REFERENCES

1. Agency for Health Care Policy and Research: *Acute pain management: operative or medical procedures and trauma,* Washington, DC, 1992, US Department of Health and Human Services.
2. Agency for Health Care Policy and Research: *Urinary incontinence in adults,* Washington, DC, 1992, US Department of Health and Human Services.
3. Agency for Health Care Policy and Research: *Pressure ulcers in adults: prediction and prevention,* Washington, DC, 1992, US Department of Health and Human Services.
4. American Nurses' Association: *Nursing's social policy statement,* Washington, DC, 1995, American Nurses' Association.
5. American Nurses' Association: *Nursing: a social policy statement,* Kansas City, Mo, 1980, American Nurses' Association.
6. American Nurses' Association: *Standards of clinical nursing practice,* Kansas City, Mo, 1991, American Nurses' Association.
7. Greve P: Documentation: every word counts, *RN* 55:57, 1992.
8. Mager RF: *Preparing instructional objectives,* Palo Alto, Calif, 1984, Fearon.
9. McCloskey JC, Bulechek GM: *Nursing interventions classification (NIC),* ed 2, St Louis, 1997, Mosby.
10. Redman B: *The process of patient education,* ed 7, St Louis, 1993, Mosby.
11. Shamansky S, Clausen C: Levels of prevention: examination of the concept, *Nurs Outlook* 28:104, 1980.

Suggested Readings

Ackley B, Ladwig G: *Nursing diagnosis handbook,* St Louis, 1997, Mosby.

This convenient reference helps nurses make a nursing diagnosis and write a care plan with ease and confidence. It correlates nursing diagnoses with known information about clients based on assessment findings, established medical or psychiatric diagnoses, and the current treatment plan.

American Nurses' Association: *Nursing's social policy statement,* Washington, DC, 1995, American Nurses' Association.

This official statement defines nursing and is an important public and professional document that should be read by all nurses.

American Nurses' Association: *Standards of clinical nursing practice,* Kansas City, Mo, 1991, American Nurses' Association.

This pamphlet should be owned by all nurses. It contains the standards of care and professional performance.

Bellack J, Edlund B: *Nursing assessment and diagnosis,* Boston, 1992, Jones and Bartlett.

This text describes a comprehensive biopsychosocial nursing approach to assessment and diagnosis. Detailed, clear, and very thorough.

Carlson J et al: *Nursing diagnosis: a case study approach,* Philadelphia, 1991, WB Saunders.

This book helps students and clinicians by providing current information and detailed case examples of how nursing diagnosis—as a part of the nursing process—can be used in a variety of clinical situations.

Carpenito L, editor: *Nursing diagnosis: application to clinical practice,* ed 4, Philadelphia, 1992, JB Lippincott.

Nursing process, in this useful text, is addressed in its utilization and organization around nursing diagnosis. Specific diagnostic categories are explored and presented in a very practical way.

Christensen P, Kenney J: *Nursing process: application of conceptual models,* St Louis, 1995, Mosby.

This text applies theoretical approaches used in the nursing process and is organized around individuals, families, and communities. Highly recommended.

Mager RF: *Preparing instructional objectives,* Palo Alto, Calif, 1984, Fearon.

This is a classic text on the art of writing behavioral objectives. It is written in a programmed learning format and is easy to read, but at the same time it is very informational. This is highly recommended for inexperienced objective-writers.

McCloskey JC, Bulechek GM: *Nursing interventions classification (NIC),* ed 2, St Louis, 1997, Mosby.

This book represents the first attempt by nurses to categorize nursing interventions. It is an ambitious effort and warrants the review and response of all nurses. It clearly communicates the many activities that make up nursing.

Meintz SL, Shaha SH: Our hand-held computer beats them all, *RN* 55:53, 1992.

The authors compare the relative effectiveness of traditional written documentation, centralized computers, bedside computer terminals, and a handheld computer. They provide a concise description of the state of the art in documentation systems.

Mottley BW: Dialogues with excellence: bringing Stanley back, *Am J Nurs* 92:34, 1992.

The author describes application of the nursing process to the care of a client who was considered to be "difficult." This is a good example of the importance of periodic reassessment and the establishment of specific expected outcomes.

Murray R, Zentner J: *Nursing assessment and health promotion through the life span,* ed 6, Stamford, Conn, 1997, Appleton & Lange.

This text presents detailed information of the normal, well individual through each stage of the development process. It incorporates physiologic and psychosocial concepts needed by the nurse to complete an assessment and interview to promote or maintain health.

Pender N: *Health promotion in nursing practice,* Stamford, Conn, 1996, Appleton & Lange.

A model of health promotion is described and applied to nursing practice in this excellent text. Highly recommended.

Phaneuf M: *The nursing audit: self-regulation in nursing practice,* New York, 1976, Appleton-Century-Crofts.

This book is a classic presentation of one approach to nursing audit. The author was a pioneer in the area of quality assurance. This methodology is applicable to many health care settings. The book also provides a profile of essential elements of client care.

Redman B: *The process of patient education,* ed 7, St Louis, 1993, Mosby.

>   *The author presents a comprehensive approach to health teaching. Of particular note in the context of this chapter is the discussion on the writing of objectives. Also of interest is the section on evaluation.*

Schumaker S, Schron E, Ockene J, editors: *Handbook of health behavior change,* New York, 1990, Springer-Verlag.

>   *Behaviors for disease prevention and disease management are described, including issues for specific populations.*

Snyder M, Egan EC, Nojima Y: Defining nursing interventions, *Image J Nurs Sch* 28:137, 1996.

>   *This article reviews the history of efforts by nursing scholars to define and categorize nursing interventions. It includes a discussion of the reasons that nursing needs to continue to pursue a unified nursing classification system.*

US Department of Health and Human Services: *Healthy People 2000,* Washington, DC, 1990, US Government Printing Office.

>   *This report is the national strategy for improving the health of the nation over the next decade. It addresses the prevention of chronic illnesses, injuries, and infectious diseases.*

Wilkinson J: *Nursing process in action: a critical thinking approach,* Menlo Park, Calif, 1992, Addison-Wesley.

>   *This text promotes professional practice and critical thinking skills of beginning and experienced nurses by integrating professional standards of care, ethical issues, wellness, and nursing frameworks into each phase of the nursing process.*

CHAPTER

2 *The Emergence of the Self*

Perhaps
it is the way
that seasons
change
that makes life
seem so simple
running from childhood
to old age
in what seems
a single bound.

Lawrence Craig-Green
Perhaps

LEARNING OBJECTIVES

After studying this chapter, the student should be able to:

- Compare and contrast the developmental theories of Freud, Sullivan, and Erikson, including the basic assumptions underlying each theory.
- Define the meaning of the term *epigenetic sequence* as described by Erikson.
- Describe the developmental tasks identified by Freud, Sullivan, and Erikson for each of the eight stages of an individual's growth.
- Analyze the role of parents in meeting the changing psychosocial needs of the child from infancy through adolescence.
- Identify threats to the developmental process that may occur at each of the eight stages of an individual's growth.
- Assess the developmental level of a client according to the theories of Freud, Sullivan, and Erikson.

---

* This is footnote text this is footnote text this is footnote text this is footnote text

Understanding the nature of the self is both the basis and realization of the nursing process. Fundamental to this understanding is the idea of self-awareness. As nurses, our behaviors, communications, and interactions are influenced by our unique perceptions, and it is only by understanding ourselves that we are able to begin to understand the private world of another. Knowledge of self, therefore, should first be incorporated into the personal world of the nurse. The nurse who is aware of her own dynamic being can then intervene more therapeutically in enhancing the health of another person, and this is the goal of the nursing process. As a primary theoretic basis for nursing, knowledge of the self must be founded on the study of the development of the self, its present dynamics, and its unfolding potential. This chapter and Chapter 3 expand on these areas.

The concept of the self has fascinated humans for centuries. We have sung about it, questioned it, written about it, and marvelled at it. There are personality tests of all descriptions to examine it more closely, but each new insight reveals the depth and complexity of the question "Who am I?" In fact, there is no universally accepted definition of the self. How one defines it reflects one's background—philosophy, theology, behavioral sciences, humanities, and so on. It also depends on one's vantage point—whether one is a participant or an observer. Think of yourself for a moment as stepping outside of your body and observing yourself objectively. You might describe your attitudes, beliefs, coping mechanisms, and what you think about yourself. Now, slip back inside, and you are a participant once more, involved in perceiving, thinking, remembering, and feeling. Together, these make up your dynamic self—dynamic because you are constantly in a state of becoming, and to this degree you can never fully know "Who am I?"

Self-awareness begins in infancy and proceeds through childhood, adolescence, adulthood, and old age, with each one of the new stages of life building on the one past. Many psychologic theorists have divided the life cycle into similar developmental stages and then described the tasks of each stage. The focus each theorist assumes in describing the developmental stages varies, depending on one's orientation and perspective. Because each theorist might isolate one particular aspect of development, it is often necessary to become familiar with more than one theorist to truly understand how the self develops. This chapter incorporates the concepts of three particular theorists, each of whom approached the developmental tasks from a unique perspective—the intrapsychic approach of Sigmund Freud, the study of interpersonal relations by Harry Stack Sullivan, and the analysis of cultural forces by Erik Erikson. In bringing together the significant contributions of these particular theorists, one's learning evolves from that of the individual to significant others and, ultimately, to society (Fig. 2-1).

CRITICAL THINKING *Question* ················

List five adjectives that describe yourself. Compare these to five adjectives that would have described you at age 10. Think about how you have changed over the past years and the adjectives you hope would describe yourself 10 years from now.
··

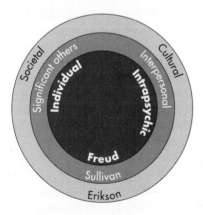

Fig. 2-1 Evolution of theories of personality, including those of Freud, Sullivan, and Erikson.

Sigmund Freud (1856–1939) was a physician by profession and lived most of his life in Vienna, Austria. He lived during an exciting time. When Freud was 3 years old, Darwin published *Origin of the Species,* and when Freud was 4, the science of psychology was founded. Simultaneously, the study of physics and energy transformations led to vital achievements for society. All of this greatly influenced Freud. He was the first person to apply many of the laws of the physical sciences to man's personality. His focus of study was intrapsychic—examining the conscious and unconscious processes within the individual, focusing on predetermined biologic needs. He viewed behavior as a product of interaction between the id, ego, and superego. Throughout his long lifetime he continued to develop his theory, and he is considered today to be the founder of modern psychiatry.

Two Freudian principles are important to his theory, and they caused a great public reaction when he initially shared them.[1] The first is Freud's belief in the unconscious. People found it hard to accept the idea that man is not the supreme master of his fate but is sometimes ruled by this unknown and fearful force that Freud called the unconscious. The second Freudian principle is that of infantile sexuality. Freud believed that children undergo a course of sexual development that in many ways parallels that of the adult. These two ideas led Freud to believe that the first few years of life are crucial to the foundation of the personality, and his work on the history of the early years of life became a cornerstone of his theory.

He analyzed specific developmental events of the early years and called them the *phases of psychosexual development.* His stages of development, which begin at birth and proceed through puberty, are based on the prominence of various organ systems and particular zones of the body. Thus Freud viewed the mouth, excretory organs, and genital organs as filling both biologic and psychosexual needs, and they became the basis for the particular phases of psychosexual development. It is important to note that each of Freud's stages is not abandoned but progress and overlap to form the developing self.

Recently, many developmental theorists and clinicians have criticized the work of Freud. His theory has not been confirmed by research studies, which has led some to believe that his theory is incorrect. Others believe that it is difficult to investigate psychoanalytic propositions. At present, there is a movement away from the traditional psychoanalytic viewpoint to one that incorporates a more interactional and cultural frame of reference.

Harry Stack Sullivan (1892–1949), also a physician, was born in the state of New York and worked mainly in the Washington, D.C.–Baltimore, Maryland area at St. Elizabeth's Hospital, the University of Maryland, Sheppard and Enoch Pratt Hospital, and Chestnut Lodge. Sullivan was trained in the Freudian psychoanalytic school, but he disagreed with some of Freud's ideas and theorized about phenomena not described by Freud—in particular, the patterns of interaction that occur between people. He is known as the founder of the interpersonal theory of psychiatry, which studies the communication and relationships between people. His view was that personality is "the relatively enduring pattern of recurrent interpersonal situations which characterize a human life."[10] During his lifetime Sullivan published only one book describing his theory,[9] but he kept many notes and lectured frequently. Since his death these have been gathered into additional publications.

Sullivan's ideas about the formation of personality were not based on the inner needs of the child but on the child's developing capabilities. Unlike Freud, Sullivan did not focus on the biologic or sexual demands of the person but on acquiring new capacities that would provide greater awareness of the interpersonal environment and greater ability to deal with it. He did, however, accept the importance of heredity and biologic growth, because he believed that a certain amount of physical development is necessary to be successful in social living. The unifying theme of Sullivan's developmental framework is interpersonal relationships and being secure in the social environment. According to Sullivan, when security is threatened, the individual will take steps to reduce the anxiety he is experiencing. Thus his stages, which begin in infancy and end in late adolescence and maturity, progress and grow in a way that reflect changes in interpersonal relationships. Sul-

livan did not believe that personality is set early in life but believed in the individual's potential for change in response to people and culture. His theory of socialized learning requires the successful negotiation of all stages of development before maturity is attained. With maturity, Sullivan's developmental framework is completed and the infant animal organism transformed into an adult human person.

Erik Erikson (1902–) was born of Danish parents and became interested in psychoanalysis after pursuing a career as an artist. He trained in Vienna under Anna Freud and came across the ocean to study at Harvard in 1934. He was greatly influenced by anthropology and man's cultural traditions. Erikson's theory incorporates Freud's ideas, but Erikson moves beyond these in his work on child analysis, developmental tasks, and man's ability to live within his particular social environment. As a social psychoanalyst his focus is cultural, and he applies the theory of psychoanalysis to social and anthropologic data to comment on broader areas of human functioning.

Erikson's work on the development of the self is most noted for the theme he assigns to each stage, the relationship of each stage to the previous and future ones, and the part each stage contributes to the total development of the personality. Erikson views the newborn as a generalist who becomes more specialized with growth through the steplike stages. His first five stages are reformulations of Freud's psychosexual stages, but unlike Freud, Erikson continues the developmental process through three additional stages of adulthood. This is Erikson's unique contribution, because most developmental theorists omit or neglect the adult years or analyze them only in relation to childhood. Erikson's stages reflect growth and movement. In each stage a central problem or task is identified; the problem is that of two opposing forces that must be brought together and integrated in the individual's experiences. Erikson states that these tasks are universal, although the particular culture defines the specific situation facing the individual. So too the specific tasks are the same for both males and females, but the content of what each gender deals with will be dif-

CULTURAL CONSIDERATIONS

The theories of personality described in this chapter have as their foundation the work of white males from the dominant culture of the time. Although these theories are clearly important and have stood the test of time, many other theories have been proposed in recent years that elaborate on, challenge, extend, or refute previous ideas. Some of these theories reflect a feminist, ethnic, or cultural perspective on human growth and development. Select a contemporary theory that reflects divergent thinking based on age, gender, belief system, or social values and analyze its contribution to understanding human development.

ferent, depending on both biology and the way the culture brings out the tasks. The challenge is mastery of the problem. With this resolution and the appropriate biologic, psychologic, and sociologic readiness, the person moves on to the next stage.

Erikson believes that life follows an *epigenetic sequence.* By this he means that there is a basic regularity of life and that the personality structure of the growing child gradually unfolds when the child's own readiness is met by his social environment. Thus development is a continuum in which each stage has a part and is related to all other parts, and the tasks of each stage must be completed for the individual to grow and move toward maturity. Finally, Erikson views the quality of parental care and family organization as crucial factors in personality development, and his theory reinforces the mutual interdependence of the individual and society.

INFANCY: BIRTH TO 1½ YEARS

*The self is a sea boundless
and measureless.*

Kahlil Gibran
The Prophet

At birth human children emerge from their mothers' wombs as separate beings with their own potentials and futures. Each receives a name, a family, and a home in which to live and grow. His world is very egocentric because it is interpreted in relation to his own needs and desires. As infants, however, each is also weak, helpless, and in many ways a reflection of his environment. Infants depend on other people to provide for virtually all their needs, and the most important physical needs at this time are for food and nourishment.

Freud calls this first psychosexual stage of infancy the oral stage in which the principal source of pleasure for the infant is the mouth and oral activities. This idea is easily seen when one watches a baby gurgling, blowing small bubbles, or attempting to put everything in his reach into his mouth. In the beginning the child experiences pleasure by putting things into the mouth, taking in food, and sucking from the mother's breast. The infant's first pleasure is in eating, but soon the child learns that the act of sucking itself gives pleasure. This pleasure is due to the excitation of the mouth and lips, and Freud views the act of sucking as the infant's first expression of the sexual instinct. The act of nursing, therefore, satisfies both the hunger and sexual instincts, and thus a link is established early between the taking in of food and sexual pleasure.

In later periods of life there are other oral activities, such as smoking, drinking, or nail biting, that may also serve to provide this pleasure sensation. Later on in this period of infancy the child develops teeth and learns the importance of biting in providing a new type of aggressive pleasure.

Basically, the Freudian view holds that the mouth has five primary functions: (1) taking in, (2) holding on, (3) biting, (4) spitting out, and (5) closing.[7] Each of these functions is a prototype or model for certain personality traits: *taking in* is associated with acquiring, *holding on* with determination and tenacity, *biting* with destructiveness and hostility, *spitting out* with rejection, and *closing* with refusal or negativism. Freudians believe that whether these traits become part of an individual's character later in life depends on the amount of frustration and anxiety that the infant experiences during this phase. For example, if someone does not consistently respond to the infant's cry for food or does not fully satisfy his hunger, he might later in life have a need to acquire material things to prevent a repetition of his frustration in early life.

During infancy, the baby is undifferentiated from his environment and has no concept of objects distinct from himself, such as "mother," or "crib," or "breast." He views the world as an extension of himself. He also reacts as a single unit to the stimuli provided by the environment. Because physical and emotional well-being are closely linked together, the baby's whole body responds to any stimulus. This is seen in the reflex response present in the infant, and especially in his total body responses to hunger, noise, touch, and so on. The baby continues to learn about his body and later during this stage experiments in holding, reaching, sitting, crawling, and, finally, walking.

The most important person for the infant is the mothering one. Research has shown that infants do not react to faces, but to the *gestalt,* or total configuration, of the person. The infant associates his mother with the person who supplies a soft breast, the sweet milk, and a warm embrace. The child begins to depend on her and becomes anxious and upset when she is gone. The mother, in turn, begins to look for a smile from the infant as a sign of contentment, and the infant begins to relate mother with pleasure and respond to her. A smile, therefore, is really a sign of beginning relatedness. With the child's emerging recognition, memory, and responsiveness, the ego begins to develop.

Sullivan, while building on Freud's description of the infant's oral needs, develops this concept of beginning relatedness. He calls the "nipple in lips" or infant-mother nursing experience the first and most crucial interpersonal situation. Included in this experience is the taste of the milk, the warmth of the touch, and the smell of the mother's body. Throughout this phase the satisfaction of what Sullivan terms the baby's need for tenderness requires the cooperation of the mothering one. The mother's complementary desire to meet her baby's needs or to supply this tenderness establishes tenderness as the infant's primary interpersonal need.

Sullivan identifies a close emotional bond between the mothering one and the child by which attitudes are communicated empathetically. Although difficult to define, this concept of empathy is an important one. It is a process of conveying feelings through physical touch and the sound of the voice rather than through direct verbal communication. It is a sensitivity to the mood of another. The mothering one can convey to the infant either tenderness or tension, and the infant will in turn react to this feeling. For example, feeding the infant is a particular time of closeness for mother and child. If the mother is upset, she will convey this to her nursing baby. The baby will respond to this and perhaps begin to fuss or cry. This increases the anxiety of the mother, and the child also becomes more upset and anxious. The concept of anxiety now develops for the infant as a feeling associated with unpleasantness or a vague dread of something without a specific object.

The infant, meanwhile, takes in all these experiences and attempts to incorporate them into his world by creating two ideas of the mother—the "good mother" and the "bad mother." The "good mother" conveys warmth, understanding, and relaxation; the "bad mother" conveys anxiety, coldness, and tension. In time, these two ideas are blended to eventually form the infant's "real mother," but this is the first explanation of the infant's interpersonal experience.

In a similar way infants begin to assimilate their own personal experiences, even though they have not formed a concept of "my individual body." They begin to develop a "good me," consisting of experiences of tenderness, approval, and general good feelings, and a "bad me," related to anxiety and tension. The "not me" is a part of the personality that evolves slowly and comes from the experience of intense anxiety. It is a vague area that includes poorly understood aspects of living, such as horror or dread. These experiences are not easily absorbed into the personality structure and can later account for serious disturbances of personality.

The "good me" is seen as more desirable by the child, who tries to support it. But how the infant sees himself is basically a reflection of how other significant people respond to him. Children who receive praise and support from parents will see themselves as good and worthwhile; in the same way, children who are criticized, scolded, or ridiculed will perceive themselves as bad, unacceptable, and without value.

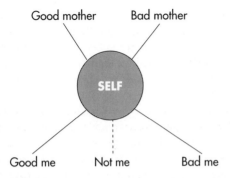

Fig. 2-2 Sullivan's concept of the infant's beginning self-system.

My mother loves me,
*   I feel good.*
I feel good because she loves me.
I am good because I feel good.
I feel good because I am good.
My mother loves me because I am good.
My mother does not love me.
*   I feel bad.*
I feel bad because she does not love me.
*   I am bad because I feel bad.*
I feel bad because I am bad.
I am bad because she does not love me.
She does not love me because I am bad.

R. D. Laing*
Knots

As the infant grows, therefore, he is sometimes "good me" and at other times "bad me." Together these notions describe what Sullivan calls the infant's self-system.[10] Figure 2-2 illustrates this idea. Finally, Sullivan points out that the origins of the infant's self-system rest not only with his significant others but also in a large part on the characteristics of the culture and society.

Erikson summarizes the primary task of maternal care in this phase as developing basic trust while overcoming basic mistrust. As Erikson states:

The firm establishment of enduring patterns for the balance of basic trust over basic mistrust is the first task of the budding personality, and therefore first of all a task for maternal care. But it must be said that the amount of trust derived from earliest infantile experience does not seem to depend on the absolute quantities of food or demonstrations of love, but rather the quality of the maternal relationship.*

Thus Freud, Sullivan, and Erikson all stress the importance of proper maternal care as a necessary condition for adequate physical and emotional development of infants. The mothering figure, however, does not necessarily have to be the biologic mother. It is, rather, the person who cares for the child, meets the child's needs, and becomes the child's significant other. Erikson continues to explain that this maternal care includes not only food but also the way the child is fed by the mothering one—with a firm sense of her personal trustworthiness and with a sensitivity to the baby's individual needs. Indeed, this is a large task for the mother, but the mother is not alone in this undertaking.

The quality of maternal care depends to a degree upon the support that the mother receives from other adults in the household—usually the husband—the family into which the child is born, the society's recognition of the family as one of its basic institutions, and the culture's guarantee for the continuation of fundamental societal mores and values.[8]

Erikson reaffirms that the infant's first socialization is in the nursing experience, when the infant perceives "I am what I am given." Then the infant interacts with society through the action of grasping, followed by the activity of biting and gripping. The basic learning of the infant at this stage is that "I can trust the world in the form of my mother." He achieves this by relying on the mother for consistency and continuity. The infant is then able to let the mother out of his sight, knowing that the mother will return when needed. This process helps infants to begin also to trust themselves and their own capabilities, and they thus acquire the virtue of hope. The bond between mother and child, therefore, "permits a mother to respond to the needs and demands of the baby's body and mind in such a way that he learns once and for all to trust her, to trust himself, and to trust the world."[4]

---

*From Laing RD: *Knots,* New York, 1970, Pantheon Books. Copyright The RD Laing Trust.

*From Erikson E: *Identity and the life cycle: selected papers,* New York, 1967, WW Norton.

The acquisition of basic trust, however, does not mean the complete loss of basic mistrust. A person needs a degree of mistrust to function in society. The infant learns that this basic mistrust provides him with anticipation of discomfort, readiness for danger, and a realistic fear of the unknown. Thus the infant is striving for a balance between trust and mistrust, and this balance will allow him to grow psychologically and accept new experiences openly.

CRITICAL THINKING *Question* ....

Do you think that the "mothering one" as described by these developmental theorists can also be the "fathering one"? Defend your position based on the tasks and challenges related to infancy and the context of contemporary American life.
••

TODDLER YEARS: 1½ TO 3½ YEARS

Trust thyself: every heart vibrates
to that iron string.

R. W. Emerson
Self-Reliance

While still an infant, the child has no self-imposed limits, but as the infant grows to be a toddler, his world changes. He becomes more occupied with eliminative activities and products, inspiring Freud to call this the anal stage of development. The primary sources of pleasure for the child are elimination and retention. The child interacts more and more with the environment and at this time discovers his first crucial limit, which centers around the act of elimination. The battleground is the voluntary control of involuntary reflexes, or toilet training. It is a battle of wills between the mother and the child, because the child wishes to please the mother but also gains pleasure from feces. Toilet training is not the only conflict at this time. Other issues could arise between mother and child, such as conflicts over eating. Toilet training, however, is a popular concern in America, and the emerging dimensions of the conflict are those between the child's desire for self-control, instinctual drives, and the requirements of the outside world represented by the mothering figure. It is the child's first contact with discipline and authority, and it is a time of assertiveness, anxiety, and self-doubt.

The resolution of this particular conflict is important, because it sets the pattern for solutions of later conflicts. According to Freud, the outcome can affect later personality development and character traits. Thus the methods used and the mother's attitudes take on particular importance. If the mother is strict and punitive and forces the child to conform, the child may willfully retain feces. This type of reaction might later be evident in an obstinate or stingy personality. Or the child may spontaneously expel feces in acts of rage that might later reappear in traits of destructiveness, impulsiveness, and violence. If on the contrary the mother encourages the child and praises his attempts, the developing child might have pleasurable associations and become creative and productive in life. Because this is an especially trying time for the child, he might revert to oral satisfactions, and regressive behavior might include baby talk, thumbsucking, or demanding a bottle.

Freudian theory holds that another of the child's activities is also important during this stage—his relationship with objects (Fig. 2-3). At this time

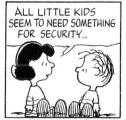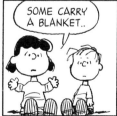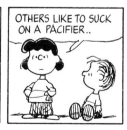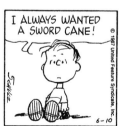

Fig. 2-3 Lucy demonstrates the importance of objects to Linus, particularly during this stage of development. (Peanuts ® reprinted by permission of United Feature Syndicate, Inc.)

the child is becoming aware of the objects and possessions in his world, and certain objects begin to take on particular value. The prized blanket, pillow, or stuffed animal becomes an extension of the child's self, and it serves to decrease anxiety. Linus with his blanket has made this idea a familiar one. Unlike Linus, who is still not ready to give up his blanket, the prized object will lose its importance to the child when his sense of trust allows him to feel more secure and less afraid in the absence of the loved one.

The child's relationships with people are also expanding, and he is now incorporating the father and other adult figures into his life. Sullivan identifies the child's chief interpersonal need at this stage as that of participation with adults. His interpersonal growth is accomplished by parental expectations. Nothing is really expected of an infant. He is the center of attention, and if he eats and sleeps, everyone is content. In the toddler stage, however, the child begins to talk and reason and is expected by the parents to answer to his name, smile when called on, and begin to conform to their family life. Sullivan sees these events as greatly influencing the child's self-image, and his self-system now begins to rapidly enlarge and expand. He sees the use of rewards and punishments associated with approval and disapproval, and begins to develop a picture of self as competent and healthy or as timid, scared, and shy.

Sullivan stresses the importance of the acculturation of the child during this stage. As Freud pointed out, the parents first begin training the child in the habits of eating, cleanliness, and so on. Then the idea of education is introduced, and the child begins to assume some duties and responsibilities. Through example and the use of storytelling, the parents attempt to pass on their cultural heritage, including social values and ethical judgments. Children, seeing themselves as an active force, learn readily at this time. In mastering the use of language, the child realizes the tremendous power of words.

To communicate better, the child begins to use words that have been consensually validated.[10] This means that the child uses the right word for a situation—one that means the same thing to the mother, family, and so on. This allows him to move from his private world of personal meanings into society and culture. The child pantomimes the actions of others

as a part of imitative learning and also begins to understand people better. He notices their responses, inconsistencies, and weak points and uses this knowledge to sometimes violate their authority. The child is still unable, however, to challenge them directly. He is not yet at a point where he can say, "mother said I was bad, but I don't think that what I did was so bad." Instead, he learns to neutralize the fear-provoking situation by the release of anger.

> Especially in circumstances in which children are punished by an angry parent—but in all cases sooner or later . . . everyone learns the peculiar utility of anger . . . Children invariably in their play are angry with their toys: and later they are angry with their imaginary companions . . . From this beginning, almost everyone . . . comes to use anger very facilely, very frequently: and they use it when they would otherwise be anxious. In other words, it comes to be the process called out by mild degrees of anxiety in a truly remarkable number of people [p. 212].*

Finally, Sullivan says that toddlers are developing skills in playing with their peers. The toddler's world, however, remains largely egocentric. This can be seen in the imaginary playmates who appear at this time or in his parallel play activities with other children. Each child, in the presence of other children, plays his own game in his own fantasy with his own monologue. Toward the end of this stage of development children show the beginning of cooperative activity in playing with children of their own age.

Erikson unifies and expands Freud's views on the anal activities of the child and Sullivan's insights into the child's relationships with others. He agrees with the importance of the anal zone at this stage but applies the concept to the child's experimentation with the social modalities of holding on and letting go. *Holding on* refers to the child's wish to return to the dependency of infancy, whereas *letting go* refers to the child's desire to use initiative in asserting himself. At this time the child perceives "I am what I give." Both parents now are significant figures for the child, and the task is the acquiring of autonomy while overcoming a sense of shame and doubt.

---

*From Sullivan H: *The interpersonal theory of psychiatry,* New York, 1953, WW Norton.

Autonomy exists when children see themselves as individuals in their own right, distinct from their parents. Shame is a feeling of being self-conscious and is associated with the child's learning to blush at this age. Doubt is a fear of failure or a fear of being in a situation he cannot handle. The goal is for the child to develop a sense of self-control without loss of self-esteem.

Having previously learned to trust the mother and his world, the child now tests this trust to see what he, as a separate person, can do. Children will try to do things on their own, such as dressing themselves or exploring new places. The crucial interplay is between the parents' control and the child's own will. Whether the child will cooperate willingly or willfully disobey is the issue, which rises above the specific conflict of toilet training. It will determine whether the child feels pride in his own independence and autonomy or shame and doubt because of lack of self-control and parental overcontrol. Everyone has some degree of shame or self-consciousness. It is impossible to develop without any. But if a child does not acquire a greater sense of autonomy, he will act and feel inferior in relationships with others.

The physical aspects of elimination and retention now take on broader significance in the process of becoming a person and relating to others. The ingredients necessary to complete the tasks of this stage are guidance and care and the child's trust in self, which was acquired during infancy. The role of the parents is to set safe limits for the child for protection, gradually granting independence and allowing him to learn tolerance, self-confidence, and appropriate releases of tension, anger, and frustration.

Successful completion of this stage results in the virtue of will, in which the child exercises free choice and self-restraint in spite of occasional feelings of shame and doubt.

CRITICAL THINKING *Question* ················

In clinic, a mother expresses her concern to you that her 3-year-old son has had an imaginary playmate for over a year. What information would you seek from her, and how would you respond to her concern?

EARLY CHILDHOOD: 3½ TO 7 YEARS

Who in the world am I?
Ah, that's a great puzzle!

Lewis Carroll
Alice in Wonderland

From early in life the child experiences genital feelings, but sexuality blooms at the age of 3 or 4 years, when genital feelings become stronger and more important. Freud associates the principal source of pleasure during early childhood with the genital organs, and he calls this the *phallic stage of development* (Fig. 2-4). It is an important stage in determining one's responses to people later in life.

The child retains the special relationship with his mothering one but also identifies with other members of the family and begins to learn sex roles. There is a natural curiosity at this time, which extends into sexual matters as well. The child becomes interested in where babies come from. Masturbation is a common learning experience. The child also compares his organs with friends and notices sexual differences for the first time. This exploration can result in some confusion, and girls may desire a penis whereas boys may want breasts or babies. Both also fear that something might be wrong with their genital organ or that their gender might be changed. When the child has some conception of his own gender, he enters into the *oedipal phase of development.*

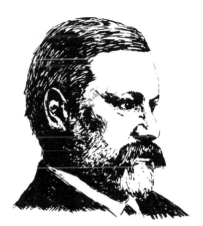

Fig. 2-4 Sigmund Freud (1856–1939).

For the boy, this phase is characterized by the Oedipus complex, in which the boy desires possession of his mother figure and is resentful of his father figure. Freud derived the name Oedipus complex from a Greek tragedy in which Oedipus, king of Thebes, killed his father and married his mother. In this complex the young boy remains faithful to his first love object—his mothering one. He desires to possess her completely and have her all to himself. He wishes to have all her love and attention and may fantasize about marrying her. The special privileges his father receives from his mother make him jealous, and the boy regards his father as his rival—wishing to remove him from the house and sometimes even wishing that his father would die. At the same time, however, he also admires and respects his father and sees him as an ideal male figure. These strong feelings and conflicts create fear and guilt in the boy. He fears what his father might do to retaliate and fantasizes his father hurting him, especially by cutting off his penis. The boy sees that a girl does not have a penis, and he imagines that someone cut hers off. Freud calls the boy's fear of losing his penis *castration anxiety.*

Freud proposes that a similar process occurs in girls that is sometimes referred to as the Electra complex, taken from a Greek myth in which the daughter contrives to murder her mother. In this complex the young girl discovers that she does not have a penis and feels that her mother is responsible. She sees that her father has this organ and becomes envious of him. Freud terms the girl's desire for the penis she fears she lost *penis envy.*

Because of these beliefs, she turns her love from her mother figure, whom she wishes to displace, and directs it primarily toward her father figure, whom she desires to possess. Again, she is ambivalent in her feelings toward her parents, because she continues to seek out her mothering one to supply her needs and provide tenderness. This ambivalence provokes her fears of being deserted by her mothering one, who she fears will no longer love or care for her.

The ages of 4 and 5 years, then, are highly excitable ones for children. They realize that masturbation is not fully satisfying, and they direct their energies into aggressive activity and play, such as running, jumping, and yelling. Gradually, because of the boy's fear of castration and guilt for wishing his father dead, he with-draws or represses his sexual wishes toward his mother. His fear and hostility toward his father also decline, and he begins to identify with his father as a strong male figure. The girl's sexual fantasies are similarly modified, and she identifies with her mother. The resolution of the complexes emphasizes Freud's theory of the bisexual nature of people. Recalling the child's early ambivalent feelings toward his parents, Freud states that each person is attracted to both their own gender and the opposite gender. According to Freud, each person has both masculine and feminine components in his constitutional framework. Biology supports this theory, because all people have both male and female sex hormones.

When boys and girls internalize the values of their parents, their consciences begin to develop. This oedipal phase can be a constructive one for the child if the child identifies with a gentle but firm parent who is in harmony with the culture. If there is not an adequate parent during this process, children may not fully develop their consciences and this will influence their later adjustment and lifestyle. This stage, therefore, is a crucial one for the child's development of good interpersonal relationships later in life.

Sullivan notes that during this stage of development, the child's form of play is evolving. In earlier stages play was very personal and private, and the child was unable to share with others. Now he continues to validate thoughts and ideas, and instead of playing alone, begins to play around and with other children.

The child manifests a shift from contentment in an environment of authoritarian adults and the more or less personalized pets, toys, and other objects, towards an environment of persons significantly like him. If playmates are available, his integrations with them show new meaningfulness [p. 38.]*

There is still no mutual effort by the children to work together for a common cause, but this task will be learned in time.

A most important event occurs during this stage—the beginning of school. To the child, this means further socialization and a new opportunity to discover how the rest of the world lives. The child

_____

*From Sullivan H: *Conceptions of modern psychiatry,* Washington, DC, 1953, WW Norton.

sees new types of authority figures, such as teachers and principals, and learns how to obey them. The teacher is a significant person for the child, because this is another adult with whom the child can compare and contrast his own parents. Thus the teacher can affect the child in a positive and supportive way or in a negative and detrimental way.

Sullivan stresses that another group of people becomes important to the child at this stage—peers, or children of the same gender who are like himself. They are allies, and together they compare facts about their parents and families. For the first time children see more clearly the limitations, strengths, and peculiarities existing in themselves and their families, and they learn to accept the differences among people. This peer group is important, and the child strives to receive support from them. Every child runs the danger of not being accepted or of being ostracized from the peer group, and the resulting loneliness is a real problem for the child at this age.

Sullivan identifies some other skills the child should acquire in forming relationships with peers during this stage—competition, cooperation, and compromise. Each one of these skills is valued by society. The child needs to compete with others fairly, to cooperate with them, and to be able to compromise without feeling hopeless. Mastering these tasks without losing self-esteem will prepare the child for more mature relationships with others.

Erikson describes the child at this stage of development as brighter, more active, and more loving than at any previous time. The child tends to forget failures quickly and freely approaches new and uncertain situations. His actions show a degree of self-confidence and a great curiosity.

Having found a firm solution of his problem of autonomy, the child of four or five is faced with the next step—and with the next crisis. Being firmly convinced that he *is* a person, the child must now find out *what kind* of a person he is going to be.*

Erikson describes the crisis of this stage as that of acquiring initiative while overcoming a sense of guilt.

While building on Freud's description of the child at this age, Erikson assumes a larger view and says that what the child is really learning about is life and the sequence of generations from birth through death. The child is identifying with adults and is beginning to see the purpose in life. At this time the child perceives "I am what I can do." Initiative plays a necessary part in determining how the child learns and what the child does. "Initiative adds to autonomy the quality of undertaking, planning, and 'attacking' a task for the sake of being active and on the move."[3] It is, therefore, a very positive force.

There are also some dangers of this stage, and these involve the child's guilt over things he has thought about or actually done. In having initiative, children violate the trusting dependency they had in infancy. They feel guilty about their oedipal fantasies and when they believe their initiative may be interfering with someone else. Mistrust of parents, self-doubt, and fear of harm all create misgivings and guilt. At this time the family unit has a very obvious impact on the child, who absorbs what his parents have taught and observes what they actually do. The child then begins to act in place of the parents through the development of his own conscience.

In summary, the child during this stage is striving to balance the forces of initiative and guilt. This will provide him with a beginning purpose in life and assist him in learning moral responsibility.

CRITICAL THINKING *Question* . . . .

Day care is commonly used in other countries but has often been the subject of criticism in the United States. Review some of the latest research findings about day care and discuss how it can have a positive effect on helping children meet the developmental tasks of early childhood.

. . . .

MIDDLE CHILDHOOD: 7 TO 12 YEARS

"Then you shall judge yourself," the king answered. "That is the most difficult thing of all. It is much more difficult to judge oneself than to judge others. If you succeed in judging yourself rightly, then you are indeed a man of true wisdom."

Antoine de Saint Exupéry
The Little Prince

As the child continues to grow, he more actively participates in the surrounding world. Socially, the child

---

*From Erikson E: *Identify and the life cycle: selected papers*, New York, 1967, WW Norton.

has entered school and meets all types of new people and experiences. Physically, he adds inches to his height and fullness to the frame. Freud describes this stage as one in which there is a decrease in sexual urge. He calls this the *latency stage,* in which the child is "desexualized" or "neutralized." This time of diminished sexuality continues until puberty, when the sexual urge is reawakened.

This particular stage of development is somewhat neglected by Freud. He does emphasize that through the resolution of the Oedipus or Electra complex of the previous stage, the child more completely identifies with the same-gender parent. Thus the child's character continues to develop along with the ego and superego. He channels sexual energy into school, projects, and clubs, and this is an active time for learning, reading, and peer play.

Sullivan notes that during this stage the child expresses a new type of interest in another person. Moving from the need for playmates during early childhood, he now becomes intimate with one particular friend. This is an important event because it shows the child's movement away from egocentricity and toward social participation. To take this step, the child must have a firm sense of self-respect and a beginning level of maturity. He must also have met the tasks of the previous stages and be ready to interact with people in a new way.

Thus the child's capacity for love begins to grow. Sullivan describes love as the belief that the satisfaction and security of the loved one are as significant to the person as his or her own satisfaction and security. It involves a sensitivity to the needs of another, and the child begins to demonstrate this.

The appearance of the capacity to love ordinarily first involves a member of one's own sex. The boy finds a chum who is a boy, the girl finds a chum who is a girl. When this has happened, there follow in its wake a great increase in the consensual validation of symbols, of symbol operations, and of information, data about life and the world [p. 43].*

Because boys know boys best and share common interests, it seems only natural that a boy should select another boy as his best friend in the same way that a girl would select another girl. Together, these friends compare experiences and share knowledge. Each learns to value the other's needs and also learns that he or she, too, is valuable as a friend to some other person. Therefore the greatest need of the middle childhood years is for interpersonal intimacy. Sullivan defines intimacy as person closeness, not as physical contact or lust.

And so I trust that you will finally and forever grasp that interpersonal intimacy can really consist of a great many things without genital contact; that intimacy in this sense means, just as it always has meant, closeness, without specifying that which is close other than the persons. Intimacy is that type of situation involving two people which permits validation of all components of personal worth [p. 246].*

In summary, Sullivan sees the child as becoming more fully human. The child learns tolerance and concern as he begins to perceive the common humanity of people. During this stage the child has the opportunity to apply what has been learned about interpersonal relationships, and the future is bright with possibilities.

Erikson emphasizes the child's transition during middle childhood from the family and into society. During this stage the child perceives "I am what I learn" and takes great pride in acquiring skills and performing tasks. Erikson states the major task of this stage as that of acquiring industry while overcoming a feeling of inferiority.

And while all children need the hours and days of make-believe in games, they all sooner or later, become dissatisfied and disgruntled without a sense of being useful, without a sense of being able to make things and make them well and even perfectly; this is what I call the sense of industry.†

Erikson interprets industry to mean the child's desire to complete something—to eagerly engage in productive activity. The child's activity gradually

---

*From Sullivan H: *The interpersonal theory of psychiatry,* New York, 1953, WW Norton.

---

*From Sullivan H: *Conceptions of modern psychiatry,* New York, 1953, WW Norton.
†From Erikson E: *Identity and the life cycle: selected papers,* New York, 1967, WW Norton.

turns from play toward accomplishing tasks. Children acquire a sense of competence as they learn to obtain pleasure from work and see it as a form of self-improvement. The child's sense of industry also incorporates the desire for knowledge of the world. As previously mentioned, this is the stage of formal education for the child. He is subject to training and teaching, becomes literate, and begins preparation for his eventual career in life. Finally, education has another purpose for both the growing child and society—it serves as a vehicle for transmitting the culture. Thus through acquiring a sense of industry, children begin to learn their place in the adult world.

While struggling for a sense of industry, the child is also striving to balance feelings of inferiority. Children feel inferior when they become aware of their own inadequacies or fail to master some tasks or skills. To relieve this inferiority, the child looks toward peers, with whom he can compare skills and accomplishments. In this sense the child needs peers to maintain self-esteem. Balancing the traits of industry and inferiority will provide the experience and maturity necessary to move into adolescence.

CRITICAL THINKING *Question* ....

Drug experimentation is on the rise among youth in middle childhood. Design a school-based intervention program for preventing drug use, incorporating knowledge of the developmental needs of this age group.

ADOLESCENCE: 12 TO 19 YEARS

A man is least known to himself.

Cicero
De oratore III

The teenage years mark a transformation from a pleasure-seeking child who is preoccupied with love of self to a reality-oriented, socialized adult who demonstrates love of others. This period of adolescence is a baffling and confusing one for the growing child. It is a time of rapid physical growth and maturation. The adolescent's body, which is suddenly changing, becomes unfamiliar. The body image shifts as he becomes reacquainted with his body. He begins

to experience sexual feelings that are both unfamiliar and enjoyable. Based on these changes, Freud calls this, his last stage of development, the *genital phase.*

The most striking process of puberty has been selected as its most characteristic; it is the manifest growth of the external genitals. . . . Simultaneously, the inner genitals develop to such an extent as to be able to furnish sexual products or to receive from them for the purpose of forming a new living being. A most complicated apparatus has thus been formed for future use [p. 605].[6]

Adolescents are unsure of themselves; they struggle with feelings of independence and dependence. Anxiety is created by new sexual desires. General confusion also affects relationships with parents, which may now become stormy and chaotic. The culmination of this phase, according to Freud, is in the adolescent's sexual choice and union as he strives for stability in life.

Sullivan elaborates on this period of development by identifying three needs of the adolescent (Fig. 2-5). The first is for personal security, which the adolescent can gain from positive appraisals from others. Thus the adolescent's self-concept continues to depend on the way other significant people see him. The second need is for intimacy, and by this, Sullivan means that the adolescent needs a close relationship with one other person. During this stage, however, the adolescent changes from

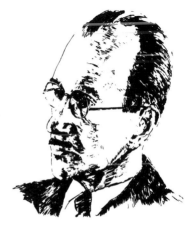

Fig. 2-5 Harry Stack Sullivan (1892–1949).

seeking a same-gender chum to desiring a close relationship with someone of the opposite gender. The third need is that of lust or genital interest. During these years there is a powerful need for genital activity in pursuit of orgasm. It arises from the adolescent's desire to feel confident in his ability to give and receive sexual gratification. The problem is that cultural expectations often conflict with the natural sequence of these needs, particularly the needs for intimacy and lust. At present, society discourages premarital intercourse, but also disapproves of early marriage. Thus the adolescent may find it difficult to meet these needs in culturally acceptable ways.

If, however, these needs are met, the adolescent's self-esteem is increased, and he can more competently enter adulthood. If adolescence is

successfully negotiated, the person comes forth with self-respect adequate to almost any situation, with the respect for others that this competent self-respect entails, with the dignity that befits the high achievement of competent personality, and with the freedom of personal initiative that represents a comfortable adaptation of one's personal situation to the circumstances that characterize the social order of which one is a part [p. 27].*

A major task of the adolescent is finding his identity. Erikson has devoted a considerable amount of time to developing this idea. By identity, he does not mean merely genital maturity or identification with the same-gender parent. He means that adolescents must find their own identities based on their own experiences, perceptions, and career desires. Doing this involves the mastery of the problems of childhood and a readiness to face the challenges of the adult world as a potential equal. Although this is the major task of the adolescent stage of development, it began in the very first stage of infancy and continues to be developed throughout life.

The specific task of this stage, then, as identified by Erikson, is acquiring a sense of identity while overcoming identity diffusion. It contains the promise of finding oneself and the threat of losing oneself. Identity is the integration of inner and outer

demands and directions to discover who one is and what one can become. It is a search for self that includes sexual and occupational choice. Thus identity should provide personal consistency and suggest one's place in the community.

This search for self is complicated by the many roles in society that can cause identity diffusion or role confusion. Identity diffusion is instability resulting from conflicting possibilities, demands, or choices; this instability creates outer isolation and an inner vacuum. Associated with a sense of identity diffusion are an overwhelming sense of shame, an inability to obtain satisfaction from any activity, a feeling of isolation and mistrust, a questioning of one's sexual roles, and the feeling that one is an object or observer in life and not an active participant. It is obvious that identity diffusion is a frightening experience. Rather than suffer in this state of nonidentity, some adolescents take on a negative identity or an identity opposite to the one society suggests. Delinquency is a form of negative identity. Because the individual cannot assume a positive identity, he or she becomes successful in a negative way. Thus negative identity reflects "a desperate attempt at regaining some mastery in a situation in which available positive identity elements cancel each other out."[2]

Adolescence is, therefore, a busy time. The adolescent has much to master in a relatively short time span. He is aided in this work by what Erikson calls a *psychosocial moratorium.* Because adolescents require time to integrate themselves into adulthood, society grants this time. A psychosocial moratorium is a socially authorized delay of adulthood because the adolescent is not yet ready to meet his obligations. It is provided for by institutions of the society, such as colleges, the armed services, or apprenticeship programs. This moratorium includes a selective permissiveness of youth by society, a playfulness of youth, short but deep commitments by youth, and adolescent experimentation with various patterns of identity. This experimentation with patterns of identity encompasses many aspects of the adolescent's life—lifestyle may range from apathy to deep commitment; dress may be characterized by great vanity or extreme unconcern; he may try out various social roles; involvement in work may include purposeful activity or work paralysis; sexual behavior

---

*From Sullivan H: *Conceptions of modern psychiatry*, New York, 1953, WW Norton.

may be bisexual, homosexual, or heterosexual; he may decide to lead others or follow authority; and the search for a philosophy of life may include drugs, religious movements, or political activity.

The end of this moratorium may or may not bring success. If the moratorium ends too early or before the adolescent is adequately prepared, the young adult will feel like a failure and feel lost as a person. If the outcome is successful, he will be able to handle the various roles of adulthood; will identify with his or her own gender and be comfortable with the opposite gender; will be considering or committed to a specific occupation; and will have developed his own unifying philosophy of life.

In attempting to meet the tasks of this stage, the adolescent has various aids. Speech or talking becomes very important. Adolescents begin to talk things over endlessly with friends. Here, speech is not only communication, it is thinking aloud, and it is a means of searching for identity. Cliques, gangs, and crowd behavior are also important to the adolescent. Sometimes, these cliques can be intolerant of others. Erikson sees this as a protective mechanism of adolescents, whereby they overidentify and tend to stereotype themselves, their enemies, and their ideals.

It is difficult to be tolerant if deep down you are not quite sure that you are a man (or a woman), that you will ever grow together again and be attractive, that you will be able to master your drives, that you really know who you are, that you know what you want to be, that you know what you look like to others, and that you will know how to make the right decisions without, once and for all, committing yourself to the wrong friend, sexual partner, leader, or career.*

So cliques, too, are mechanisms of self-expression, and tolerance of others arises only when one is secure in oneself. Finally, the adolescent uses significant others from society at large to identify with, and peers replace parents as essential supports and conveyers of values.

In summary, the adolescent is searching for something and somebody to be true to and acquiring a sense of identity, and the virtue of fidelity provides a place in his corner of society.

---

*From Erikson E: *Identity and the life cycle: selected papers*, New York, 1967, WW Norton.

CRITICAL THINKING *Question* ················

How might access to others through the Internet aid an adolescent's search for personal security, intimacy, and identity? How might it impede an adolescent's important developmental tasks?
···

ADULTHOOD

Beside our need for a meaning, also a need for human intimacy without conventional trappings—for the experience of a circle where power expresses itself in meaningful and beautiful forms.

Dag Hammarskjöld
Markings

Childhood and youth have now ended, and the adult must stand ready to take one's place in society. Although Freud omits a discussion of the adult years of life, Sullivan summarizes his theory with an analysis of mature adulthood. He regards maturity as the integration of various needs and believes that well-rounded maturity is a scarce commodity.

Sullivan defines the components of a mature person. The first is self-respect. Self-respect has its roots in infancy, beginning with the dynamics of empathy and anxiety. It is a basic and essential ingredient of a healthy personality. Next, the individual must have the ability to validate his thoughts and communicate meanings. This task is primarily learned during the early childhood years, and it is carried over into adolescence and adulthood. Thus the adult should be able to appraise a situation and report on it without the use of understatement or exaggeration. Incorporating the learning of the early childhood years, the next component is the ability to compete fairly, cooperate harmoniously, and compromise with satisfaction. Another major criterion of maturity is the ability to form healthy interpersonal relationships. This would include forming, maintaining, and terminating good, close friendships with people of both the same and the opposite gender. These interpersonal contacts encourage the mature adult to be increasingly sensitive to the needs, anxieties, and feelings of others. Finally, Sullivan's last component is self-awareness of the various aspects of one's own personality and motives for relating to others.

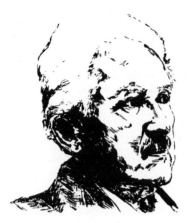

Fig. 2-6 Erik Erikson (1902–   ).

Sullivan's mature adult, therefore, is a person who has successfully met the challenges of previous developmental stages. The mature adult has confidence in his own abilities and is open to sharing himself with other people. And it is at this stage that Sullivan's developmental theory is completed.

Erikson, unlike most theorists, expands and adds depth to the psychosocial description of the years between adulthood and death (Fig. 2-6). He identifies the primary task of adulthood to be that of attaining intimacy while overcoming a feeling of isolation. He describes intimacy as a closeness both to oneself and to others. An adult is obliged to first examine and accept his own resources, ideas, and potential—all of which make up identity. Then he can experience intimacy with others through the commitment of close friendships and the fulfillment of sexual unions.

Thus, the young adult, emerging from the search for and the insistence on identity, is eager and willing to fuse his identity with that of others. He is ready for intimacy, that is, the capacity to commit himself to concrete affiliations and partnerships and to develop the ethical strength to abide by such commitments, even though they may call for significant sacrifices and compromises [p. 263].*

The adult now has the freedom and responsibility to participate in a career of choice, a close relationship with another adult, and governmental and societal affairs as a citizen. Each of these areas in life pro-

vides a sense of involvement and intimacy, but before the adult can be really intimate, he must have a sense of identity and thus be psychologically ready. "Intimacy is really the ability to fuse your identity with somebody else's without fear that you're going to lose yourself. It is this development of intimacy which makes marriage possible as a career choice."[5] So the adult gathers his accomplishments from previous years and now transforms them into the reality of mature, unselfish love.

Some adults avoid this closeness with others. They retain a safe, social distance or may reject relationships involving potential closeness. Erikson sees this avoidance activity as a dangerous one, because it will lead the adult into isolation and self-absorption. Such an adult is lonely and lives in the emptiness of his own world. This is the danger of this stage of development. Achieving a balance between intimacy and isolation is, therefore, the next logical challenge to a positive identity that establishes a basis for future growth.

CRITICAL THINKING *Question* ················

Some adults may unconsciously marry in order to complete aspects of themselves, escape from their world, or fill a void in their lives. If these couples decide to have children, discuss the impact this could have on their ability to be effective parents.
···

MIDDLE AGE

To know oneself one should assert oneself.

Albert Camus
Notebooks 1935–1942

In the middle-age stage of development the adult emerges as a teacher and learner. A new dimension is added to life, which Erikson calls the balance between generativity and self-absorption. By generativity he means concern for the next generation expressed through one's guidance, interest, and encouragement of others. This responsibility is shared by the individual and his mate as they pass on to the next generation their hopes, virtues, and wisdom.

It is not necessary to have children of one's own to meet the task of this stage. The world of an adult includes work, ideas, and relationships with others, and learning in these areas can be passed on to the

---

*From Erikson E: *Childhood and society,* New York, 1963, WW Norton.

many children of society. In this sense the idea of generativity moves beyond procreation to include productivity and creativity. The individual now becomes involved with the duties and tasks of maintaining the social system of the world. If generativity triumphs at this stage, a person develops the basic strengths of caregiving.

The challenge now is whether the adult will accept the new generation as his responsibility; and if so, whether the adult will help this new generation to develop the basis of life—trust. If he does not meet this challenge, the adult faces a life of stagnation and self-absorption. The exclusive self-love and self-concern will remove him from the life of society and leave the adult alone and impoverished. Generativity, however, will involve the adult in the development and perfection of society's many products. This parental responsibility for that which society generates has no limits to its accomplishments. Thus education, child care, new ideas, works of art, and scientific developments are given new meaning and value because of the learning of this stage of development.

CRITICAL THINKING *Question* ⋯⋯⋯⋯⋯

How might a career as a nurse help an individual face the middle-age challenge of generativity versus self-absorption? Consider other careers and decide whether it is the nature of the work or the way in which the individual approaches the work that is most important to personality growth.

⋯⋯⋯⋯⋯⋯⋯⋯⋯⋯⋯⋯⋯⋯⋯⋯⋯⋯⋯⋯

OLD AGE

Grow old along with me!
The best is yet to be
The last of life, for which the first was made:
Our times are in his hand
Who saith, "A whole I planned.
Youth shows but half; trust God: see all,
    nor be afraid!"

Robert Browning

The final years of life allow the individual to gain a fuller perspective of his own life and the life cycle of humanity (Table 2-1). The individual struggles for a

sense of integrity while overcoming a sense of despair. About this last stage of development, Erikson has said:

Only in him who in some way has taken care of things and people and has adapted himself to the triumphs and disappointments adherent to being, the originator of others or the generator of products and ideas—only in him may gradually ripen the fruit of these seven stages. I know no better word for it than ego integrity [p. 268].*

Integrity is acceptance of the life cycle and a more profound love for mankind. It provides a successful solution to the conflicting demands of despair so commonly characteristic of old age. A despairing person complains that life is too short, and he bemoans the many unfinished tasks. This person is disgusted and remorseful and, above all else, fears death.

Integrity, however, implies wisdom. From the lessons of life the individual has adopted a philosophy of life that transcends his own life and reunites the generations of mankind. There is no need for a person to fear death if he has acquired integrity. In addition, this last stage sees the fullest development of trust.

Because trust is the first virtue of infancy, the life cycle becomes complete as a unifying whole.

Webster's Dictionary is kind enough to help us complete this outline in circular fashion. Trust (the first of our ego values) is here defined as "the assured reliance on another's integrity," the last of our values. . . . It seems possible to further paraphrase the relation of adult integrity and infantile trust by saying that healthy children will not fear life if their elders have integrity enough not to fear death [p. 269].*

Thus integrity is the realization of all previous stages of development and the goal of life.

CRITICAL THINKING *Question* ⋯⋯⋯⋯⋯

Think of an older person you greatly admire. Evaluate this individual based on his or her progression through the eight stages of development identified by Erikson.

⋯⋯⋯⋯⋯⋯⋯⋯⋯⋯⋯⋯⋯⋯⋯⋯⋯⋯⋯⋯

---

*From Erikson E: *Childhood and society*, New York, 1963, WW Norton.

TABLE 2-1   Comparison of developmental theories

	THEORIST		
	S. FREUD	H.S. SULLIVAN	E. ERIKSON
Background	1856-1939 Founder of psychoanalysis	1892-1949 Founder of school of interpersonal psychiatry	1902- Social psychoanalyst
Basis of theory	Behavior is a product of interaction among three systems—id, ego, and superego. "Intrapsychic"	Personality is viewed in the context of interpersonal relationships. "Interpersonal"	Applies theory of psycho-analysis to social and anthropological data to comment on broader areas of human functioning. "Cultural"
Developmental stages			
1. Infancy	*Oral (0-1½ yr)* 1. Primary source of pleasure is the mouth.	*Infancy (0-2½ yrs)* 1. Important concepts are empathy, anxiety, and the "self-system." 2. Chief interpersonal need is for tenderness.	*Trust vs. mistrust (0-2 yr)* 1. Oral needs are of primary importance. 2. Adequate mothering is necessary to meet the infant's needs. 3. Acquisition of hope.
2. Toddler years	*Anal (1½-3 yr)* 1. Primary sources of pleasure are through elimination and retention. 2. First experience with discipline and authority. 3. Development of object relationships.	*Childhood (2½-4 yrs)* 1. Further development of the "self-system." 2. Use of consensual validation and interaction with peers. 3. Chief interpersonal need is for adult participation.	*Autonomy vs. shame (1½-3 yr)* 1. Anal needs are of primary importance. 2. Father emerges as an important figure. 3. Acquisition of will.
3. Early childhood	*Phallic (3-6 yr)* 1. Primary source of pleasure is genital. 2. Emergence of Oedipus and Electra complexes.	*Juvenile (4-8 yr)* 1. Socialization of the child as competition, coopera-tion, and compromise are learned. 2. Chief interpersonal need is for individuals of the same gender who are like himself.	*Initiative vs. guilt (3-6 yr)* 1. Genital needs are of primary importance. 2. Family relationships contribute to an early sense of responsibility and conscience. 3. Acquisition of purpose.
4. Middle childhood	*Latency (6-12 yr)* 1. A basically quiet stage of development marked by expanding peer relationships.	*Preadolescence (8-12 yr)* 1. First intimate inter-personal relationship occurs with a peer of the same gender.	*Industry vs. inferiority (6-12 yr)* 1. An active period of socialization for the child as he moves from the family and into society. 2. Acquisition of competence.
5. Adolescence	*Genital (12+ yr)* 1. Sexual desires and urges become prominent and the individual seeks fulfillment of them.	*Late adolescence (12+ yr)* 1. The individual experiences needs for personal security, intimacy, and lust.	*Identity vs. identity diffusion (13+ yr)* 1. Search for self in which peers play an important part. 2. A psychosocial moratorium is provided by society to aid the adolescent.

TABLE 2-1   Comparison of developmental theories—cont'd

	THEORIST		
	S. FREUD	H.S. SULLIVAN	E. ERIKSON
Developmental stages—cont'd			
5. Adolescence—cont'd		*Late adolescence (12+ yr) —cont'd* 2. Marks the establishment of a love relationship and the ability to live and share with another.	*Identity vs. identity diffusion (13+ yr)—cont'd* 3. Acquisition of fidelity.
6. Adulthood		*Maturity* 1. Characterized by interpersonal growth of the human person who has the capacity for happiness, self-awareness, and self-respect.	*Intimacy vs. isolation* 1. Characterized by the increasing importance of human closeness and sexual fulfillment. 2. Acquisition of love.
7. Middle Age			*Generativity vs. self-absorption* 1. Characterized by productivity, creativity, parental responsibility, and concern for the new generation. 2. Acquisition of care.
8. Old age			*Integrity vs. despair* 1. Characterized by a unifying philosophy of life and a more profound love for mankind.

DISCUSSION QUESTIONS

1. Why would Freud's belief in the unconscious and infantile sexuality be shocking to European society in the 1930s? What cultural norms prevailed at this time, and how did society react to his formulations?

2. Erikson believes his stages of development are universal and not bound to any particular culture. Accept or reject his beliefs based on your own analysis of his theory applied to another cultural group you have studied.

3. Both Sullivan and Erikson were trained in the Freudian psychoanalytic school but moved beyond the basic Freudian tenets. What other aspects of the individual were focused on by these two theorists?

4. Describe the physical, psychologic, and social benefits that the infant and mother receive from breastfeeding.

5. Fairy tales play an important role in a child's early acculturation. Analyze three popular fairy tales for the messages they convey regarding sex and family roles, morality, personal fulfillment, and mortality.

6. Trace the importance of relationships with a peer of the same gender through each developmental phase according to Sullivan.

7. Critique the images of MTV in light of the developmental tasks of adolescence and young adulthood.

8. Today, many women, particularly feminists, are critical of Freudian theory. What aspects of this theory might they object to, and what evidence do they have to support their criticisms?

9. Explain how a country's economic recession and high unemployment can negatively affect the successful resolution of the tasks of adolescence, adulthood, and old age.

10. Compare the individual's perception of his sexuality during the middle childhood, adolescent, and adult years. What particular problems regarding sexuality occur in each of these stages, and how are they positively resolved?

11. Describe personal incidents in your life as they relate to the various stages of development. Identify which stage you are in, and state supporting behaviors.

12. Think of a client with whom you are working and assess his or her developmental level according to Freud, Sullivan, and Erikson.

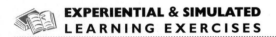

EXPERIENTIAL & SIMULATED LEARNING EXERCISES

Behavioral observation

PURPOSE: To develop skills in the observation of behavior and familiarity with the normative behaviors of various age groups.

PROCEDURE: Assign students to locate individuals representative of various developmental stages: an infant, a preschool child, a young adult, and so on. The student should observe the person for 5 to 10 minutes and record the behavior that is observed. Each student should collect several samples of behavior from a variety of age groups.

DISCUSSION: Students should compare their observations of behavior for each assigned group with each other and with established norms. Particular attention should be paid to differences in observations. Another focus for discussion is the location of the people who were observed. For instance, where did students go to find a young adult, an elderly person, and so on? Why did they look in these particular places? Does this reveal anything about the student's perception of that particular age group?

REFERENCES

1. Brill A, editor: *The basic writings of Sigmund Freud,* New York, 1938, Random House.
2. Erikson E: The problem of ego identity, *J Am Psychoanal Assoc* 4:88, 1956.
3. Erikson E: *Childhood and society,* ed 2, New York, 1963, WW Norton.
4. Erikson E, Erikson J: The power of the newborn, *Mademoiselle* 6:101, 1953.
5. Evans R: *Dialogue with Erik Erikson,* New York, 1967, Harper & Row.
6. Freud S: *New introductory lectures on psychoanalysis,* New York, 1933, WW Norton.
7. Hall C: *A primer of freudian psychology,* Cleveland, 1954, World Publishing.
8. Maier H: *Three theories of child development,* New York, 1969, Harper & Row.
9. Sullivan H: *Conceptions of modern psychiatry,* New York, 1953, WW Norton.
10. Sullivan H: *The interpersonal theory of psychiatry,* New York, 1953, WW Norton.

Suggested Readings

The following books are some of the original works of the three major theorists included in this chapter.

Erikson E: *Childhood and society,* ed 2, New York, 1963, WW Norton.

Erikson E: *Identity: youth and crisis,* New York, 1968, WW Norton.

Erikson E: *Insight and responsibility,* New York, 1964, WW Norton.

Erikson E: *Life cycle completed: a review,* New York, 1982, WW Norton.

Erikson E, Erikson J, Knick H: *Vital involvement in old age,* New York, 1986, WW Norton.

Freud S: *A general introduction to psycho-analysis,* New York, 1935, Garden City.

Freud S: *Collected papers,* New York, 1959, Basic Books.

Freud S: *The interpretation of dreams,* New York, 1933, Macmillan.

Freud S: *Three essays on the theory of sexuality,* London, 1949, Image.

Sullivan H: *Conceptions of modern psychiatry,* New York, 1953, WW Norton.

Sullivan H: *The interpersonal theory of psychiatry,* New York, 1953, WW Norton.

It is sometimes helpful to use secondary sources to increase one's understanding of the concepts developed by a particular theorist. The following texts are recommended to the reader for their clarity, synthesis, and ability to concisely describe a particular theoretic viewpoint.

Blos P: *On adolescence: a psychoanalytic interpretation,* New York, 1962, Free Press.

Brill A, editor: *The basic writings of Sigmund Freud,* New York, 1938, Random House.

Brown I: *Freud and the post-freudians,* Baltimore, 1961, Penguin Books.

DeLevita D: *The concept of identity,* New York, 1965, Basic Books.

Evans R: *Dialogue with Erik Erikson,* New York, 1967, Harper & Row.

Hall C: *A primer of freudian psychology,* Cleveland, 1954, World Publishing.

Maier H: *Three theories of child development,* New York, 1978, Harper & Row.

Mullahy P: *Oedipus—myth and complex,* New York, 1948, Hermitage Press.

Mullahy P, editor: *A study of interpersonal relations,* New York, 1949, Hermitage Press.

Mullahy P, editor: *The contributions of Harry Stack Sullivan: a symposium on interpersonal theory in psychiatry and social science,* New York, 1925, Hermitage Press.

Stevens R: *Erik Erikson, an introduction,* New York, 1983, St Martin's Press.

For those individuals who wish to study the developmental process in more detail, the following journals and books are recommended.

Adolescence, Age and Aging, Aging and Human Development, Child Development, Child and Family, Developmental Psychology, Human Development, Journal of Aging and Health, Journal of Gerontology, Journal of Youth and Adolescence, and Pediatric Clinics of North America.

These journals are rich sources of information on the various aspects of human development.

Anderson C: *The stages of life,* New York, 1995, Atlantic Monthly Press.

 Builds on previous work in the field to put forth a new "maturational theory" of how a human develops psychologically. Thought-provoking reading.

Barron McBride A: *The secret of a good life with your teenager,* New York, 1987, Times Books.

 A nurse-author explores the key developmental themes that characterize the experience of parents when their children are teenagers. This is a warm, insightful, and balanced book.

Field T: *Infancy,* Cambridge, Mass, 1990, Harvard University Press.

 An enjoyable review of the motor, perceptual, cognitive, social, and emotional processes of infant development.

Freiberg K: *Human development: a life span approach,* Boston, 1992, Jones and Bartlett.

 This book is an excellent overview of physical, cognitive, and psychosocial development throughout the life span.

Gilligan C: In a different voice, Cambridge, Mass, 1982, Harvard University Press.

 Developmental theorists have usually focused on men's behaviors and values. This book explores relatedness in women and its impact on empathy, intimacy, and moral choices.

Santrock J: *Life-span development,* Madison, Wis, 1997, Brown & Benchmark.

 Up-to-date presentation of research in the three primary domains of human development: biologic, cognitive, and socioemotional processes. Excellent resource.

Woods R: *Handbook of the clinical psychology of aging,* New York, 1996, Wiley.

 Comprehensive coverage of the psychologic aspects of aging written as a reference for practitioners, teachers, and researchers.

CHAPTER

3 *The Dynamics of Self-Growth*

This above all—to thine own self be true
And it must follow, as the night the day,
Thou canst not then be false to any man.

William Shakespeare
Hamlet, Act I, Scene 3

LEARNING OBJECTIVES

After studying this chapter, the student should be able to:

- Define the following terms: *body image, self-ideal, self-concept,* and *self-esteem.*
- Describe how each of these concepts of the self is formed and developed in the individual.
- Discuss factors and experiences throughout the life cycle that influence these concepts of the self.
- Describe the characteristics of a healthy personality.
- Analyze why knowledge of the self is an important part of each phase of the nursing process.
- Identify ways in which a nurse can first assess and then enhance a client's body image, self-ideal, self-concept, and self-esteem.
- Initiate the process of self-awareness and self-growth in oneself.

Studying the development of the self provides a theoretic framework for nursing but does not, in itself, ensure the success of the nursing process. Quality nursing care depends on the *therapeutic use of self.* This means that the nurse must first grow in self-knowledge and then apply this self-knowledge in the nurse-client relationship. The self, however, is neither spontaneously discovered nor dramatically unmasked. Rather, it is slowly revealed by thinking about and understanding the stages of development. It involves questioning one's own feelings and actions, understanding one's motivations, and accepting and trusting one's capabilities. It is an attempt to know the kind of person one is and to become conscious of one's values and goals. Once this base is established, helping relationships can be formed with others.

Through these helping relationships the nurse can better assess the client and his world. Understanding the person in light of his own point of view and own unique experiences is the most real way of knowing someone. To see the person as he sees himself, through his own self-expressions, is one purpose of the nurse's assessment. With this knowledge, the nursing process can be implemented while the client's identity is maintained and self-esteem enhanced. Knowledge of the self also facilitates the evaluation of the nursing process as the nurse asks, "Did I enhance the physical, psychologic, and social growth of my client and myself?" Understanding one's self, therefore, is a difficult task that requires the application of one's emotions and reason to the challenge of becoming a more mature person and a more effective nurse.

It is necessary for the education of nurses to provide more time and opportunity for the student to explore the dynamics of the self—both the student's own and her clients'. The nurse must be able to examine her own behavior as well as see how it appears to others. The nurse should analyze the behavior of clients and seek out their feelings and perceptions. Some concepts, such as body image, self-ideal, self-concept, and self-esteem, describe important aspects of the personality. Understanding them and their influence on the individual will aid the nurse in providing quality professional care.

VARIABLES OF THE SELF

The self operates much like a drawbridge. It can raise its beams and separate us from others as unique individuals, or it can lower its defenses and join us with other people around us. It is a complex mechanism that may initially seem very difficult to assess. As a nurse, one assesses feelings, thoughts, and actions, and most important in this assessment is the value the individual places on the various qualities of the self. In response to "Tell me about yourself," you may say, "I am a fairly attractive woman in my late teens who does pretty well in school. Right now, I'm a little overweight and I'm worried about my next exam." Most people describe themselves in terms of good or bad, pretty or ugly, fat or thin, adequate or inadequate. Some qualities, such as seeing oneself as a man or woman, are central to the person and are strongly defended and resistant to change. Some are easily and clearly described, whereas others are vague or inexpressible. It is from verbal statements and nonverbal behaviors that assumptions are made about the self. Unlike physical data, however, these are inferences or abstractions and need to be validated with the client.

As an individual, no one ever completely knows his inner self. The Johari Window[11] shown in Fig. 3-1 illustrates this idea.

Quadrant 1 is an open quadrant that includes the behaviors, feelings, and thoughts known to the individual and those around him. Quadrant 2 is called a blind quadrant, because it includes all those things that others know but that the individual does not know. Quadrant 3 is the hidden quadrant and includes those things that only the individual knows. This is a secret and protected area of the self. Quadrant 4 is the unknown quadrant that contains aspects of the self unknown to the individual and others. Altogether, these quadrants represent the total self. Three principles help one understand how the self functions in this representation:

1. A change in any one quadrant will affect all other quadrants.
2. The smaller the first quadrant, the poorer the communication.
3. Interpersonal learning means that a change has taken place so that quadrant 1 is larger and one or more of the other quadrants are smaller.[9]

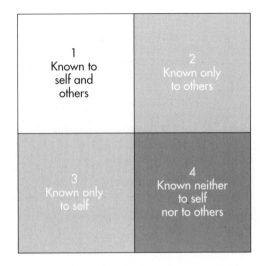

Fig. 3-1 Johari Window. Each quadrant, or windowpane, describes one aspect of the self.

Compare *A* and *B* of Fig. 3-2. *A* represents a person with little self-awareness. This person's behaviors and feelings would tend to be limited in variety and scope. *B,* however, shows an individual with great openness to the world. Much of this person's potential is being developed and realized. He has an increased capacity for experiences of all kinds—joy, hate, work, and love; he has few defenses; and can interact more spontaneously and honestly with others. Figure 3-2, *B* represents a worthy goal for the nurse to strive to attain—for the nurse and others.

To aid in this task, some specific aspects of the personality can be further explored and applied to the individual. In this chapter the concepts of body image, self-ideal, self-concept, and self-esteem are described, followed by a discussion of the effect of various interpersonal and environmental influences on the individual. These aspects are then summarized and reviewed in a definition of the healthy personality.

CRITICAL THINKING *Question* ··············

Review the quadrants of the Johari Window presented in Fig. 3-1. Draw a Johari Window for yourself, reflecting current levels of your own self-awareness and openness.

··

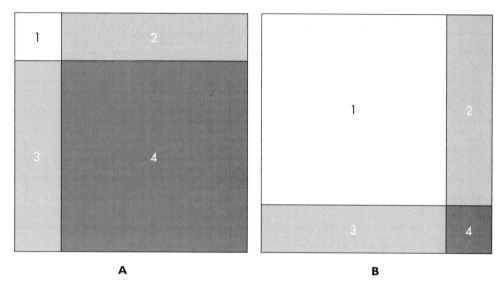

Fig. 3-2 Johari windows showing varying degrees of self-awareness (see Fig. 3-1). **A,** Person with little self-understanding. **B,** Individual with great self-awareness and openness.

BODY IMAGE

The experience of one's own body is the basis for all other life experiences.

Paul Schilder

How a person feels about himself is basically related to how he feels about his body. The body is the most visible and material part of the self and occupies a central role in the individual's perceptions. The body concept, or the body image, is the sum of the conscious and unconscious attitudes the individual has toward his body. It includes present and past perceptions as well as feelings about size, function, appearance, and potential. Body image is a dynamic entity, because it is continually being modified by new perceptions and experiences.

Developmental changes

At birth the infant does not have a body image. The infant receives input from his body and the environment but reacts to it in a global undifferentiated way. As he develops, his awareness expands and he begins to explore the parts of his body. The infant receives sensory stimulation through physical contact with others, and gradually becomes aware of the separateness of his own body from others and the limitations that his body places on him. Opportunities are also provided for the young child to manipulate the environment. Through bathing, eating, and playing, the child begins to learn to master both his body parts and the environment.

In the beginning he sees his body as similar to others but soon perceives some differences. For one thing, his own body is with him more than anyone else's. Also, when he pinches his arm, he realizes it hurts more than when he pinches that of another person. He notices that his arms and legs respond to his own wishes more often than to the wishes of others, and he realizes that when he touches himself, both parts feel—the part touching and the part being touched.

The toddler explores his genitals and becomes curious regarding the sexual anatomy of playmates. If given a mirror, he reacts with pleasure at seeing his own reflection. These discoveries allow the young child to regard his body as uniquely his own and to create a beginning body image.

With age, bodily changes increase the child's self-awareness as he focuses more on his body and the bodies of others. Studies have shown that the child begins to have a basic knowledge of his body and how it functions at approximately 9 years of age. At this age and earlier, the child's concept of himself, his body, and its function is greatly influenced by the attitudes of his parents, who express these attitudes through their actions, their explanations, and the things they fail to explain or mention. A school-age child who was given a mirror would probably analyze how he looks and what he sees about himself.

Adolescence is the next period of rapid growth, and the child commonly feels awkward and trapped inside his strangely changing body. At this time height, weight, and physical strength increase, and secondary gender characteristics begin to emerge. The development of breasts, menarche, growth of pubic and facial hair, and voice change are all new aspects of the body that must be integrated into the individual's evolving body image. The timing of this development becomes very important, as the adolescent, whether an early or late maturer, tries to conform to his peers. At the end of adolescence the disproportions that are characteristic of the growth years begin to balance out, and a more mature level of development is attained.

Early adulthood sees some stability in body growth, and the individual strives to maintain and increase body control. Gymnasts, flamenco and ballet dancers, and actors are good examples of individuals who have developed a relatively high degree of body control. Studies have shown that differences in body image exist between the genders. It appears that women have a more defined and stable body image and that this begins in childhood. Women have a clearer sense of body boundaries, sensations, and experiences and arrive at realistic concepts of their bodies. Studies also report that with a higher degree of body awareness, women also tend to have a clearer sense of identity.

These differences in body image between men and women may partly result from the different anatomic structures and functions between the male and female body, but they may also be partly caused by the different lifestyles and cultural roles of men and women. In Western culture, the socialization of women emphasizes a concern for the way their bodies impress others. They have been expected to devote considerable time to grooming themselves and adorning their bodies. Consequently, women have tended to equate self with body and to judge themselves based on body functions. Men, on the other hand, are expected to be strong and agile but not preoccupied with their bodies. Consequently, men have tended to equate self with outward achievement and accomplishment and to deemphasize their body attributes. Current changes in gender role stereotyping facilitate more honest and accurate adult body images of both men and women.

Middle age brings new challenges as different body parts age at different rates. The individual realizes that his body is not functioning as well as it had previously. With age, general metabolism and muscle tone decrease and there is a tendency to gain weight, especially in the trunk. Flabby skin and bulges are telltale signs of increased age. There are also changes in the characteristics of the hair and skin. Gray hair, receding hair lines, and balding are common occurrences. The skin of the face, hands, and arms becomes coarser, and wrinkles appear. Many people suffer presbyopia (difficulty seeing close objects), and the senses of hearing and smell may be impaired. One of the most significant changes at this time is the climacteric, which marks the termination of the individual's reproductive capacity. Because of hormonal changes, the individual becomes less feminine or masculine and must incorporate these physiologic changes into the body image.

The later years of life bring a further decline in physical abilities. When an older adult looks in the mirror, he sees his years reflected before him. The face tells his age more distinctly than any other body part. The skin is dry, coarse, baggy, and creased. Because of loss of teeth, the jaw is smaller and the chin sags. The hair on his head is probably thin and gray, and his hands are marked by veins and thick, tough nails. The shoulders may be stooped, and his stature may appear smaller. In addition, there is a decrease in the secondary gender characteristics and in the senses of hearing, vision, and taste. All of these changes are obvious in old age, but it is for the individual to decide whether they represent increased wisdom and integrity or increased regret and bitterness.

Effect on self-conceptions

Throughout life body awareness serves as an anchor for self-knowledge, and this is an important part of self-concept (Fig. 3-3). Studies have shown that the more a person accepts his body or likes it, the more secure and free from anxiety he feels. There is also evidence to suggest that one's appearance is an important determiner of self-esteem. People who accept their bodies are more likely to have higher self-esteem than people who dislike their bodies. In addition, the general form of the body image tends to be idealized. For instance, we tend to think of ourselves as younger or more attractive than we are.

Most people also tend to think of themselves as clothed, not naked, which suggests the importance of clothing in one's body image. To maintain body image and self-esteem, a person will tend to camouflage faults. The millions of dollars spent in the United States on makeup and fashions attest to this. One can dye one's hair, cream it, cut it, blow it, straighten it, curl it, or shave it off. If one is unhappy with one's face, one can try cream, suntan oil, surgery, paint, or facial masks. Through clothes one can try to look taller, thinner, sexier, or richer.

Many people may believe that physical appearance is a superficial characteristic with little influence on our lives. However, research indicates that appearance is the means to many highly valued ends in our society, and its influence may begin at a very early age. Thus physical attractiveness may play a major role in the social development of the child. Nor are the effects of physical attractiveness limited to early in life. Studies suggest that attractive adults are seen as possessing other fine qualities—they are friendlier, more intelligent, and more socially graceful. Perhaps this is true because they are treated more favorably. In any case it would appear that the physical attractiveness stereotype may serve as a self-fulfilling prophecy.

Physical attractiveness also seems to be a crucial standard by which we form our first impressions. Many people first saw Richard Nixon and John Kennedy competing for the presidency in their televised debates. Some believe that Nixon lost that campaign because he did not have a good makeup man and did not appear to be as attractive as John Kennedy to the television audience. In a similar way it has been observed that part of Ronald Reagan's success in his presidency can be attributed to his ability to project an attractive media image. More recently, Bill Clinton appeared more relaxed and open than Bob Dole in the presidential debate, and this helped to turn the tide of his campaign.

In an initial encounter the first thing people notice is the gender, age, race, appearance, and clothing of the person. Clothing and appearance serve as cues to our social status and wealth, and they may also lead others to assume some facts about the attitudes, characteristics, or values of the person. Consider meeting a young person with short hair who is dressed in a tailored suit; how might your impressions of this individual differ from those of an individual dressed

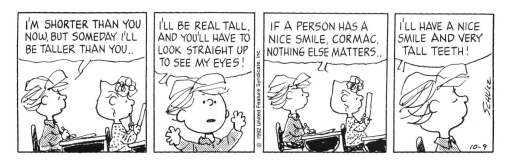

Fig. 3-3 One's perceptions regarding body image can greatly influence behaviors and interpersonal relationships in both positive and negative ways. (Peanuts ® reprinted by permission of United Feature Syndicate, Inc.)

in jeans, hiking boots, turtleneck sweater, and down vest? You might assume one is going to work while the other is a student or is relaxing outdoors.

Although an individual's style of dress provides information, standards for dress change over the years. In the 1960s young people in jeans and sandals were considered radical, hip, or antiestablishment. Now, however, jeans are an accepted style of dress for people of all ages. Uniforms also provide information. Medical people in white and police in blue are associations made by a majority of Americans. Other examples might include the individual who links baldness with virility or the once-popular belief "If you know one area, you know what to expect of the other. For instance, the better the brain, the smaller the breasts; and vice versa: the bigger the breasts, the lower the IQ." The fact that these are all unvalidated and biased assumptions does not mean that they might not occur to the individual or be influencing the individual's relationship with others.

Many of a person's feelings about body image are related to the fact that he has a fairly clear image of how he would like to look (i.e., the body ideal). If the actual body closely resembles the ideal body image, this person is more likely to think better of both the physical and nonphysical parts of his self. One's body ideal is greatly influenced by cultural standards. In the pioneer days of America women who were heavier and stronger in physique were thought to be more attractive. During the flapper era, small, flat-chested women were considered most desirable. In the early 1960s the *Playboy* woman, with large, firm breasts and a small waist, was the American ideal. Currently, the trend is toward admiring women with trim, well-toned bodies reflecting the national preoccupation with exercise and fitness. The emergence of the sport of women's body building is a good example of changing cultural conceptions of ideal body types. Body consciousness continues to dominate the American way of life, but it appears that attitudes are becoming more flexible and individual differences more widely accepted.

Another aspect in understanding an individual's body image is the idea that different parts of the body may have different values to different individuals. The loss of a big toe may be taken more casually by an office worker than by a ballerina. Gaining 5 lb may

be an inconvenience to a construction worker but career threatening to a jockey. The value of body parts, like all aspects of the self, is fundamentally individual in nature.

CRITICAL THINKING *Question* ················

Do an informal survey of your friends and family members. Ask them what aspects of their body appearance are most satisfying and most dissatisfying to them. Also ask them to identify which body part is of most importance to them. See whether there are similarities in the answers based on gender, age, occupation, or cultural background.

··

Nursing assessment

There are various ways a nurse can assess the body image of another. The person's posture, makeup, cleanliness, and clothing all provide data. In addition, talking with the patient provides more clues. In an indirect way people reveal feelings about their body parts by the use of such common descriptive phrases as "brokenhearted," "eyes popped out of my head," "lost my head," "teeth would fall out," "hair stood on end," "yellow-bellied," and so on. More directly, the nurse can draw out her client's feelings by asking: "What is his perception of health? Is the client satisfied with his appearance? What is the body ideal? What importance is attached to the body parts and functions? Age, occupation, and cultural background are also important information. Knowing these things about the client will help the nurse to recognize the meaning that health and illness have for the client and the effect that change will have on his self-concept and life activities.

Another useful way of communicating is the drawing (Fig. 3-4). When an individual is asked to "draw a person," the image created may be a kind of self-representation that includes his perception of himself and his conception of a person. Examining the various parts of the body as well as the facial expression may provide clues to the person's body image. The drawings can also be used to evaluate knowledge and personal perceptions relative to the body.

Human figure drawings are particularly helpful in understanding children's perceptions, especially when they are unable or unwilling to talk. Drawings

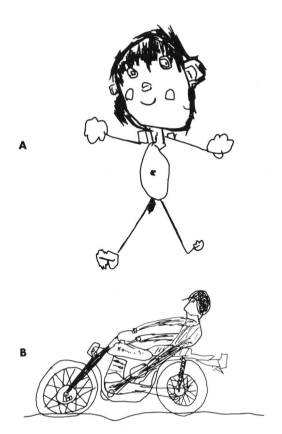

Fig. 3-4 Self-image drawings by two boys. **A** was drawn by a 7-year-old and **B** by a 13-year-old. Differences related to age, body perceptions, and interests are evident.

by well-adjusted children are very similar, but those by children experiencing physical or emotional stress are strikingly different and may provide insight into the perceptions of the particular child.[8] It is important to remember, however, that serious interpretation of these drawings should be done by someone with educational preparation in the use of the testing procedure and should be built on knowledge of the child as a whole.

Related problems

In dealing with people of various backgrounds, the nurse will have an opportunity to assess a wide range of body perceptions. In addition, she will have her own concepts of body ideal and body image. Overriding all of this is the broader cultural norm. At pre-

sent the United States appears to be committed to youth, wholeness, beauty, and health. This cultural norm gives rise to some common body-image problems. Probably the number-one appearance problem is obesity, as evidenced by the many reducing clubs and diet books now popular. In America obesity is a public health problem, and for the individual overeating can have adverse effects both physically and psychologically. Physically, high blood pressure and heart disease are more prevalent in obese adults and contribute to shorter life spans. Psychologically, studies have indicated that overweight people may be unable to derive satisfaction from their relationships with people or their work, so they attempt to find satisfaction through food.

An equally serious problem is that of being underweight. Unhealthy preoccupation with excessive thinness has led to the increasing incidence in this country of the eating disorders of anorexia and bulimia nervosa. These disorders occur most frequently, although not exclusively, among female adolescents and young adults. People with anorexia nervosa perceive that they are fat and literally starve themselves to achieve their goal of being thin. However, because of the distortion in their body image that they experience, the goal is unattainable. Even when emaciated to the point that their appearance is skeletal, they will maintain that they are fat and persist in their attempt to lose weight. People with bulimia nervosa consume large amounts of food and then purge through vomiting, laxatives, or excessive exercise. These disorders document that the relentless pursuit of excessive thinness in a society can be as destructive to individuals as ignoring the effects of obesity.

Signs of aging, including wrinkles, graying hair, and balding, are another area of body anxiety. Many people panic at the first sign of a gray hair, and hundreds of "special preparations" or "external youth creams" have been advertised for front-line duty in the war against wrinkles. Sagging muscles, receding hairlines, and loss of teeth all mark the passage of time and are often met by varying negative reactions—denial, anger, regret, or deep depression. In our youth-and beauty-oriented culture there often appears to be little value in getting older, and too many people overemphasize the importance of appearance as a primary basis for security and self-esteem.

If older people worry about aging, younger people worry about skin problems. The teenager with acne is the source of many jokes, and this group spends millions of dollars each year to keep their cheeks free from blemishes. The latest worry everyone over 12 can share is related to body odor—not just underarm odor, but also mouth odor, vaginal odor, and even foot odor. It has been suggested that the cosmetic industry continues to create areas for bodily concern to sell more products and make more money.

Some people are even less secure in their body image and actively strive to change or improve their natural endowments. Surgery on the nose or breasts and hair transplants reflect a strong desire to satisfy a body ideal that is much different from the reality. Finally, a much more serious body image problem is experienced by the transsexual, a person who psychologically identifies with the opposite sex. These individuals experience internal conflicts between their self-perceptions and their bodies. Some even attempt to resolve this problem by undergoing surgery or hormone treatments to change their gender and eliminate the conflict between their feelings and their bodies.

In addition to these common body image problems the nurse will also be exposed to specific disturbances related to the health-illness continuum. Many medical procedures invade the body integrity of the client—blood tests, catheterization, suctioning, injections, and so on. Even an ear examination or taking a temperature can be an invasion of body privacy. These procedures are particularly threatening to a child who is just beginning to master his body and who takes pride in control over it. Undergoing surgery is even more traumatic, and the loss of a body part or function can lead to serious body-image disturbances. The Vietnam War resulted in many young men who returned home as amputees or paraplegics; they had to start their lives over again while simultaneously adjusting to their new body images. Until recently the removal of a breast because of cancer was regarded as something tragic, personal, and hidden by women. With the operations of movie stars, politicians and other celebrities, however, mastectomies have been exposed to the public forum.

Breast self-examinations have been nationally televised. Now more women are aware of the disease and perhaps seek help sooner.

Growth, illness, trauma, and surgery all change the body and require adjustments of one's body image. The nature of the adjustment will partly depend on the type of body change and the developmental level of the client. For instance, an illness that limited a young child's mobility or ability to master the environment would be more threatening to this child than a disfiguring illness, but a teenager would find disfigurement very difficult to cope with because teenagers are very concerned with attractiveness and acceptance. Also related to body changes is shame. Loss of body control or damage to body integrity may provoke a feeling of failure within the individual. Adaptation to body change requires, therefore, that the individual adjust the body ideal, regain a sense of autonomy, and obtain satisfaction in life by a new balance of his physical, psychologic, and social experiences.

In summary, a person with a healthy body image shows appropriate concern for his health and appearance. If he is ill, he will seek help and try to restore his health. He will include proper diet and sufficient sleep in his daily activities and not dwell on or continuously worry about his health. He will try to look his best and will then take his appearance for granted. He will be able to make friends, form loving relationships, and be successful at work not because of his appearance alone but also because of his personal warmth and genuine achievement. An individual with an unhealthy body image will be preoccupied with health and overconcerned by daily aches and pains. He will be extremely anxious about his appearance, because he views his body as his primary means for gaining attention and acceptance. This preoccupation with his body will lead him to neglect other areas of his life, such as work and interpersonal relationships. Most unfortunately, it will also divert him from analyzing and solving the basic problems that have created his body anxiety and concern.

Because one's body image is continually changing and evolving, it is important to assess the body to ensure the accuracy of one's body image. Accuracy is achieved through observing, validating, and expanding one's knowledge. Even though doctors and nurses routinely care for people's bodies, they are notoriously neglectful of their own. "Do I get enough sleep each night?" "Do I eat well-balanced meals?" "Do I provide time for rest, relaxation, and exercise?" These are the questions each person must answer. If the answers are yes, one's body image is probably accurate as one strives to look one's best and then accepts nature for what it is.

CRITICAL THINKING *Question* ....

Given what is known about exposure to the sun causing skin cancer, how would you explain the fact that many people continue to value and pursue suntans? What issues does this raise regarding health knowledge, health beliefs, and health behaviors?

....

SELF-IDEAL

The self-ideal is the second important aspect of the personality. Each individual has a certain standard by which he judges his behavior. The standard may be either an image of the kind of person one would like to be or a number of aspirations, goals, or values that one would like to achieve. These ideals are based in part on society's norms, and the individual strives to attain them. The individual compares who he is or what he is doing to his personal picture of who he would like to be or what he would like to be doing. The self-ideal, therefore, is the individual's perception of how he should behave, and it is represented by his saying, "I should be . . . ." It creates self-expectations to which the individual tries to conform.

The formation of the self-ideal begins in childhood and is influenced by significant others. Initially, the child tries to conform to the parent's expectations and demands, even if they are too great. For his behavior the child is either rewarded or punished. In this way he learns what is "right" and "wrong" and when he is being "good" or "bad." With time the child internalizes the parental ideals, and they form the basis of the child's own self-ideal.

One's self-ideal may be clear and realistic and facilitate personal growth and relations with others, or it may be vague, unrealistic, and demanding. For example, if a person's self-ideal includes an intact

body and independent control over all aspects of the body, it may be difficult to adjust to the dependency and restrictions of aging.

In general, congruence between one's self and one's self-ideal is an important determiner of mental health. This has been supported by studies of people undergoing psychotherapy. The characteristic person who enters therapy has been shown to have a self-image that is far removed from, or even negatively correlated with, his self-ideal. At the conclusion of therapy, however, there has been evidence of significantly greater congruence between real self and self-ideal. This indicates that the adequately functioning individual is one who sees himself as being very much like the person he would like to be.

It is also true that a person's self-ideal is resistant to change. This is an important point, because sometimes one's self-ideal may be inappropriate and lowering the standards would lead to more satisfaction for the individual. Everyone can probably recall friends who throughout school worried greatly about grades. Their self-ideals were probably those of *A* students, but because they were unable to earn an *A*, they were frequently depressed or discouraged. It would certainly have been better if these students had learned to lower their expectations a little. However, perhaps because their parents valued grades also, they could not successfully readjust their standards.

In addition, one's self-ideal influences one's relationships with others. For instance, there is evidence that a person tends to select friends that resemble more closely his self-ideal rather than self-concept. This may cause one to more closely examine one's friends as a mirror of what one would like to become.

It is evident that one's self-ideal is an important determinant of personality and that a person's ongoing self-evaluation is based on his self-ideal. When working with a client, therefore, it is important that the nurse ask: "What is this person's self-ideal? Does he conform to his self-ideal? Does fulfillment of his self-ideal bring him satisfaction? Is his self-ideal compatible with the norms of society regarding health? How is his self-ideal different from mine? How can I help him conform to his self-ideal?" If the individual does not meet his expectations, he perceives himself as a failure and feels guilty and ashamed. If, however, he can attain his self-expectations, he experiences greater self-esteem and a more positive self-concept.

SELF-CONCEPT

The individual's self-concept consists of all the aspects of himself of which he is aware. It includes all of the self-perceptions—feelings, values, and beliefs—that direct and influence behavior, and it is represented by saying, "I am . . . ." It is the frame of reference through which the individual interacts with the world. No one is born with a self-concept; it is not genetically determined. Rather, it is learned by every individual, throughout one's lifetime from experiences with oneself, other people, and the realities of the changing world. Developmental theorists such as Freud, Sullivan, and Erikson have examined how it is derived from intrapsychic, interpersonal, and cultural experiences. It grows with one's perception of the world; it matures as one's body matures; and it changes as one evaluates oneself and one's social interactions and as one gains more self-knowledge.

Developmental changes

Self-concept begins at an early age. Although it has been considered to be a uniquely human characteristic, this is being questioned by some researchers. In a series of experiments chimpanzees exhibited self-directed behavior when exposed to a mirror. That is, they reacted as if they realized that the image in the mirror was a representation of themselves and not another chimp. Babies are usually approximately 10 months old when they show signs of recognizing themselves in mirrors. Children who have had little exposure to mirrors take longer, and some retarded people may never show signs of self-recognition. The young child who has established a beginning sense of body image continues cognitive development and further differentiates himself from others.

The acquisition of language is an important factor in this process, and the child's own name is a major linguistic aid. Pronouns do not provide the beginning sense of identity in the same way names do. This is illustrated in the following dialogue between a bright 4-year-old and his teacher as reported by Margaret Mead:

STUART: *Me* is a name, you know. My name.
TEACHER: *Me* is my name, too.
STUART: No, it is mine. How can it be yours? I am *me*.
TEACHER: I am, too.
STUART: No, you are not *me*. You are you. (after a pause). I am *me* to me, but you are *me* to you.[13]

By responding to his name, however, the child perceives himself as someone special, unique, and independent.

As the child becomes aware of his separateness, he also becomes aware of the behavior of others toward him. Research has supported Sullivan's belief that children's self-concepts are greatly influenced by "significant others" and that their self-concepts are very similar to the way they believe their parents view them. If a parent holds the child in high regard, the child is also likely to perceive himself as worthwhile. If he is frequently criticized and ridiculed by his parents, he might develop a self-concept in which he views himself as inadequate and unlovable. Consider the case of 9-year-old Jeffrey in the Clinical Example.

This example demonstrates the importance of the parent's behavior toward the developing child. Studies have also indicated that when parents have healthy, positive self-concepts, their children's self-concepts also tend to be positive.

When the parent has a wholesome, consistent self-concept, he can provide a more secure environment in the form of love, attention and respect for his child. When this occurs, the child can like, value and respect himself, and face the world with greater strength, security and confidence. When both parents provide this kind of nurturance, the child's self-concept is even stronger. With additional reinforcement provided by significant others, the self-concept is further strengthened. In each instance, the child tends to identify and model himself after the people who have positive value for him [p. 35].*

Studies have indicated that children are the most uncertain about their self-concepts and that their insecurity reaches a peak during the high-school years. This would support the crisis of acquiring a

---

*From Fitts W et al: *The self concept and self actualization,* Research monograph 5, Nashville, Tenn, 1971, The Dede Wallace Center.

CLINICAL EXAMPLE

Jeffrey came to the pediatric clinic because of his frequent behavioral outbursts. He could not seem to get along with boys his own age, and when things did not go his way, he had violent temper tantrums. Jeffrey would not cooperate with his teacher and always talked in a belligerent and arrogant manner. He described himself as "dumb" and frequently complained that "no one would ever want to be my friend." When the clinic nurse talked with his family, she realized that Jeffrey was a very insecure and lonely child. After some discussion it became clear that each parent handled Jeffrey differently. His father was a very conscientious person who had high self-ideals and expectations for his family. He did not believe in praising Jeffrey for things that Jeffrey did well, but he was quick to point out things that Jeffrey did wrong. Jeffrey's mother tried to mediate between her husband and son and reacted by giving in to all of Jeffrey's demands. The nurse assessed that both of these approaches could be making Jeffrey feel as though he could not do anything right. She inferred that with his father's criticism and his mother's pacification, Jeffrey could not learn to feel competent or secure within himself. To cover up for his low self-concept and feelings of inferiority, he acted like a bully with his peers. Because he was not making friends by his behavior, this reinforced his feelings that he was not important and that no one could ever like him.

sense of identity that Erikson has identified as the developmental task of adolescence. Research has shown that the self-concept becomes clearer during the college and adult years and is most pronounced and differentiated among the elderly.[18]

A person's view of oneself, however, is not only a collection of the views, expectations, and desires of others. Each individual can observe his own behavior the same way that others do and form opinions about himself. In addition, as the Johari Window (see Fig. 3-1) illustrates, there are some feelings and thoughts not known to others that can extend one's self knowledge and contribute to one's self-concept. The individual has more knowledge about himself than does anyone else. Whether he uses this knowledge is based on his own maturity and desire to grow. As he matures, hopefully, the individual becomes more self-directed and able to achieve the feeling that he is in control of his own life.

Although one's self-concept is continually developing and changing, there is also a degree of consistency and stability. Relative inner consistency gives unity to life and predictability to behavior. Erikson has described the acquisition of a firm identity as the realization of personal consistency and a gaining of self-direction. This is not to imply that a person wears only one mask. In fact, a person wears slightly different masks in response to different roles and situations.

Each new experience provides the individual with the opportunity to explore new aspects of the self and to grow through this increased self-knowledge. As the individual internalizes this new information, self-concept develops and this learning becomes a part of his new behavior pattern. The individual's ability to be open and accepting of new situations and ideas can, therefore, enhance self-concept.

The personality component of self-concept has been the subject of a large body of research over the years. Psychology and sociology have accounted for over 2000 publications on the self, including research related to social deviance, interpersonal attraction, psychopathology, and psychotherapy. However, there are frequent contradictions among the findings, and this area of the personality continues to be one of much interest and controversy.

As a nurse it is important that one realize a positive self-concept is directly related to mental health for both adults and children. Emotionally disturbed children express lower self-concepts than more normally functioning children. Psychotherapy with adults appears to produce positive changes in self-concept, and this in turn appears to produce positive changes in behavior. Therapeutic intervention allows the individual to grow in self-understanding, self-responsibility, and self-esteem. Also, a positive or well-integrated self-concept has been found to be correlated with good interpersonal communication.[18]

Nursing assessment

Every nursing assessment, therefore, should include data related to the client's self-concept: How does the client describe himself? What strengths does he think he has? What does he see as his areas of weakness? How does he feel about his relationships with others? How does he react to compliments and criticism? After interacting with the client, the nurse should then objectively examine his behavior: Are his statements contradictory? Is his behavior congruent with his statements? Data related to the client's self-concept are an essential part of the nurse's assessment. She can then incorporate her analysis in the planning and implementing of care in relation to the total needs of her client.

CRITICAL THINKING *Question* ....

Obtain copies of the nursing assessment forms used in the health care facilities of your clinical rotations. Evaluate the information obtained from the client related to self-concept based on the following criteria: Is it adequate, appropriate, efficient, and effective? What changes in the nursing assessment forms, if any, would you recommend based on your evaluation?
....

SELF-ESTEEM

Self-esteem is a personality variable that has attracted the attention of psychologists and philosophers alike. Philosophers such as Pascal, Locke, and Rousseau have believed that the individual's desire for approval and esteem is the primary social motivator of his behavior. The psychologist William James once said, "What every person craves most is praise."[7] For the individual, self-esteem is the product of self-confidence and self-respect. It is the belief that one is competent to live and worthy of life.

There is no value judgment more important to man—no factor more decisive in his psychological development and motivation—than the estimate he passes on himself. This estimate is ordinarily expressed by him not in the form of a conscious verbalized judgment, but in the form of a feeling, a feeling that can be hard to isolate and identify because he experiences it constantly; it is part of every other feeling; it is involved in every emotional response. . . . The nature of his self-evaluation has profound effects on a man's thinking processes, emotions, desires, values and goals. It is the single most significant key to his behavior. To understand a man psychologically, one must understand the nature and degree of his self-esteem and the standards by which he judges himself.[2]

Self-esteem can be defined as the individual's personal judgment of his own worth, obtained by analyzing how well he matches up to his own standards and how well his performance compares with others. It evolves through the comparison of the individual's self-ideal and self-concept and is represented by his saying "I can . . ." If the individual's self-concept does not conform to his self-ideal, he will experience low self-regard or low self-esteem (Fig. 3-5, *A*). If there is great conformity, he will experience high self-worth or high self-esteem (Fig. 3-5, *B*).

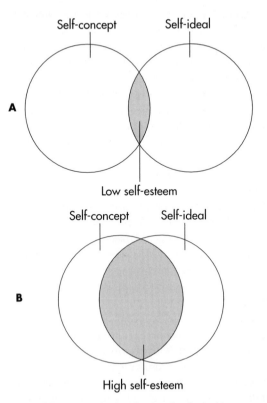

Fig. 3-5 A, Individual with a low level of self-esteem because of a large discrepancy between self-concept and self-ideal. **B,** Person with greater conformity of self-concept and self-ideal and, therefore, a person with a high level of self-esteem.

Developmental changes

Self-esteem is derived from two primary sources: the self, and others. In the same way that the child's self-ideals are initially incorporated from the expectations of significant others, the child's self-esteem is also initially an acceptance of the parents' evaluations of him.[14] According to developmental theory, it is at approximately the age of 2 years that the child actively experiences levels of self-esteem. At this time there are the first signs of the child's overt disagreement with the parents, desire for independence, and exploration of the environment. Erikson has identified the child's struggle between autonomy versus shame and initiative versus guilt as occurring at this age. When the child is approximately 6 or 7 years, self-esteem is increasingly related to competition with others.

Coopersmith suggested that success in certain areas of life is essential for the development of high self-esteem.[3] In establishing and maintaining self-worth, one needs a feeling of significance—success in being accepted and approved by others; a feeling of competence—ability to cope effectively with life; and a feeling of power—control over one's own destiny.

This last aspect of feeling control over one's own destiny is also referred to as self-efficacy. Self-efficacy refers to a person's belief in one's ability to organize and implement actions that will bring success.[1] This may include regulating one's motivation, thought processes, affective states, and activities, or it may involve changing environmental conditions. Self-efficacy has been found to influence the course of action people choose to pursue, how much effort they put forth, how long they will persevere in the face of obstacles and failures, how resilient they will be to adversity, whether their thought patterns are positive or self-defeating, how much stress they experience in coping with taxing environmental demands, and the level of accomplishment and pleasure they will realize.

Coopersmith identified notable antecedents of high and low self-esteem.[3] He asked, "What are the conditions that lead an individual to value himself and to regard himself as an object of worth?" The answers he received were parental acceptance, respect, and limits. The parents of the children with high self-esteem demonstrated warmth, acceptance of their children, and a democratic family process. The children were allowed to voice their own opinions and question their parents' opinions. They had close rela-tionships with their parents and shared activities and discussions with them. The parents of the children with high self-esteem also had clearly defined and enforced limits or rules. They were less permissive and more consistent, and they used rewards more often than punishments in dealing with their children. The combination of realistic and consistent limits plus respect for the child's opinion enhanced the child's ability to succeed. Coopersmith also found that the children of parents who expected them to live up to the standards that they (the parents) had set were more successful. Thus in Coopersmith's opinion the four best ways to promote a child's self-esteem are to:
1. Provide the child with successes
2. Instill ideals
3. Encourage aspirations
4. Help build defenses against attacks on the child's self-perception

Having successful experiences as a child adds to the individual's self-esteem and helps him cope with the difficult tasks of adolescence. Adolescence is a time of idealism, insecurity, and changing self-concepts. It is not until adulthood that some stability is obtained. Then the person is more realistic, has learned to cope with his deficiencies, and emphasizes his strengths. In later life, the problem of self-esteem again arises because of the aging process and the norms of society.

A number of threats to the self-esteem of the aged can be identified. The first threat is the tension between young people and the aged—that the young people desire to lead and dominate the older ones. The second threat is the result of society's emphasis on youth and beauty—a norm that devalues the physical process of aging. The third is that of reduced interpersonal relationships because of the death of friends and relatives and lack of a peer group provided through employment. The fourth is the physiologic process of aging, which limits emotional and physical resources, and the fifth is caused by the psychologic restrictions of aging, which influence memory, sensation, speed, and activity. These problems of aging require new coping behaviors because all people need a stable, positive evaluation of themselves for self-respect, self-esteem, and esteem from others. This evaluation leads to feelings of adequacy, achievement, competence, importance, mastery, and integrity (Fig. 3-6). A successful level of self-worth is well represented in the prose by Satir (see box on p. 68).

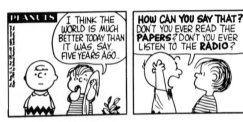 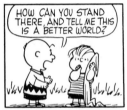 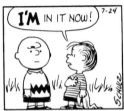

Fig. 3-6 Linus is able to trust himself and see himself as worthwhile. With his feelings of significance, competence, and power, he is a good role model for Charlie Brown. (© 1959 United Feature Syndicate, Inc.)

My Declaration of Self-Esteem

I am me.

In all the world, there is no one else exactly like me. There are persons who have some parts like me, but no one adds up exactly like me. Therefore, everything that comes out of me is authentically mine because I alone chose it.

I own everything about me—my body, including everything it does; my mind, including all its thoughts and ideas; my eyes, including the images of all they behold; my feelings, whatever they may be—anger, joy, frustration, love, disappointment, excitement; my mouth, and all the words that come out of it, polite, sweet or rough, correct or incorrect; my voice, loud or soft; and all my actions, whether they be to others or to myself.

I own my fantasies, my dreams, my hopes, my fears.

I own all my triumphs and successes, all my failures and mistakes.

Because I own all of me, I can become intimately acquainted with me. By so doing I can love me and be friendly with me in all my parts. I can then make it possible for all of me to work in my best interests.

I know there are aspects about myself that puzzle me, and other aspects that I do not know. But as long as I am friendly and loving to myself, I can courageously and hopefully look for the solutions to the puzzles and for ways to find out more about me.

However I look and sound, whatever I say and do, and whatever I think and feel at a given moment in time is me. This is authentic and represents where I am at that moment in time.

When I review later how I looked and sounded, what I said and did, and how I thought and felt, some parts may turn out to be unfitting. I can discard that which is unfitting, and keep that which proved fitting, and invent something new for that which I discarded.

I can see, hear, feel, think, say and do. I have the tools to survive, to be close to others, to be productive, and to make sense and order out of the world of people and things outside of me.

I own me, and therefore I can engineer me.

I am me and I am okay.

From Satir V: *Peoplemaking*, Palo Alto, Calif, 1972, Science and Behavior Books.

Every day people experience threats to their self-esteem. Maybe one does poorly on an examination, makes an embarrassing remark, or dresses inappropriately for a dinner party. How insecure or ashamed one feels may depend on whether one's mistake is a typical behavior or an isolated incident, as well as on what defense mechanism one uses in response to the threat. There are certain ways that everyone can maximize or maintain his self-esteem.

Each person selects his particular life goals or self-ideals. By so doing, he identifies certain areas in which he would like to succeed, as seen in the following Clinical Example.

 CLINICAL EXAMPLE

*T*wo *third-year college students enroll in the same course on foreign governments. Both receive a B in the course. One student is a nursing major; she took the course as an elective. It is not her main area of interest, but she wanted to expand her knowledge. She is very pleased with the grade, because it is better than she thought she would do and it enhances her self-esteem. The other student is a political science major. She feels that the course is very important and expected to do better, because government is her major. Consequently, she is disappointed and experiences decreased self-esteem.*

Not all people value the same goals. Research suggests that people tend to set goals that they believe they can accomplish. Thus the more realistic the self-ideal, the greater the chance of accomplishment and the resulting self-esteem.[14] It is not the type of goal one sets but accomplishment that leads to self-esteem. Learning to swim may be as important for one person as passing a test is for someone else. The crucial factor is that society create sufficient opportunities to allow each individual the opportunity of achieving his goal. This applies to opportunities for advanced education, as well as adequate jobs and cultural stimulation.

Hamachek has identified additional ways of maintaining self-esteem.[6] One way is by selecting one's environment so that one is more likely to have positive experiences. If one is successful in dealing with people, one should choose a more active and involved job rather than a job requiring solitary analysis or work. Another way is by selecting as friends people with whom one agrees. Selecting people with similar values may reduce the interpersonal defenses one uses. Finally, one's appraisal or personal interpretation of events or statements allows one to interpret things in a less threatening manner. All of these mechanisms defend the self by limiting our awareness to some degree, however, and thus they may also limit our growth.

What happens if someone experiences low self-esteem? Low self-esteem has been found to be associated with depression, anxiety, substance abuse, and social deviance. People seeking psychologic help usually have two things in common: poor interpersonal relations and low self-esteem. Jourard has referred to those events in life that result in low self-esteem as "dispiriting" events; he believes that there is a connection between "dispiritization," suicide, disease, and death.[10] Therapeutic intervention by doctors, nurses, and psychotherapists, therefore, should involve a change in the client's level of self-esteem to effect a change in his level of wellness.

CRITICAL THINKING *Question* ....

Are you surprised to learn that in North America more people die by suicide than by homicide? Do you think that this fact requires a reallocation of social resources? If so, in what way?
••

Nursing assessment

Thus the area of self-esteem is an additional part of the nurse's assessment. She inquires: "What does my client think about himself as a person? How well does he meet his self-ideal? Does he value his strengths? Does he view his weaknesses as important personality deficits, or are they relatively unimportant to his self-concept?" Coopersmith has presented the following monologues that might be helpful examples to the beginning student. The first is of a person with high self-esteem:

I consider myself a valuable and important person, and am at least as good as others of my age and training. I am regarded as someone worthy of respect and consideration. . . . I'm able to exert an influence upon people and events, partly because my views are sought and respected and partly because I'm able and willing to present and defend those views. I have a pretty definite idea of what I think is right . . . and have a fairly good understanding of the kind of person I am. I enjoy new and challenging tasks and don't get upset when things don't go well right off the bat [p. 47].[3]

A person with low self-esteem reports:

I don't think I'm a very important or likeable person, and I don't see much reason for anyone else to like me. I can't do many of the things I'd like to do or do them the way I think they should be done. I'm not sure of my ideas and abilities, and there's a good likelihood that other people's ideas and work are better than my own. Other people don't pay much attention to me and given what I know about myself, I can't say I blame them. I don't like new or unusual occurrences and prefer sticking to known and safe ground. . . . I don't have much control over what happens to me and I expect that things will get worse rather than better [p. 47].[3]

One role of the nurse in her therapeutic use of self is to intervene in ways that enhance her client's self-esteem. If she remembers that every person needs a feeling of significance, competence, and power, she will add to the client's growth and level of self-esteem.

INFLUENCES ON THE SELF

Building on knowledge of developmental theory and insight into the variables of the self, we can now examine some of the factors influencing an individual's self-perceptions throughout his life. Basically it may be stated that:

$$Heredity + Environment = Personality$$

Thus prenatal influences are quite significant. The mother's physical health—whether she suffers from nutritional inadequacies, genetic defects, or diseases such as rubella, smallpox, acquired immunodeficiency syndrome, syphilis, diabetes, or high blood pressure—influences her child in many ways. Drugs such as narcotics, barbiturates, quinine, alcohol, and cocaine may have reversible or irreversible effects. Maternal emotional stress and the mother's attitude toward the pregnancy also influence the developing fetus. Thus genetic factors and the maternal environment are responsible for many characteristics of the individual at birth.

Once the child enters the world he is assaulted by numerous physical and interpersonal stimuli. The parents in turn react to his appearance as they analyze who he looks like most. They also react to gender—how does a father feel about his new daughter when he was hoping for and dreaming of a son for so long? The parents' initial reactions are conveyed to the child and influence how they meet the infant's dependency needs.

As the child grows older he begins to explore his own body. He then receives more parental messages from their reactions to his naked body and from their responses to his masturbation. When he asks for sexual information, he may get any of a number of responses. Some parents change the subject, and the child gets the impression that either the parent doesn't know or the information is too terrible to tell. Another parent may respond, "You're too young . . . I'll tell you when you get older." With this response the child might feel inferior or inadequate. Still another parent may give the child a high-level crash course on the nature of the sexual response that completely baffles and overwhelms the child. Finally, many parents tell their child about "a seed growing in the ground that becomes a flower . . . soon a bee comes along . . ." The child enjoys the lovely story but has no more knowledge or information than when the question was asked. A straightforward, simple, and accurate answer that provides the required information enhances the child's knowledge and body image.

At this time the child's body begins to take on a certain shape, and physique as well as other people's assessment begin to influence self-concept. Research has indicated that body physique influences not only one's view of self but also one's personality traits, temperament, and behavior patterns. One theory classifies individuals according to three basic components: endomorphic, ectomorphic, and mesomorphic, defining each one of these and correlating each with certain behavioral characteristics.[16,17]

Endomorphy refers to the dominance of the digestive organs and is seen as a predominance of fullness or roundness throughout the body. The endomorphic body type is associated with a viscerotonia temperament, which includes general relaxation, love of comfort and eating, sociability, and attraction to food, people, and affection. For this individual "the digestive tract is king and its welfare appears to define the primary purpose of life."[17]

Ectomorphy refers to the dominance of the brain and central nervous system. The ectomorphic individual is tall, thin, and fragile and has the greatest sensory exposure to the outside world. This person has a cerebrotonia temperament, which is characterized by restraint, love of privacy, secretiveness, hypersensitivity, and inhibition. He shies away from people and avoids attracting attention to himself.

Mesomorphy refers to the predominance of muscle and bone, and the physique is compact and rectangular. The corresponding somatotonia temperament is assertive, energetic, risk taking, powerful, and competitive and is dominated by activity. Figure 3-7 illustrates the physiques associated with each of these three body types.

Everyone can recall thin, muscular, and heavy individuals who match these descriptions. At times, however, one's body ideal, body image, and cultural norms can come into conflict and produce behavior inconsistent with one's feelings. For instance, a child may be greatly overweight and feel miserable and rejected by everyone, but this child may feel forced to act jolly and easygoing because the parents believe that an obese child is a happy and affectionate one. So the child soon learns that appearance elicits a positive or negative social response that affects the self-concept.

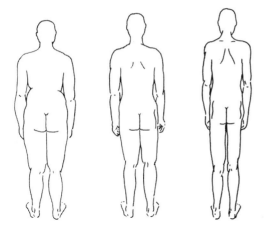

Fig. 3-7 Body physiques that are examples of endo-morphy (*left*), mesomorphy (*middle*), and ectomorphy (*right*), as described by Sheldon.

Family and social relations

Another influence on the child is ordinal position in the family. First-born children tend to be brighter or more intelligent.[14] This is evidenced by the predominance of first-born children enrolled in college and by the number of American presidents who have held first-born ordinal positions in their families. First-born girls and boys have been found to be more ambitious and achievement oriented in comparison with middle children. Furthermore, first-born children tended to identify with their parents, whereas younger children identified more with their peers. Toman has postulated that certain personality characteristics are associated with the type of family constellation that the individual experienced as a child, such as being the youngest and the brother of sisters or the oldest brother of brothers. His theory further suggests that new interpersonal relationships will be codetermined by earlier ones.[19]

Parental discipline has also been shown to be a factor affecting the child's self-esteem. There are two major influences on a parent's child-rearing practices: the practices used by his parents, and the accepted child-rearing practices currently being advocated in his society. Most parents behave toward their children as their own parents behaved toward them. Often this is not a conscious process but an "acculturation" of their parents' style. The person-

Children Learn What They Live— Parent's Creed

If a child lives with criticism, he learns to condemn.
If a child lives with hostility, he learns to fight.
If a child lives with ridicule, he learns to be shy.
If a child lives with tolerance, he learns to be patient.
If a child lives with encouragement, he learns confidence.
If a child lives with praise, he learns to appreciate.
If a child lives with fairness, he learns justice.
If a child lives with security, he learns to have faith.
If a child lives with approval, he learns to like himself.
If a child lives with acceptance and friendship,
He learns to find love in the world.

ality and methods of his parents can have a significant influence on the child's self-concept. A cold, rejecting, or demanding parent might convey to the child that he is not lovable or worth very much. An inconsistent parent does not provide the child with secure limits from which to develop his self-ideal. The overprotective parent may create a dependent child who has little self-esteem and feels that he must always rely on others, not himself. A parent who provides clear limits and positive reinforcement tells the child that he is a capable, worthwhile person and thus adds to the child's self-concept. This can become a self-fulfilling prophecy when the child meets his parents' expectations and experiences success. Positive child-rearing is reflected in the verse by Dorothy Law Nolte (see box above).

CRITICAL THINKING *Question* ....

About one third of women in America report having been sexually abused before age 18. Discuss the impact this trauma can have on a child's or an adolescent's self-esteem, interpersonal relationships, and sense of competency.
••

The family unit itself also influences the child's self-concept. Freud has discussed the importance of the same-gender parent for the developing child. Even if the actual parent is not present, boys need a father figure and girls need a mother figure to integrate their perceptions regarding their gender and self-concept. How do broken family units affect the child? Certainly death, separation, and divorce require adjustment, but it cannot be assumed that a traditional, intact family unit is necessarily better than a single-parent or blended family structure. Research indicates that both active family discord and lack of parental affection are associated with juvenile antisocial behavior. Goode has noted

that a family in which there is continued marital conflict, or separation, is more likely to produce children with problems of personal adjustment than a family in which there is divorce or death . . . [The] choice usually has to be between a continuing conflict or divorce. And the evidence suggests that it is the conflict of divorce, not the divorce itself, that has an impact on the children [p. 455].[5]

What appears to be important, therefore, is the quality of the home life and the self-esteem of the parents rather than the number of family members living together.

Outside the home, school emerges as a major part of the child's life. It provides the opportunity for the child to receive praise, confidence, and self-respect as well as rejection, criticism, and self-doubt. One study has indicated that high-achieving students have more positive self-concepts than do low-achieving students, even though they do not differ in intelligence.[4] Furthermore, high achievers have better peer relationships and emotional adjustment. The question that arises is which comes first—positive self-concept or high academic achievement? The question has no definite answer, but one fact appears certain: increase one and the other will also improve. That is, better school performance will lead to a more positive self-concept and vice versa.

Within the school the teacher becomes the child's significant other and thus actively influences the child's self-concept. Hamachek[6] has summarized five generalizations that explain how effective teachers differ from less effective ones:

1. They seem to have a more positive view of others.
2. They see themselves as potentially friendly and worthy in their own right.
3. They have a favorable view of democratic classroom procedures.
4. They are able to see things as they seem to others or from someone else's point of view.
5. They see students as people capable of doing things for themselves once they feel trusted, respected, and valued, not people you "do things to."

Many aspects of school influence the child's self-perceptions. If expected to succeed, given praise, and seen as valuable, the child will grow into adolescence feeling competent.

Adolescents are strongly influenced by their peer group. They strive for acceptance from the group, and the opinions of their friends greatly affect their self-concept. Also at this time adolescents are striving for freedom from their families. Overly strict parental restraints tell them that they are not capable of making their own decisions. Parents fear the mistakes their children might make, yet by setting rigid rules, they provoke rebellion and their children meet their worst expectations. Adolescents are also struggling with their biologic impulses and views of morality. Their sexual activities are influenced by peer pressure and by their fears of rejection. The moods of adolescents seem to fluctuate frequently, and their self-concept often changes with each mood.

The evolution of one's personality does not stop at adolescence but continues throughout life. The self-esteem of adults is derived from external, as well as internal, sources. Religion, social class, job, and salary all reflect the worth of adults. Are they happy with their jobs? Are they performing well? Are the jobs valuable in the eyes of society? Are they paid well? Can they support their families? Interpersonal, marriage, and family relationships are also important. Is spending time with one's family a rewarding and ego-building experience or an embarrassing, conflictual, and self-deflating one? Increasingly, adults look toward society to confirm their self-concepts. They are exposed to books, television, movies, and newspapers, all of which convey the values of society, and they evaluate themselves against society's norms to determine their self-worth.

The development sequence of the adult years suggests the following phases of adulthood: between the ages of 22 and 28 years, people strive to become more self-reliant and concentrate their energies on building for the future, both personally and professionally; between the ages of 29 and 34, adults become more self-reflective and money, marriage, and children become increasingly important; between the ages of 35 and 43, marital comfort decreases and adults view time as passing too quickly; between the ages of 44 and 50, adults come to terms with time and with themselves as individuals; by the age of 50, death becomes more of a reality and adults are increasingly concerned with their health and with experiencing the fullness of life.

Old age brings on additional stress to the self-perceptions of individuals. They have experienced the change of life, their children are grown and have left home, and their careers have ended. They may now have limited financial resources, failing health, and fewer living friends and family. Whereas early in adulthood they took pride in their independence, they may now be experiencing role reversal and increasing dependency on others.

Earlier research of the aged painted a rather bleak picture of how the aged viewed themselves. Recent research, however, has revealed some interesting facts concerning the aged and their self-perceptions. Findings seem to negate the stereotype that older persons are lonely, unhappy, concerned about being old, and preoccupied with their aches and pains. Furthermore, income, social contact, and perceived health are closely associated with the self-concept. The following are some characteristics of "successful agers." They continue to be involved socially with others, to engage in activities that give them a sense of worth (part-time jobs, housework, volunteer activities, or hobbies), and to operate within relatively unconfined life spaces that meet personal needs and social expectations. This picture of the elderly is quite different from the stereotype that many people hold. It suggests that many of the elderly are living a fulfilled life and are experiencing what Erikson has described as the virtue of wisdom arising from ego integrity.

THE HEALTHY PERSONALITY

Freud devoted much of his time to describing neurosis and abnormal behavior, but basically he would view an individual as healthy if that person were not afraid of his feelings or emotions. The healthy person would have sufficient energy to do productive work and would have the freedom to express himself in loving relationships with others. Sullivan's view of a healthy personality would be a person with a clear understanding of himself, the people around him, and how he related to others. He would have a realistic concept of other people and an ability to love.

 CULTURAL CONSIDERATIONS

Self-conceptions include both personal or individualistic and group or collective aspects, although their relative influence will depend on the type of culture in which people are raised. People live their lives in sociocultural environments that differ in their shared values, social practices, and opportunity structures. Cultures that are individualistically oriented tend to favor self-initiative and pursuit of self-interest, whereas those that are collectively oriented place group interest and shared responsibility above self-interest. However, these global classifications mask much diversity and variability and rest on a questionable assumption of cultural uniformity. Specifically, collectivistic systems, such as East Asian ones founded on Confucianism or Buddhism, favor a communal ethic, but they differ significantly from each other in particular values, meanings, and customs. Nor are individualistic cultures a uniform group—Americans, Italians, Germans, and the British differ in their particular brands of individualism. Even within an individualistically oriented culture such as the United States, the New England brand of individualism is quite different from the Californian version or that of the Southern region of the nation. In addition to the diversity within and between cultures placed in the same category, even members of the same national culture adopt different orientations depending on circumstances. Thus cultural orientations must be treated as multifaceted dynamic influences in explaining how self-conceptions develop within independent and interdependent social systems.

Erikson would equate health with the successful completion of the stages of development and with the resolution of the crises associated with each. Thus a healthy adult would have established a sense of trust, autonomy, initiative, industry, identity, intimacy, generativity, and integrity. His life would have meaning, and his relationships with others would be rich and fulfilling. These are general descriptions, however, that may be difficult to apply when assessing a client.

Maslow's hierarchy

Another psychologist, Abraham Maslow, has developed a theory of human behavior based on the individual's needs and potentialities. Maslow has created a hierarchy of basic needs that must be gratified for the individual to reach his fullest capability. They are

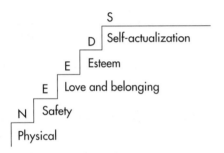

Fig. 3-8 Maslow's hierarchy of needs as they progress in steplike fashion from the physical need to the need for self-actualization.

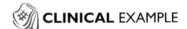

CLINICAL EXAMPLE

After assessing Mr. G. in his home, the community health nurse has determined that:

Mr. G. appeared apathetic and hostile.

Mr. G. had discontinued his involvement with his church group.

Mr. G. had no visitors within the month from family or friends.

Mr. G. did not respond to the nurse when she talked to him and appeared to be experiencing a hearing loss.

Mr. G.'s love and belonging needs were not being met, but this may be directly related to his hearing loss. The most therapeutic nursing approach, therefore, may be to give priority to his physical auditory needs. Once these needs are more adequately met, he may then regain interest in other people and his environment and thus satisfy his love and belonging needs.

progressive needs—the basic ones must be met before those of the higher levels can be attained. Figure 3-8 visualizes these needs in a steplike progression from lowest to highest.

Physical needs include physiologic requirements such as food, water, and air. Safety needs pertain to the necessity of a secure physical environment that is free from threat. Love and belonging needs include the desire for intimacy and relationships with other people. Esteem needs refer to the desire for self-respect and recognition from others that one is a worthwhile, valuable person. Self-actualization needs include the desire for self-fulfillment as one concentrates on realizing one's own potential.[12] Maslow has said that to reach the higher levels of functioning, the individual must have met his more basic lower needs. For example, a person will not be able to engage in tasks that serve to increase self-esteem (esteem needs) if worried about keeping a job and meeting monthly mortgage payments (safety needs). A person will not be able to develop interpersonal relationships (love and belonging needs) if concerned about getting enough food to eat (physical needs).

The nurse may find Maslow's hierarchy of needs useful in analyzing her client's needs and in setting mutual priorities. In doing this it is essential that she validate her observations with the client. One behavior may have many different causes and may arise from any one of Maslow's needs. All physical problems, therefore, do not necessarily originate from physical needs as defined by Maslow. They may instead be related to a higher-level need. All

interpersonal behaviors do not necessarily originate from love and belonging needs but may be related to physical needs. One can solve the problem only by identifying the proper need. For example, if the behavior of constipation is assessed, the nurse should not automatically place it in the category of physical needs and assign it top priority; rather she should collect additional data and see if it is a behavior related to another need, such as the need for self-esteem. A client experiencing low self-esteem may experience constipation, anorexia, and other physical complaints. In this instance the need for self-esteem should be given priority and supportive treatment should be given to the physical complaints. The nurse must also examine all of the facts carefully in assessing and formulating the plan of care, as seen in the Clinical Example above.

Only by mutual interaction with the client can the nurse determine the meaning behind the behavior and the basic unmet need.

Maslow's hierarchy presents a holistic view of a person's needs and can help the nurse organize and set goals with her client. Once the client has satisfied his lower needs, he can then devote his energies to self-actualization. Because this implies self-fulfillment and the maximizing of human potential, Maslow did a study of self-actualized people and attempted to describe them. His group includes Lincoln, Jefferson, Walt Whitman, Beethoven, Franklin D. Roosevelt, Einstein, and Eleanor Roosevelt. The characteristics of the self-actualized individuals he has described include:

• Accurate perception of reality
• A high degree of acceptance of self, others, and human nature
• Spontaneity
• Problem centered as opposed to self-centered
• Need for privacy
• High degree of autonomy and independence
• Freshness of appreciation
• Frequent "mystic" experiences
• Identification with mankind
• Intimate relationships with a few significant others
• Democratic character structures
• Strong ethical sense
• Unhostile sense of humor
• Creativeness
• Resistance to conformity[12]

Maslow's theory of the healthy personality describes a self that is continually seeking, growing, and facing new challenges. The healthy or self-actualized self is spontaneous and natural as the individual actively experiences life and expresses his own uniqueness.

Rogers has further developed a description of the individual who is moving toward self-growth and fulfillment.[15] He refers to a "fully functioning person" who has the psychologic freedom to move toward becoming more fully himself. Such a person displays the following behaviors:

1. He moves away from facades and self-images that are not true to himself.
2. He moves away from others' expectations of what he "ought to be" and society's pressures for conformity.
3. He moves away from pleasing others who wish to impose artificial goals on him.
4. He moves toward becoming autonomous, self-directing, and self-responsible. He chooses the goals he wishes to move toward.
5. He is more open to change and exploring his own potential.

6. He desires to experience all of himself and hide nothing. He is more open to his own self and the lives of others.
7. He trusts and values himself and dares to express himself in new ways.*

CRITICAL THINKING *Question* ················

How do you compare with the behaviors identified by Rogers[15] as characteristics of a fully functioning person? Which behaviors would you focus on as important areas for your own future growth and development?
··

Dynamics of the self

It is possible to describe the healthy personality according to developmental theory and the dynamics of the self. This description may help to give perspective to the many aspects of the self previously discussed. An individual with a healthy personality would experience:

1. A positive and accurate body image. *Body image* is the sum of the conscious and unconscious attitudes the individual has toward his body. It includes present and past perceptions as well as feelings about size, function, appearance, and potential. A healthy body awareness would be based on self-observation and appropriate concern for one's physical well-being.
2. A realistic self-ideal. *Self-ideal* is the individual's perception of how he should behave or the standard by which he appraises his behavior. An individual with a realistic self-ideal would have attainable life goals that are valuable and worth pursuing.
3. A positive self-concept. *Self-concept* consists of all the aspects of the individual of which he is aware. It includes all of his self-perceptions, which direct and influence his behavior. A positive self-concept implies that the individual expects to be successful in life. It includes the negative aspects of the self as part of the individual's personality. Such a person believes he can master his environment. He does not fear rejection but feels

---

*From *On Becoming a Person* by Carl R Rogers. Copyright © 1961 by Carl R. Rogers. Used by permission of Houghton Mifflin.

secure and accepted. He has the courage to face life openly and realistically and affirm his own existence.

4. A high self-esteem. *Self-esteem* is the individual's personal judgment of his own worth, obtained by analyzing how well he matches up to his own standards and how well his performance compares with others. It is evolved through the comparison of the individual's self-ideal and self-concept. A person with high self-esteem views himself as someone worthy of respect and dignity. He believes in his own self-worth, and he approaches life with aggressiveness and zest. The individual with a healthy personality is one who sees himself to be very much like the person he would like to be.

5. A clear sense of identity. *Identity* is the integration of inner and outer demands in the individual's discovery of who he is and what he can become. It is the realization of personal consistency. The individual with a clear sense of identity experiences a unity of personality and perceives himself to be a unique individual. His "sense of self" gives his life direction and purpose.

6. An openness to people. *Relating to others intimately* is the final characteristic of the individual with a healthy personality. Through open and honest communication he can trust others and enter into mutual and interdependent relationships. His capacity for sharing enables him to enter into an authentic relationship with another person and experience love, freedom, and interdependence.

An individual with these qualities is able to perceive himself and his world accurately. His insight into himself creates a feeling of harmony and inner peace.

NURSING AND SELF-AWARENESS

Self-knowledge is best learned
not by contemplation, but action.
Strive to do your duty and you will
soon discover of what stuff you are made.

Goethe

In learning about the nursing process it is essential that the nurse learn the dynamics of the self. The nurse who cares for the biologic, psychologic, and sociologic needs of her clients will be exposed to a broad range of human experiences. She must learn to deal with anxiety, anger, sadness, and joy in helping clients at all intervals of the health-illness continuum. Her goal is the attainment of authentic, open, and personal communication. In her nursing care she must be able to examine her own feelings and reactions as a person, as well as her actions as a professional provider of care. A firm understanding and acceptance of her own self will allow the nurse to acknowledge a client's differences and uniqueness.

It is commonly assumed that because a nursing student has taken some courses in the behavioral sciences, she is able to use herself in a therapeutic manner in the clinical setting. Most nursing textbooks that describe the nursing process include a paragraph or two stressing the importance of self-awareness in quality nursing care. The process and components of self-growth for the nurse are never described. The self-concept of the client is treated in a similarly cursory and general way. These omissions convey an implicit message to the nursing student: self-analysis is commendable, but a token assessment will suffice. To further reinforce this message, the student's curriculum is burdened with tasks and papers that allow little time for quiet contemplation leading to self-growth.

All of the previously described components of self-awareness—body image, self-ideal, self-concept, and self-esteem—make up the nurse's "sense of self." They influence all of her actions and interactions with others, although it is often difficult to isolate and analyze them. Yet in many daily experiences, they merge and coexist, as seen in the Clinical Example.

It is necessary that nurses have the time to explore and define the many facets of their personalities. If nursing does involve perceiving, feeling, and thinking, nursing students should have the time and opportunity to study the basics of their experiences. Authenticity in relationships must be learned. For the nurse to do this, it is first necessary that she experience openness and authenticity in her relationships with instructors and supervisors. The student and instructor can mutually participate in a human-to-human relationship that accepts and respects individual differences. By acting as role models, instructors can facilitate students' self-awareness, increase their level of functioning, stimulate more

CLINICAL EXAMPLE

Imagine that you are taking an examination in nursing. You stay up late studying the night before and miss some needed sleep. On the day of the exam you toss on some old jeans and a shirt, skip breakfast, and hurry to take the test. You arrive looking tired and sloppy and feeling hungry (body image). Running through your head is the pressure of wanting to be a good nurse. You feel that you ought to know the content to give good nursing care. You might even be considering graduate school some day (self-ideal). Of course, you realize that so far you are doing well in the nursing course. You really enjoy the clinical experience, and both you and your instructor agree that your performance is very good (self-concept). It is still true, however, that whether you leave feeling good about yourself or somewhat guilty will partly depend on how well you do on the test (self-esteem).

self-direction, and enable them to cope more effectively with the stressors of life.

Authenticity also involves being truthful and open to exploring one's thoughts, needs, emotions, values, defenses, actions, communications, problems, and goals. In the process of becoming a nurse the student has many new experiences providing opportunities for self-learning. Feelings about them should be focused on and discussed. The student might enter her clinical settings with high ideals and unrealistic images. Perhaps she views nurses as "miracle workers" who are all-knowing and all-caring in their mission. During her initial encounters she may feel fearful, anxious, and inadequate, and she may wonder how she will ever acquire the necessary knowledge. The student might devalue her ability and feel that she is imposing on her clients. Both her expectations and abilities should be analyzed to raise her self-esteem and reinforce her capabilities. At another time she may identify closely with the client and feel anger at the impersonal system and unresponsive personnel. The student may feel the need to quickly master many technical skills and react with impatience and hostility at a learning program

that is structured to develop her expertise in a more thoughtful and progressive way. Her anger should be identified, verbalized, and accepted. Only then can she analyze how she expresses anger and how she can resolve her feelings in a constructive manner.

It is not easy to embark on a career in nursing while still in adolescence, because as a nurse the student will be faced with many adult responsibilities. The care of infants, as well as adults, will be required. The student will be forced to face disease and death when most of her friends are focusing on youth, enjoyment, and the future. This might alienate her from some friends and trigger feelings of despair and self-doubt. Her feelings of loneliness and sadness should be shared, so that she can experience the benefit of an interpersonal relationship in working through her own needs.

The development of self-awareness by the nurse must be a self-initiated process. She is an active participant in analyzing her thoughts, communications, and relationships with others. Because it is difficult to be participant and observer at the same time, other ways of collecting data should be used. Tape recordings provide an opportunity for the student to review her communications and study them more closely. Videotapes give feedback regarding nonverbal messages, as well as tone and inflection. Maintaining a diary allows for the expression of feelings, the description of perceptions of the student's self-concept, and comments on the student's level of self-esteem.

This introspection should also be accompanied by self-disclosure. Sharing perceptions with others allows the nurse to gain new information and evolve new insights. The interaction with the analysis may be written in the form of a processed recording. This disciplines the nurse to look beyond the obvious and to take the time to explore her own feelings. Her instructor can review the recording with her and identify areas that the student overlooked or blocked. Throughout her growing process the student needs the support and guidance of her instructor. Together they can analyze the student's behavior; the student can then assess her own strengths and limitations. It is often helpful to share these experiences with a peer group. Because students are all in a similar situation they are able to empathize, criticize, and support each other as they learn, together, more about themselves.

Finally, the process of self-awareness is a painful one. It is not easy or pleasant to objectively examine one's self, particularly when what one finds conflicts with one's self-ideal, but like many painful experiences it presents a challenge: accept these limitations of the self, or change the behaviors that support them. Choices such as this are the catalysts for growth and stimulate new responses to the question "Who am I?"

DISCUSSION QUESTIONS

1. Discuss your perception of the meaning of "being a professional" in relation to nursing. What kind of behavior and attitude does the phrase imply? Is it evident in nursing practice today?

2. Use Piaget's theory of cognitive development to describe how a child's perception of his body changes from 3 to 13 years of age.

3. Consider your own body appearance. What aspects of it satisfy you most and least? What body parts are most important or valuable to you? What aspects of aging are of most concern to you?

4. Pregnancy results in many physical changes. Describe the influence these changes may have on a woman's body image.

5. Analyze the self-portraits painted by Vincent van Gogh in relation to his changing body image and self-perceptions throughout his lifetime.

6. Describe why a routine physical examination may be threatening to a 4-year-old child. How can it be modified to reduce the threat?

7. Breast self-examination should be a routine part of every woman's health care practices. Take an informal survey among your friends. How many of them regularly perform a breast self-examination? What reasons are given by those who don't?

8. Identify at least five of your own self-ideals. Evaluate these ideals on the following criteria. Are they clearly defined? Realistic? Based on your own expectation or that of others? How could they be modified to increase your self-esteem?

9. Nicknames have significant influence on one's self-concept. Discuss how the nicknames of people you know influence their views of self.

10. Select a peer and identify all the behaviors you can observe in relation to this person's level of self-esteem. Describe with a rationale the level of self-esteem you believe this person is experiencing. Validate your assessment.

11. Single-parent families are becoming more common in this country. What threats does this phenomenon pose to the growth and development of the selves of the children in these families? What measures could society implement to help prevent problems?

12. Select a client with whom you are working and compare this client's self-concept and self-ideal to determine the level of self-esteem. Validate your analysis. Identify possible ways to enhance his self-esteem.

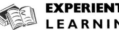 **EXPERIENTIAL & SIMULATED LEARNING EXERCISES**

1. Describing feelings 1

PURPOSE: To experience the sharing and mutual understanding of feelings.

PROCEDURE: Have the group form pairs. Have one member of the pair share his or her high and low experience of the week. The other person should then paraphrase these experiences and try to describe the feelings associated with them. Switch roles and repeat.

DISCUSSION: Ask the group members to reflect on the experience of talking about feelings. Was it difficult? Easy? Is it something that they do seldom? Frequently? Are there feelings that they have more difficulty expressing? What are they? Which feelings are most difficult to respond to? Why?

2. Describing feelings 2

PURPOSE: To share immediate feelings with peers.

PROCEDURE: Select a group of photographs that elicit an emotional response; for instance, pictures of the birth of a child, a handicapped person, or an elderly couple. Show a photograph to the group, then ask each student to share the feeling that the picture evokes.

DISCUSSION: One area of focus is the student's own experience in sharing feelings. Another is the differences in the feelings of different people in response to a single stimulus and the possible reasons for the differences.

3. Presentation of self

PURPOSE: To enhance self-awareness and communication skills.

PROCEDURES:

1. In the group ask all participants to line up on one side of the room in relation to each other on the basis of their:
   a. Physical attractiveness
   b. Intellectual capabilities
   c. Professional skills
   d. Self-confidence
2. Break the group into pairs. Have one member of each pair describe himself or herself to the other. The listening partner then introduces the member to the larger group. Switch roles and repeat.
3. Break the group into pairs. Have each partner take turns completing the following sentences:
   a. "In introducing myself, I would say . . . ."
   b. "If I could change one part of my body, it would be . . . ."
   c. "The most attractive part of my body is my . . . ."
4. Break the group into triads. One person talks, one listens, and one records. Each takes turns at each position. The task is to talk for 1 minute about yourself. After each person has spoken the discussion assignment is made.

DISCUSSION:

1. Describe the ease or discomfort felt in describing self.
2. Were some of the sentences relatively easy or difficult to complete? Why?
3. Which type of references were frequently used in describing self?
   a. Past, present, or future
   b. Negative or positive attributes
   c. Gross generalities, specific references
   d. Self/other references

4. Self-awareness 1

PURPOSE: To use the Johari Window for increased self-awareness.

PROCEDURE: Select one member of the group and ask another group member to list three positive and three negative aspects of that individual. Then have all of the members share their perceptions. Do this for all group members.

DISCUSSION: Ask the group to discuss how the quadrants of the Johari Window were changed for each individual participant. Students may also want an opportunity to share the feelings they experienced during the exercise.

5. Self-awareness 2

PURPOSE: To grow in awareness of self-concept and to gain feedback from others about their perception of oneself.

PROCEDURE: Ask the participant to imagine that there is a large body lying on the floor. Identify the location of the head and the feet. Then ask each member to stand at the location of the body part that he or she believes is more representative of his or her usual role (i.e., a person who sees himself or herself as a thinker might stand in the area of the brain). Each person should then explain the meaning of the chosen position. After all group members are located and have explained their choices, the group may discuss whether they agree with the placements or if they would like to move anyone based on their actual performance in the group.

DISCUSSION: The class should be encouraged to talk about the amount of congruence between self-perception and group perception. This may be related to the concept of the Johari Window. Members will need an opportunity to share the feelings evoked by the exercise and the applicability of the awareness gained to other life experiences.

REFERENCES

1. Bandura A: *Self-efficacy: the exercise of control* , New York, 1997, WH Freeman.
2. Branden N: *The psychology of self-esteem,* Los Angeles, 1969, Nash.
3. Coopersmith S: *The antecedents of self-esteem,* San Francisco, 1967, WH Freeman.
4. Fitts W et al: *The self-concept and self-actualization,* Research monograph 5, Nashville, Tenn, 1971, The Dede Wallace Center.
5. Goode W: Family disorganization. In Merton R, Nisbet R, editors: *Contemporary social problems,* New York, 1966, Harcourt Brace Jovanovich.
6. Hamachek D: *Encounters with the self,* ed 4, New York, 1991, Holt, Rinehart & Winston.
7. James H, editor: *The letters of William James, part II,* Boston, 1920, Atlantic Monthly Press.
8. Johnson B: Childrens drawings as a projective technique, *Pediatr Nurs* 16:1, 1990.

9. Jourard S: *Personal adjustment: an approach through the study of the healthy personality,* New York, 1963, Macmillan.
10. Jourard S: *The transparent self,* New York, 1971, Litton Educational.
11. Luft J: *Of human interaction,* Palo Alto, Calif, 1969, National Press Books.
12. Maslow A: *Motivation and personality,* New York, 1970, Harper & Row.
13. Mead M: *New lives for old,* New York, 1966, William Morrow.
14. Mruk C: *Self-esteem research, theory and practice,* New York, 1995, Springer.
15. Rogers C: *On becoming a person,* Boston, 1961, Houghton Mifflin.
16. Sheldon WP: *The varieties of human physique,* New York, 1970, Harper and Brothers.
17. Sheldon W: *The varieties of temperament,* New York, 1942, Harper and Brothers.
18. Thompson W: *Correlates of the self-concept,* Research monograph 6, Nashville, Tenn, 1972, The Dede Wallace Center.
19. Toman W: *Family constellation,* New York, 1969, Springer.

Suggested Readings

Bandura A: *Self-efficacy: the exercise of control,* New York, 1997, WH Freeman.

Important and inclusive text that explores how human actions are affected by people's beliefs in their abilities to produce desired effects by their efforts. Comprehensive review of the concept of self-efficacy with clinical applications and understandings.

Birren J, editor: *Handbook of mental health and aging,* San Diego, 1992, Academic Press.

Authoritative reviews of the scientific and professional literature on mental health and aging. Definitive reference work in the area.

Burnard P: *Learning human skills: an experiential guide for nurses,* Oxford, 1990, Heinemann Nursing.

Uses case studies and learning exercises to help nurses know themselves better and thus be of greater help to others. A most useful book for nurses who wish to expand their self-conception.

Cash T, Pruzinsky T: *Body images: development, deviance and change,* New York, 1990, Guilford Press.

This volume describes diverse concepts of body image, body-image development, deviations from normal appearance, and ways to facilitate body-image change.

Coopersmith S: *The antecedents of self-esteem,* San Francisco, 1967, WH Freeman.

Extensive and valuable research was conducted by this author into causative factors related to self-esteem. Some of the research studies are classics in the field and have applications for both primary and secondary prevention activities.

Gaylin W: *Feelings, our vital signs,* ed 4, 1991, New York, Harper & Row.

The author believes that feelings serve a purpose for us as warning signals that can help us move closer to our ideal. He analyzes such common feelings as anxiety, guilt, shame, and pride in a descriptive and enjoyable way.

Hamachek D: *Encounters with the self,* New York, 1971, Holt, Rinehart & Winston.

This book is about self-concept—how it grows, develops, changes, and expresses itself in behavior. The scope of the book is broad, and it is based on extensive research but written in a simple, explanatory manner. It is an excellent resource for learning about the self.

Johnson C: *Life beyond 85 years: the aura of survivorship,* New York, 1997, Springer.

Based on research, this text captures the insights, adaptations, competencies, and capacities people over age 85 need in order to manage their physical and social environments and sustain a sense of well-being.

Johnson J: *Mothers and their children,* London, 1994, Sage.

Presents a feminist sociology of child rearing that reveals the diversity of women's views and the cultural understandings and social context of contemporary Western child rearing.

Jourard S: *Personal adjustment, an approach through the study of healthy personality,* New York, 1963, Macmillan.

This classic text describes healthy personality or positive mental health. It is organized into two major sections. The first eight chapters deal with the person; the last five chapters explore the human in relation to his fellow human.

Jourard S: *The transparent self,* New York, 1971, Litton Educational.

This book proposes that an individual can attain health if he gains courage to be himself with others and when he finds goals that have meaning for him. The concept of self-disclosure is developed, and three chapters are specifically addressed to nurses. This is highly recommended reading for students and practitioners.

Mruk C: *Self-esteem research, theory and practice,* New York, 1995, Springer.

Most inclusive resource on research, theory, and practice related to self-esteem. Synthesizes content and presents it in an understandable and useful way.

Satir V: *Peoplemaking,* Palo Alto, Calif, 1972, Science and Behavior Books.

According to the author, the family is the "factory" where human beings are made. This is a book written for families about family process. It analyzes self-worth, communication systems, and family rules in a most enjoyable way.

Strasen L: *The image of professional nursing,* Philadelphia, 1991, JB Lippincott.

This book outlines strategies that novice and experienced clinical nurses, nurse managers, and nurse executives can implement to enhance their self-image and performance.

4 *The Communication Process*

I wanted to hear you, understand you.
I tried to be there to listen to your words.
I tried to understand what you were not able to say,
But still we could not communicate.

Perhaps they are right, there is a generation gap
   that can not be crossed.
But I refuse to believe that you can not hear
   my most important message—
I care for you. I love you my child.

Ann Carmel

LEARNING OBJECTIVES

After studying this chapter, the student should be able to:

- Define communication.
- Compare and contrast the verbal and nonverbal communication levels.
- Identify congruent and incongruent communication.
- Identify the functional components of the communication processes.
- Recognize communication patterns used by self and others.
- Discuss negative and positive factors that influence the communication process.

For centuries human beings have been concerned with the topic of communication. Its importance in the maintenance of human contact is seen in the Old Testament story of the Tower of Babel. When the builders of the tower to the heavens were punished by being given different tongues, they separated according to their languages. Each group went off to a different land. The New Testament story of the Pentecost also alludes to the importance of communication. The disciples of Christ were given the "gift" of tongues so that people of all languages would be able to understand them. Hence, not being able to share one's thoughts and ideas is presented as a punishment, and being able to communicate with others is viewed as a gift.

In recent years businesses have recognized the influence of communication with prospective consumers and among their own employees. Workshops and seminars geared toward increasing the effectiveness of communication are popular. Colleges and universities now offer several courses in communication. Glancing through any school catalog will reveal numerous courses in any number of departments, from business administration and psychology to speech and drama, directed toward understanding the act of communicating.

Nursing has also shown an awareness of the significance of communication behaviors—behaviors that were for many years considered "natural." Clark[7] reviewed the literature related to communication skills in nursing. She found that although the importance of communication in nursing care is recognized and its value clearly demonstrated, analysis of clinical nurse-client interactions shows that interpersonal competence is still low. Hence the teaching of communication skills remains a priority in nursing education.

In this chapter communication is examined in relationship to the nursing process. Hence the anatomy and physiology of speech production, vision, hearing, touch, and feeling are not discussed, nor are mathematic theories (such as computer language) or linguistic theories examining the spoken language across cultures included. Rather, the approach is sociopsychologic. It is an analysis of group interactions—the group being primarily that of two people: the nurse and the client.

Examining communication from a sociopsychologic approach emphasizes that it is a dynamic, ongoing process. It is not static. It does not happen and end. It is constantly becoming. It is dynamic in that it is ever changing and ongoing throughout time.

Communication viewed this way is also a unique experience—unique because of two factors: the pattern organization of the individual; and the fourth dimension, time. *Pattern organization* refers to the individual qualities of each participant—no two people are the same. Patterns are characteristic ways that individuals respond to similar stimuli or situations. An example is the client who comes to the physician for each physical ailment he perceives. Every time he has an ache or pain or notices something that may be indicative of poor health, he appears at the physician's office. His response to the stimuli of pain or body change is to seek medical attention; this is one of his patterns. All individuals have characteristic ways of responding—each somewhat different from any other. These patterns are important in the process of communication.

The fourth dimension, *time,* also makes each communication that occurs different from any other. For years human beings have viewed the world as three-dimensional—having length, width, and depth. The nurse must also be aware of time, the dimension that was previously reserved for the world of science fiction. What happens now, at this moment, can never be recaptured. It is not the same as anything that has occurred previously, nor will it be repeated in the future. The individuality of the participants and the quality of the time dimension make communication a unique experience—something that cannot be duplicated.

How, then, does one study something that is constantly changing? How does one grasp the meaning of what is being said, or share some of oneself with another? The answer is that one will probably never know exactly what another person is thinking or be able to share with another exactly what one thinks, because the system of communication relies on words and body expressions. However, an important first step is to be able to read our own thoughts and feelings, to be in touch with ourselves, and to know what we want to express. Chapters 2 and 3 were devoted to the development of this self that one seeks

to know; Chapter 12 follows a student nurse through a relationship with a client. In this relationship the student hopes not only to learn about another person but also to get to know herself better—to develop self-awareness. The student tries to become aware of her own pattern organization and how it influences that of another in the fourth dimension.

COMMUNICATION DEFINED

The definition of communication is integrally related to the purpose of communication; both definition and purpose vary among sources. *Webster's New Third International Dictionary* defines communication as "the act or action of imparting or transmitting." In this definition the conveyance of information is the primary purpose of communication.

Ruesch and Bateson[27a] define communication as "all of the procedures by which one mind may affect another." The procedures include not only verbal messages but all human behavior, including the arts. Their definition of communication implies a purpose of influencing the behavior or ideas of another.

Other theorists stress the social or interpersonal aspects of communication rather than its message transmission function. Satir[29] has limited communication to "nonverbal as well as verbal behavior within a social context."

From the definitions presented, the function of communication is seen either as primarily the means of transferring information or as a fundamental component of a relationship. Both of these functions are relevant in a discussion of the nurse-client relationship. However, when communication is defined as primarily a means of information transfer, the scope of the communication process appears more limited. In certain circumstances (such as health education, which will be discussed later in this chapter), this definition is more accurate in describing the nurse-client relationship.

In addition, the dynamic, ongoing process of communication can be viewed as the vehicle for establishing a relationship. Not only is communication involved in conveying information and influencing another throughout a relationship, communication *is* the relationship. When one examines the interaction occurring between individuals or groups, one is examining communication, the verbal and nonverbal messages between or among participants. If there is no communication, there cannot be a relationship. Therefore communication is not only the behavioral manifestation of an abstract concept ("relationship"), it *is* the relationship.

LEVELS OF COMMUNICATION

Verbal level

Basically, one communicates on two levels: the verbal and the nonverbal. The *verbal level* is associated with the spoken word. It primarily involves the physiologic and cognitive mechanisms required for speech production and reception. Although the verbal level is most commonly associated with the term *communication,* it represents only a small segment of total human communication.

Development of verbal level How an individual learns to share thoughts and ideas with others, or how a child learns the art of language, is a prime question for researchers in multiple areas, for example, semantics, syntax development, and phonology. All of these areas are concerned with the processes involved in the individual's growth from a crying neonate to a verbally competent adult.

Although historically language development has been an area of interest, research before the eighteenth and nineteenth centuries was scarce. According to Riley's historical summary, the Egyptian pharaohs were the first to investigate the origins of language.[24] Riley divided early theorists into three groups: (1) human verbal learning, (2) innateness, and (3) learning theory.

The human verbal learning group started with the research of Ebbinghaus, who studied the learning of consonant-vowel-consonant nonsense words in adults. The child was seen as a miniature adult, and the vague and meaningless nonsense words for adult learners were equated with the child's learning of meaningless words. This learning of nonsense words is essentially serial learning and free-recall learning. It is the development of word associations rather than language. The learning of nonsense words applies to the learning of language only in terms of learning a series of natural instructions or the lines in a play or a speech. Current research in this area deals with paired-association learning. In this style of learning the subject is given a word and expected to associate a word to

this given word. The multiple presentations of lists of paired words shows that the responses are first learned and then hooked to the stimulus or given words.

Riley[24] termed the second group of research as *innateness.* It is represented by the work of the early psychologist Wilhelm Wundt, who was interested in how language was used to describe sensory experiences. Chomsky's 1957 syntactic structures combined linguistics with the basic assumptions of Wundt. Linguistics as outlined by Chomsky provides a detailed set of rules to determine if a sentence is grammatic or not, and these rules describe all aspects of language. Recent research offers some support for an innate readiness to communicate. Wood[36] reviewed research in the area of nonverbal language development and verbal language development; she concluded that children are programmed for speech in the following ways:

1. Infants are able to distinguish speech from other sounds.
2. Infants are able to produce speech when the vocal mechanisms mature.
3. Biologic factors help explain the emergence and development of nonverbal language.

The third language research group identified by Riley[24] was the learning theory/conditioning camp. Initial work was based on the research of Pavlov and continued with Skinner's operant conditioning. According to this theory a child is reinforced for using grammatic rules. When a child has prerequisite skills and the environment is ready to reinforce, language learning occurs.

The French psychologist Jean Piaget's developmental theory includes qualitative cognitive changes that occur with age.[21] The thought processes and cognitive abilities of the 2-year-old are different from those of the 16-year-old. In addition, Piaget's developmental theory accepts and incorporates the behavioral conditioning theories throughout the developmental sequence and the importance of the environment in learning language. Piaget's theory questions the sufficiency of the behavioral theory in explaining language development.

Piaget contends that verbal communication begins during infancy with the child's imitation of a model. The infant is not able to differentiate the sounds of the model from those produced by the self; rather "the infant tends to repeat the activity (believed to be his own) which has already been set in motion; that is, the infant carries on the activity of making sounds in general" [p. 40].[12] Later, the infant is able to combine the visual cue of the model's lips moving with the cue of his own lips moving in imitation.

Research conducted by Trevarthen[33] examines videotaped interactions of mother-infant pairs. One conclusion drawn from the tapes is that a complex form of mutual understanding develops between the mother and infant from 2 to 3 months of age. This interaction is regulated by the infant. The mother adapts to the infant, with each mother-infant pair developing a unique communication style. The mother's behaviors are seen as subordinate to the actions of the infant, and there is a close imitation of the baby by the mother. According to Piaget, toward the end of infancy the child has the capacity to mentally represent and imitate the model without the model's physical presence.[12] However, words used at this time do not symbolically represent an absent person, place, or thing; rather, they are concretely related to objects present in the environment, the actions of the child, or both. Word meanings are flexible and personalized by the child. By 2 years of age the child uses words symbolically; however, these meanings are still personalized.

Piaget's work with children between the ages of 4 and 11 shows that the preschool child's language is primarily egocentric and noncommunicative. "He talks either for himself or for the pleasure of associating anyone who happens to be there with the activity of the moment."[21] The child's communication lacks the purpose, appropriate to adult communication, of influencing the listener.

There are three categories of egocentric speech: repetition, monologue, and collective monologue. The following interaction between two 4-year-olds in a nursery school setting is an example of the repetitive form of noncommunicative speech:

ABE: I'm using a blue crayon. (The crayon is green.)
LES: I'm using a blue crayon. (The crayon is purple.)
ABE: I'm using a blue crayon.
LES: I'm using a blue crayon.

In this interaction the purpose of Abe and Les' statements is not to convey a message to one another;

rather, pleasure is obtained from the act of repeating the words.

The monologue form is similar to a Shakespearean soliloquy. It is as though the child were thinking aloud; there is no listener. The collective monologue is "the most social of the egocentric varieties of child language, since to the pleasure of talking it adds that of soliloquizing before others and of interesting, or thinking to interest them, in one's own action and one's own thoughts."[21] It is the most common of the egocentric language types. Although the child is still not speaking to anyone, there is an awareness of the presence of others. The following example illustrates the collective monologue, with its beginning social awareness, among 4-year-old children in a nursery school:

REE: (Looking at a book of baby farm animals: Mau and Mug are also looking at books.) A dog. (She turns the page.) I have a horse. It's a big horse. Chap has a horse. I want to see a real horse. (She turns the page.) Here's another horse. (She is looking at a lamb. She turns back to the first picture of a horse.) Here's another horse. (Mug and Mau continue to look at their own books and talk about what they are seeing.)

In this interaction, again, the purpose is not related to the transfer of information but to the pleasure of talking. However, Ree is aware of Mau and Mug's presence and speaks as though they were listening.

In the school-age child there is a gradual diminishing of egocentric speech and a corresponding increase in communicative speech. In socialized language there is a true exchange of thoughts with others. Questions, answers, and commands are some examples of socialized speech.[21]

Piaget's last stage of development is adolescence. By this stage, most noncommunicative speech has been abandoned and language has taken on the socialized forms of the adult, demonstrating the adolescent's ability to reason. Table 4-1 summarizes Piaget's work on early language development.

Limitations of verbal communication Even though a person has progressed to the use of socialized communicative speech and desires to influence another or to enter into a relationship with another, these learned skills and rational purposes do not guarantee a successful interaction. Some of the prob-

TABLE 4-1   Summary of Piaget's work on early language development

DEVELOPMENTAL STAGE	LANGUAGE DEVELOPMENT
Infancy (birth to 2 years)	Early infancy: imitation of model, unable to differentiate model sounds from those made by the self Late infancy: mental representation and imitation of a model without model's presence, personalized meaning of words concretely related to objects physically present in environment.
Toddler years (2 to 4 years)	Symbolic use of words with personalized meanings
Early childhood (4 to 7 years)	Egocentric, noncommunicative speech dominates; three types discussed: repetition, monologue, and collective monologue
Middle childhood (7 to 11 years)	Increased communicative, socialized language; corresponding decrease in egocentric speech
Adolescence (11 to 15 years)	Socialized adult communication

lems arise from the fact that within a particular language, there are numerous dialects and subdialects confusing the meaning of words. An example in the American version of the English language is the word *dynamite*. Dynamite to one group is an explosive, whereas to another it is an exclamatory word denoting interest, enthusiasm, and approval—a vague superlative. Therefore the relatively simple English sentence "That is dynamite!" has a variety of meanings. There are at least two expressed meanings: one is a simple statement naming a substance present, and the other is a more vague statement regarding the expression of an above-average thought or idea. In addition to the two meanings directly expressed by these three words, there are also a number of indirect or unexpressed messages, such as "be careful, this is dangerous," or "I want to hear more," "I'm listening," and "I approve." The possibilities are infinite.

Not only do word meanings change with cultural groups, within very similar subgroups there is often a discrepancy in the meaning of words. The denotative meaning of a word refers to some concrete description of the word; for example, the word *dog* can be defined as "any of a large group of domesticated animals related to the fox, wolf, and jackal [Webster]." However, for each denotative meaning there is a connotative meaning—a personalized meaning. The connotative meaning of "dog" to one person may be a large, furry, loving pet, whereas to another it may be a ferocious, dangerous animal. Although "dog" brings a relatively similar picture to

mind—that of a four-legged, hair-covered animal—the personalized or connotative meaning varies with past experience, present frame of reference, and other internal variables.

Even within the nursing profession words do not always have the same meaning. Burnard[6] examined the communication between nursing students and nurse educators in an experiential learning setting to develop interpersonal skills. He identified two language styles. The instructors used a language style based on humanistic psychology; it involved the use of words such as *self* and *knowledge* without adequate definitions, resulting in a communication breakdown. In contrast, students used a restricted code with a dependence on the use of personal accounts. Burnard contends that a language and values barrier exists between the students and the teachers. Both have different views regarding the purpose of the experiential learning and even the educational process. These differences are reflected in their communication. This study points out the importance of nurses in supervisory positions modeling appropriate communication skills. Additional information about the acquisition of therapeutic communication skills is presented in Chapter 5.

Usually throughout verbal exchanges participants assume, often erroneously, that words mean the same thing to all people. Because words are only symbols, they can never be the same as the specific dog, mother, or so on to which the speaker is referring. The problem intensifies as the words become more abstract. A consensus of denotative and connotative meanings for *statue* is easier to reach than is a shared meaning for a more abstract word such as *aesthetic.*

In addition, there are many parts of life that cannot be put into words, such as the sorrow felt at the death of a loved one or the sympathy felt when someone dear is in pain. This does not mean that the nurse should discard verbal communication as uncertain and therefore irrelevant. Rather, she should be aware of the denotative and connotative meanings of words and attempt to clarify with clients the meaning of their words. Clarification as a specific therapeutic communication technique will be discussed later.

Nonverbal level

The majority of communication occurs on the *nonverbal level.* Nonverbal communication includes all forms of communication that do not involve the spoken word. Perception of nonverbal communication involves all of the senses, including hearing, used on the verbal level.

The processes that underlie nonverbal communication are the same as those that underlie verbal communication. Like verbal communication, gestures and body language vary according to time, place, and social economic status. Gestures convey symbolic meaning, and some are part of a given language. Finally, there are regularities in nonverbal communication that resemble the syntactic rules of verbal communication.

Feyereisen and de Lannoy[9] outline the underlying assumptions of nonverbal communication. According to these authors, language and nonverbal communication serve different functions, with emotions and interpersonal attitudes being primarily expressed by nonverbal communication. In addition, nonverbal communication allows the individual to establish, develop, and maintain a social relationship. Argyle[1] delineates additional functions of nonverbal communication, including self-presentation, rituals, and accompaniment and support of verbal communication. According to Argyle, affiliation or liking is expressed primarily through nonverbal communication. This positive expression of affiliation is an important social skill, and individuals rated as socially unskilled are found to look, smile, and gesture less than do other people. Smiling is one of the main reinforcers given by one person to another. It is not only a powerful source of interpersonal rewards but is also an indicator of positive feelings. Self-presentation is mainly achieved by appearance and, to a lesser extent, by voice. Rituals include greetings and other nonverbal communication. The nonverbal communication that accompanies and supports speech involves an intricate coordination of pausing and looking, followed by head nods, smiles, and gazes. These nonverbal communications are highly synchronized with speech and are described by Argyle as a "gestural dance." Pauses are part of the nonverbal communication accompanying speech and function as planning time for verbal communication. If a speaker is punished for pausing in a laboratory experimental setting, the result will be decreased pause length but a significantly higher number of verbal repetitions. Gaze is intermittent, usually approximately 3 seconds in duration, and is used at the end of utterances to obtain information from the listener regarding their reaction to what was said.

Rime and Schiaratura[25] stress that gestures accompanying speech emerge from the speaker's attempt to communicate. Essentially, the speaker is trying to relate verbally the sensory and motor parts of an experience or external object. When speakers are not seen by listeners, there is no decrease in body movement. When speakers' movements are restricted in experimental laboratory settings, there is a decrease in the vividness and imagery in their speech. Thus Rime and Schiaratura conclude that gestures help speakers express their thoughts; the box below outlines the multiple functions of nonverbal communication.

Functions of Nonverbal Communication
....

Nonverbal communication has multiple purposes, including:
- The expression of emotion
- The expression of interpersonal attitudes
- The establishment, development, and maintenance of social relationships
- Self-presentation
- Rituals
- Support of verbal communication

Types of nonverbal communication Ruesch and Kees[28] divide nonverbal communication into three types: sign, action, and object. Sign nonverbal communication includes all gestures from the simple "peace sign," with the index and middle finger raised, to the complex system of sign language used by the hearing impaired. Sign nonverbal communication primarily involves the sense of sight. According to the Roman orator, Cicero, gestures represented a former, "natural" state of language. The early psychologist Wundt believed that gestures primarily expressed emotions. Research has indicated that quality of emotion is expressed by facial movement while body cues relate the intensity of emotion.[9]

Action nonverbal communication involves all body movements that are not specific signals (i.e., running and dancing). The senses used to perceive action language are sight, hearing, and touch.

Object nonverbal communication incorporates "all intentional and nonintentional display of material things."[28] Included in object nonverbal communication are furnishings and their physical arrangement, clothing and other physical adornments, and the written word. All of the senses, including smell and taste, are involved in perceiving object nonverbal communication. Figures 4-1, 4-2, and 4-3 are examples of these three types of nonverbal communication.

Nonverbal communication develops on two levels: the conscious and the unconscious, or the voluntary versus the spontaneous. The facial nerve goes to both the hypothalamus and the motor cortex in the brain. The cortical motor system specializes in learned, willfully induced facial behaviors but not emotional facial behaviors. The hypothalamus reflects the innate emotions; the cortex reflects social learning and cultural history. Experiments with clients who have cortical lesions show that they smile normally when something strikes them as funny (spontaneous or innate reaction); in contrast, clients with subcortical lesions can smile on command but are not able to smile spontaneously.[9]

Development of nonverbal communication How an individual learns to use the body, clothing, and so on to communicate nonverbally depends on

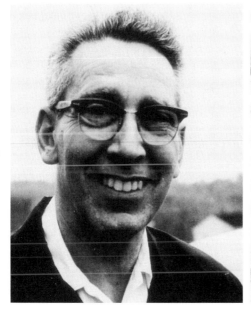
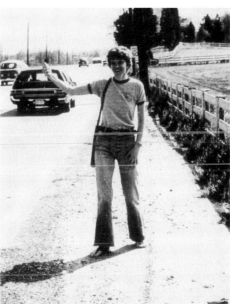

Fig. 4-1 Sign nonverbal communication. **A,** The smile is used to replace the words. The message is "Hello." **B,** The raised thumb of the hitchhiker sends the message "I would like a ride."

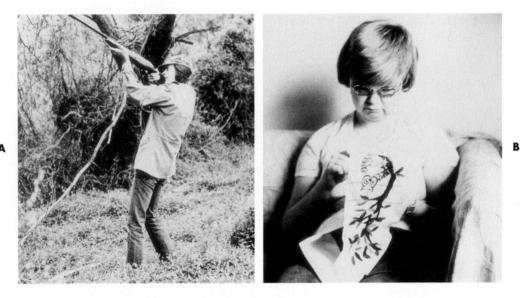

Fig. 4-2 Action nonverbal communication. **A,** The boy is shooting a shotgun for the purpose of obtaining food. At the same time he is giving nonverbal messages. "I am a hunter" is one. **B,** The act of doing needlework communicates a message, and the needlework itself is an example of object nonverbal communication.

the influence of three main factors: imitation, culture, and pattern organization. In Piaget's theory of language development, imitation is the first mode used by the infant to facilitate language formation. Imitation also plays an important role in the development of nonverbal communication. The child's imitation of the parents expands into imitation of various significant others, such as teachers, television heroes, and peers. A basic example is the preschool child who puts on the mother's makeup and jewelry, thus communicating the nonverbal message "I am grown up." Another common example is adolescent drug abusers whose use of drugs is an imitation of members of their peer group. The nonverbal message is "Chemicals make you part of the group."

Nonverbal communication is also acquired from the particular culture of the individual. Culture includes the individual's socioeconomic group, educational background, and geographic area, as well as ethnic and racial heritage. Among various cultural groups there are marked differences in the meaning of similar nonverbal messages. For example, a man and woman greet and kiss each other on the cheek. What are possible meanings for this behavior? How would the cultural background of the participants influence the nonverbal message?

Wilkens[34] reviews the nursing literature on transcultural nursing and cautions against the danger of cultural stereotyping. The differences within a culture are often as great as or greater than the differences between cultures. In trying to be culture specific, it is possible to forget the uniqueness of the individual. Culley[8] also cautions that an ethnic group is not an absolute category. It is important not to form ethnic stereotypes and to remember that ethnic groups are stratified by gender, education, occupation, and social economic status. According to both authors, nurses must be aware of cultural differences and be culturally sensitive. Nurses should seek out information about the cultural groups with whom they have regular contact. Reimer, Brink, and Saunders[23] recommend that nurses complete a cultural assessment to help understand the meaning of the client's communication.

Argyle[1] contends that cultural differences in nonverbal communication are a major source of friction, misunderstanding, and annoyance. Argyle states that there are even cultural differences in "dis-

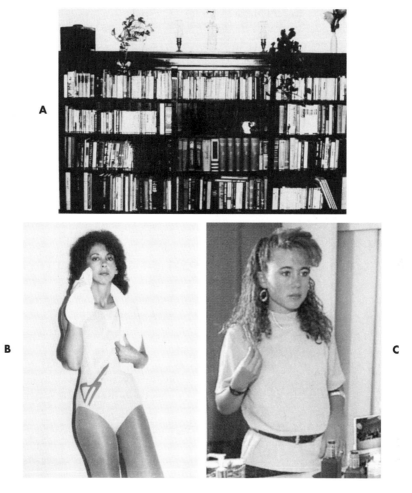

Fig. 4-3 Object nonverbal communication. **A,** How people furnish their homes, the books they read, and their use of plants and other small objects for decorations all give nonverbal messages about them. **B** and **C,** The clothes people wear, how they arrange their hair, and the perfume and jewelry worn give nonverbal messages to others. (**C** From Fortinash KM, Worret PA: *Psychiatric-mental health nursing,* St Louis, 1996, Mosby.)

play rules" or when an emotional expression should be shown. For example, the Japanese have a display rule that negative emotions should not be shown.

Cultural variations in gestures linked with speech have been studied.[1] In a comparison of Yiddish versus Italian immigrants in New York City, it was found that Yiddish gestures involved fine hand movements and marked out the direction of thought. The Italians gestured from the elbow, were expansive, and used many illustrative gestures. Level of gaze also varied among cultures. Arabs, Latin Americans, and Southern Europeans (individuals from a high-physical-contact countries) looked at their listeners more than did individuals from low-physical-contact countries. In the United States blacks looked at their listener less than did whites both while speaking and listening.

Rothenburger[26] presents an excellent case for considering cultural variations in interpreting the meaning of another's communication. According to Rothenburger, one of the erroneous beliefs in health care that hinders the therapeutic nurse-client interaction is the assumption that Western medicine is omniscient and omnipotent. In Japanese culture the physician is viewed as a skilled and sympathetic technician whose job is to help with the cure; responsibility for curing rests with clients and their families. Native Americans believe that humans live in harmony with nature and that technical medicine is not part of this harmony.

Duldt, Griffin, and Patton[8a] discuss an individual's use of space as a reflection of his culture. According to these authors, Americans typically surround themselves with 2 to 3 feet of personal space, an area that others must gain permission to enter. In contrast, Germans need a much larger area; their "privacy has been intruded upon if you can see inside the room."[8a] The English may never have a personal space of their own: children share nurseries, businesspeople share offices. To be alone the English do not need to go into their own room, but only to stop talking. Mediterranean cultures like the French eat, live, and breathe in crowds. Their homes are crowded. The cafés in which they socialize are crowded. To communicate they sit or stand close together and periodically touch the person with whom they are talking.

Another cultural group discussed by Duldt, Griffin, and Patton are the Arabic groups of the Near East. In private Arab homes there are open spaces, high ceilings, and minimal furnishings. In contrast, public areas are crowded, and it is acceptable to push, shove, and intrude on another's personal space. When speaking to another, it is acceptable to be close enough to smell the other person and to breathe on each other.

The Japanese culture is the last group discussed by these authors. To the Japanese, close physical contact is associated with family warmth, similar to that shared by an American family sitting around a fire. In Japan relationships are important in their use of physical space. To illustrate this point houses are not numbered on a block sequentially but in the order in which they were built. Awareness of cultural variations can help the nurse understand the message of the client and to deliver the intended message to the client.

Being aware of the significant others and the particular culture of an individual, however, does not guarantee shared meaning in nonverbal communication. The third factor that must be considered is individual pattern organization. Although the men in Fig. 4-4 belong to the same culture and family

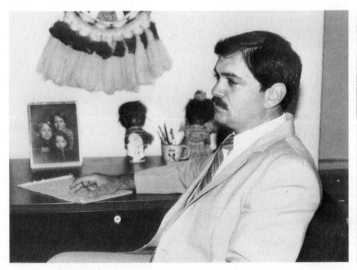
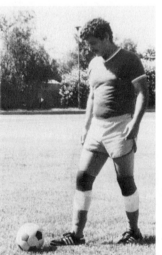

A

B

Fig. 4-4 Although both men have the same cultural influences and have significant others, their pattern organization is demonstrated in their varied object nonverbal communication. The individual's pattern organization influences the choice of clothing, posture, and other nonverbal messages.

background, their object nonverbals communicate very different messages.

One individual difference is personality, and personality is related to nonverbal communication in the literature. Individuals with a high need for relationships or who want to be approached socially often demonstrate the following nonverbal behaviors: longer gazes, increased physical proximity to others, more smiling, louder voices, higher pitch to the voice, and more talking. The nonverbal behaviors of anxious individuals compared with relaxed individuals is not as clear, according to Argyle.[1] Dominance in nonverbal communication is demonstrated by variation in speech and vocal style, as well as in gaze pattern. Dominant individuals tend to speak louder and faster and have fewer pauses. In general, they display a higher level of energy. Their gaze pattern involves more looking while talking, less smiling, and a greater physical distance between the speaker and the listener. The dominant individual generally also has a relaxed posture.

Argyle outlines several gender differences in nonverbal communication as well. Females tend to smile more while they speak, approach closer to their listener, look at their listeners more, are more expressive, and have higher judgment accuracy, especially in identifying the meaning of facial expressions. Males communicate with a louder voice and lower pitch, and their gestures are more expansive and more restless. Males also touch females more when outdoors, but this difference is related primarily to status differences.

Giving meaning to nonverbal communication

To determine the meaning of nonverbal messages it is necessary to examine the development of the individual's nonverbal communication. This includes the role models of the individual; family, peers, and significant others in past relationships; the culture of the individual; and the individual's traits, characteristics, and manifestations of self, or pattern organization. The reverse is also true. To deliver the desired message it is necessary to be aware of one's own nonverbal messages—how these three factors (imitation, culture, and pattern organization) influence behaviors in the message being sent and affect the perception of that message.

The following clinical situations are used to clarify the interrelationships among these three factors:

Ms. G. is a 35-year-old woman of English descent who comes to the medical clinic complaining of chest pain. During the initial interview Ms. G. begins to cry and sob hysterically. She pulls at a handkerchief she is holding and tells the nurse that she "can't live like this anymore." In assessing the meaning of Ms. G's nonverbal communication, the nurse relies on data previously collected. She knows that Ms. G's mother overreacts to situations and that Ms. G. has demonstrated an inability to cope with stress in the past. Although a strong display of emotions is not characteristic of her cultural group, a significant role model and the personality of the client are conducive to such behavior. What does this nonverbal communication mean? In this case Ms. G. wants someone to listen; she wants an opportunity to ventilate her feelings of frustration and inadequacy in meeting the situation.

Another client, Ms. P., with the same cultural background and with similar role models, characteristically appears calm and intellectual in stress situations. Her statement of "I can't live like this anymore," accompanied by tearful eyes, wringing hands, and clenched teeth, delivers a different message. In this situation Ms. P. is asking for help in controlling her own behavior and in meeting the stress. She is contemplating suicide.

As with the verbal level of communication, there are numerous problems in interpreting the nonverbal messages of another. One of the most significant difficulties is encountered when attempting to attach verbal meanings to nonverbal messages. This is true because of the complexity of the body messages and the lack of concepts for decoding. Because the body does not rely on the projection of sound, its messages are more rapid. In addition, body language lacks the precision of the verbal level of communication and is probably more closely related to the messages delivered by music, drama, and the plastic arts than those of verbalizations.

Another significant difficulty in attaching meaning to nonverbal behaviors lies in the complex messages that the behaviors often emit. The face and body are used not only to express inner feelings and emotions but also interpersonal transactions, such as "I don't agree with you" and "Will you please explain that?"

The interpersonal aspect of nonverbal messages leads to another area of concern. It is often impossible to examine nonverbal messages out of context. Nonverbal communication is connected to the past and future, and it therefore is often distorted or meaningless when removed from the appropriate sequence. At times the body reveals a number of feelings simultaneously. Some are expressed so clearly that they help determine the context of the interaction; others can only be given meaning from the context of the situation.

The complexity of nonverbal messages poses a particular problem to researchers attempting to identify meanings for selected body movements. Identifying such meanings has often been done by showing subjects photographs of strangers. In reviewing a series of research studies on nonverbal communication, Meyers and Meyers[18] stated that using this "stranger" method makes it impossible to study the nuances of human interactions.

Spiegel and Machotka[31] support this view that the movements of the human body apart from human activities are meaningless gestures. The meaning attached to nonverbal behaviors is often largely of a subjective nature (based on one's own pattern organization); therefore validation of meaning must be obtained. However, validation presupposes that the senders of nonverbal messages are aware of how they are feeling.

In a series of studies Spiegel and Machotka[31] examined the meanings expressed by the position of the arms. They found that the more the body was covered by the arms, the more the subject was seen as rejecting. However, when the arms were open completely, the subject was seen as exhibitionistic and immodest rather than as completely open. Spiegel and Machotka propose that the nonverbal level of communication is more closely related to the pictorial arts than to the verbal level of communication. Hence their research was based on subjects' evaluation of classical art.

Nonverbal messages are an important aspect of nurse-client relationships. Not only must nurses be aware of the client's nonverbal messages and seek to validate their meaning, they must also have an awareness of their own nonverbal communication.

In general, the meaning of nonverbal communication is more universal than is that of the spoken word with its language variations. For example, a smile means "Something pleasant is being experienced," and the wringing of hands means "Something uncomfortable is happening." However, a specific message, with its ramifications and implications for the nurse-client relationship, is dependent on the individuals involved.

METACOMMUNICATION

In addition to defining or describing communication according to whether it occurs at the verbal or nonverbal level, one can also discuss communication in a third way, as *metacommunication*. Metacommunication occurs at both the verbal and nonverbal levels. It is essentially communication about communication. Satir[29] defined metacommunication as "a comment on the literal content as well as on the nature of the relationship between the persons involved." It conveys the sender's attitude toward himself, the message, and the listener. Therefore there are two parts to all communication: the literal message (what is being said) and instructions on how to interpret or decode what is being said.[29] Verbal metacommunication can be a simple, precise statement on how to decode a message, such as "I meant that," "That was an order," or "I was only joking." Nonverbal metacommunication is usually more implied. For example, when a client says "And then my mother died," the smile disappears from the client's face and tears come to the eyes. The nonverbal metacommunication is "This sorrows me."

Metacommunication can also tell the listener how an individual processed through three representational systems: auditory, visual, or kinesthetic. An individual will usually use some combination of the three but with a definite preference for one mode of processing. Neurolinguistic programming, derived from linguistics and psychiatry, helps the nurse determine the client's favored representational system. Neurolinguistic programming evaluates the client's body position, preferred verb forms, and breathing. Knowles[15] believes that when the nurse uses the same representational system as the client, communication is facilitated. One way to determine the representational system being used is by the client's choice of verbs. Some verbs are auditory, such as *listen, hear, attend,* and *gripe;* others are kinesthetic, such as *feel, arouse, excite, itch, creep,* and *shudder;* and still others are visual, such as *see, observe,* and *behold.* Another neurolinguistic programming technique to determine the client's favored representational mode is using eye-accessing cues.[15] Eye movements of looking up are associated with the visual mode. The auditory mode is associated with looking from side to side or down at the nondominant hand. Individuals who process information through the kinesthetic mode look down at the dominant hand primarily.

Breathing patterns are also associated with different modes of information processing. Abdominal breathing is reflective of a kinesthetic mode, shallow thoracic breathing with the visual mode, and even breathing or prolonged expirations with the auditory mode. Knowles[15] suggests that the nurse should identify the pattern most commonly used by herself and practice mirroring others who use different modes of information processing. She suggests starting by imitating the breathing pattern of another and gradually trying to match other behaviors, not by using identical behaviors but rather by using behaviors from the same mode.

Table 4-2 summarizes various ways the nurse can determine the primary representational system being used by the client and gives examples of nursing statements that would be appropriate to that channel or representational system.

CONGRUENT COMMUNICATION

A basic principle of communication is that the verbal and nonverbal levels, the literal content and the metacommunication, all should be saying essentially the same thing. If they are, the communication is termed *congruent.* However, if the client is sitting in a corner of the room with eyes downcast and replies to the nurse's question "How are things today?" without eye contact by saying, "Great" in a flat tone with a depressed affect, the communication is termed *incongruent.* The nurse is receiving two different messages. The verbal level and literal content are saying, "I am fine," while the nonverbal and metacommunication are saying, "I am miserable."

The box on p. 94 provides another example of incongruent communication. In this interaction the client's message on the verbal level is "I'll allow you

TABLE 4-2 **Ways to determine primary representational system being used by client and nursing-related statements appropriate to that channel**

AREAS OF OBSERVATION	REPRESENTATIONAL SYSTEM		
	AUDITORY	VISUAL	KINESTHETIC
Breathing patterns	Even breathing or prolonged respirations	Shallow thoracic breathing	Abdominal breathing
Eye movements	Side-to-side or down at nondominant hand	Upward	Down at dominant hand
Language usage			
Use of verbs	Listen, hear	See, behold	Feel, arouse
Other terms	Noise words: blast, roar	Television, chart, design, map, graph	Touch, anger, joy, smooth, soft, rough
Slang expressions	Speak your mind, sounding board, tell him off	I see what you mean, I read your mind, show off	It's hard to tell, between a rock and a hard place
Nursing statements appropriate to representational system	Tell me more . . . I hear . . . I'd like to speak to you about How would you say you feel?	Show me where the pain is. What seems to be the problem? I see what you're saying.	Where do you feel the pain is? I am not in touch with your meaning. How are you feeling?

Example of Incongruent Communication

....

NURSE: Hello, Mr. S. Do you mind if I sit here and talk with you for a while? (Smiles and points to the chair next to Mr. S.)

VERBAL MESSAGE: I'd like to talk with you. Is this agreeable?
NONVERBAL MESSAGE: I'd like to talk with you.
METACOMMUNICATION, NONVERBAL: I am friendly and interested in you; I would like to sit in the chair next to you.

MR. S.: Yes, that is fine. I mean, I'd like that. (Doesn't look at the nurse; continues to look out the window, rocking in his chair. The nurse approaches Mr. S. and sits in the chair next to him.)

VERBAL MESSAGE: I'd like to talk with you also.
NONVERBAL MESSAGE: I'm really not interested.
METACOMMUNICATION, VERBAL: I meant what I said; it's okay to sit next to me.
METACOMMUNICATION, NONVERBAL: Stay away.

MR. S.: (His body stiffens.) What would you like to talk about?

VERBAL MESSAGE: You decide on a topic.
NONVERBAL MESSAGE: You frighten me. Go away.
METACOMMUNICATION, NONVERBAL: Go away.

---

to enter my personal space," but nonverbally the client is saying, "Stay away from me." Such incongruent or double-level messages produce a dilemma for the listener. To which level should the nurse respond? If the nurse responds to the verbal level, the client can become angry for the apparent insensitivity to his need for privacy. If the nurse responds to the nonverbal level, the client can refute by saying, "But I told you it's OK." There is no way to perform in two opposite ways at the same time; hence the nurse can feel frustrated, angry, or both by her inability to respond to the message. She is in a double-bind situation, "damned if she does and damned if she doesn't."

Research on the communication patterns of families has shown that the double-level message is often found in families of psychotic clients. What better method can one use to totally baffle, confuse, and freeze another into indecision? Whether the speaker is aware of the dual component of his message and its effects on others varies. In many cases the nonverbal level reveals the unconscious, or conscious but unacceptable, "true" message. The approach the nurse uses to decipher the message depends on the relationship formed with the client. In the beginning phases of a relationship it would probably be more effective for the nurse to reply to the nonverbal message; if the client questions the response, the nurse should explain that although the client told her to sit down next to him, the feeling she received was that he would be more comfortable if she did not. In later phases of the relationship the nurse could confront

the client with the dilemma. However, any approach used depends on the individuals involved and the particular circumstances surrounding the situation. For example, a client who constantly uses double-level messages demands a far different plan of care than a client who occasionally places the nurse in a double-bind situation.

Nurses must also be aware of the congruency of their own communication. For a nurse to walk around all day smiling and trying to act "interested in others" when in reality a friend was taken to the hospital the night before or the nurse's car was stolen during the night would hinder congruent communication. This is not to say that personal problems should become the topic of conversation with clients throughout the day, or that it is impossible to be interested in others if there is pain in one's personal life. Rather, one should be aware of internal feeling states and the resulting communication. A simple statement that "this is a bad day" may be sufficient for clients to know that the nonverbal messages of impatience or anger are not directly related to their behavior but are influenced by factors beyond their control. A further exploration of nurse and client feelings and how they affect communication is found in Chapter 12.

EXAMINATION OF THE COMMUNICATION PROCESS

As stated in the introduction of this chapter, communication is a dynamic, ongoing process. To examine this process and its functional components it is necessary to artificially punctuate or stop the process. Punctuating the process arbitrarily determines the beginning and ending of a particular interaction.

A (NURSE): Do you mean that your son has *never* come to visit you here?

B (CLIENT): No . . . not *never* never. He only comes on holidays, like Christmas and my birthday. Probably because he feels guilty.

A: He feels guilty?

In this interaction A sends a message to B: "Do you mean that your son has *never* come to visit you here?" B receives the message and returns a message to A: "No . . . not *never* never. He only comes on holidays. . . ." A receives the message and sends another message back to B: "He feels guilty?" However, all information before and after this interaction is excluded. In addition, not only is A sending the message "Do you mean that your son has *never* come to visit you here?" to B, at the same time A is receiving nonverbal messages from B. B may be shaking his head in agreement to what A is saying, may be smiling, or may be gazing out the window as if uninterested in A's message. Therefore B is not only receiving A's message, B is also sending a message to A. While A is receiving nonverbal messages from B, she is also sending a message. To identify A as the sender while A is stating the message "Do you mean that your son has *never* come to visit you here?" is to be incomplete, because A is also receiving messages at the same time; thus the process is dynamic and ongoing. It is also possible to punctuate the process and begin with B's message "No . . . not *never* never. He only comes on holidays. . . ." Starting this way arbitrarily identifies B as the sender and A as the receiver.

FUNCTIONAL COMPONENTS OF THE COMMUNICATION PROCESS

The communication process is made up of five functional components. The first is the *sender*. This includes not only the person sending the message but also the effector organs involved in sending the message. In the previous example A is using the anatomic structures necessary for speech and all the body parts involved in transmitting nonverbal communication. For instance, while saying the word

"never," A could slowly shake her head left and right or raise an eyebrow as if to question B.

The second component is the *message* itself—what is actually said and its corresponding nonverbal and metacommunication. The words used, the body language, and the tone, inflection, loudness, and pitch of the voice are all part of the message sent.

The third component is the *receiver* and all the anatomic structures necessary for receiving messages. All of the senses can be involved in receiving nonverbal messages.

The fourth component is the message B returns to A in response to A's message; this is termed *feedback*. In the example given, B is qualifying his connotative meaning of the word *never* with his feedback. "No . . . not *never* never. He only comes on holidays. . . ." This does not mean that only the receiver of the message can send feedback. While B is sending his feedback or message, he is also receiving feedback from A. A could be shaking her head in agreement or raising her eyebrows, indicating understanding of the qualification of the term *never,* or she could be twisting her brow, asking for additional qualification of the term. Also, both A and B are constantly receiving internal feedback from the self. A good example of internal feedback is silently reading a letter recently composed to see if it "sounds correct." Another example is a public-speaking situation in which the speaker realizes as soon as something is said that it wasn't exactly what was meant or how the speaker wanted to present the message. This realization comes from the utilization of internal feedback.

Internal feedback does not involve only the sense of hearing a message transmitted. A social error at a gathering may be realized when nausea, stiffness in the back of the neck, or some other internal feedback signals the enactment of a social blunder. A basic example of internal feedback is the busy professional who becomes involved in work past the normal lunch hour. The stomach does not forget lunch and begins to contract. The growling stomach is internal feedback—the system informing itself of a need, desire, anxiety, or so on. How aware the sender-receiver is of internal feedback influences the interpretations and responses that are evoked. If the busy professional does not "feel" the stomach contractions or associates the discomfort with an ulcer or some other gastrointestinal disturbance, this person may not respond to the system's need for food. Instead, he or she may complain of a vague pain, become angry and impatient with the secretary, call a physician for treatment, or make a note to bring antacids to work. This represents a failure to read, analyze, and use internal feedback appropriately.

The last functional component of the communication process is *context* —the setting in which the interaction occurs. Context is one of the most important factors involved in determining the meaning of an interaction, because it involves the fourth dimension (time) and pattern organization. Because the present moment is completely unique, it can never repeat the past or be recaptured in the future. The pattern organization of the participants adds to the uniqueness of the interaction. A performance of Shakespeare's *Antony and Cleopatra* today could never be the same as when the first Cleopatra said, "As well a woman with a eunuch play'd / As with a woman.— Come, you'll play with me, sir?" [Act II, Scene 4]. Pattern organization influences the actors playing sender and receiver, thus it influences their communication.

ADDITIONAL PROCESSES NECESSARY FOR COMMUNICATION

The functional components—sender, message, receiver, feedback, and context—are necessary for communication to occur. Figure 4-5 shows the relationship between these components. In addition, Ruesch[27] has outlined three processes needed for the sharing of information: perception, evaluation, and transmission.

Perception

Hamachek[13] has defined *perception* as "the process by which we select, organize, and interpret sensory stimulation into a meaningful and coherent picture of the world." He believes that an individual's needs, values, beliefs, and self-concept are vital factors in determining how an individual views his life space or surroundings.

Studies of hungry versus not-hungry grocery shoppers have demonstrated the influence of the basic biologic need for food on the purchaser's perception of desirable goods. Hunger, or the need for food at the time of buying, increases the value potential of food. Thus hungry grocery shoppers perceive themselves as needing more food.

Not only do an individual's basic needs for food, clothing, shelter, and love influence perceptions, a person's values and beliefs are also strong determining factors on how that person views his or her life space. For example, a person who values the acquisition of material goods above everything else may see a situation as perfectly legal, whereas another person with different values sees it as illegal.

Janzen[14] contends that an overt awareness of perceptual skills is necessary for a therapeutic interaction. According to Janzen, the screening and decoding of stimuli are perceptual skills that require an inductive thought process, from specifics to general, as opposed to a deductive process, which is usually taught in nursing. For example, a student is taught that if client A has "depression," then X, Y, and Z are normally present. The student looks for X, Y, and Z, often distorting

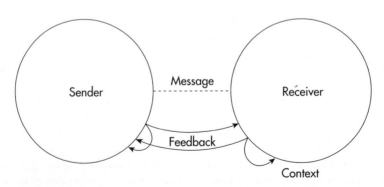

Fig. 4-5 Components of the communication process.

perceptual input to find what should be present. Janzen contends that the process of perception is just as important as or even more important than the outcome. The process of perception consists of selective attention to stimuli, organization of stimuli into categories, and perceiving relationships among the categories.

If a sender is to share information with a listener, the listener must perceive what the sender intended. This is a difficult task. The nurse can facilitate the communication process with clients by sharing perceptions, asking the client for feedback concerning perceptions, comparing perceptions, and reaching a common denominator.

For communication to occur, perception is necessary. Therefore any disorder that interferes with perception, such as blindness, deafness, amnesia, mental retardation, or psychosis, hinders the communication process.

Evaluation

Evaluation is the second process outlined by Ruesch. This involves the ability to analyze the information perceived. Many of the factors affecting perception also influence the evaluation process. Ruesch and Bateson[27a] have contended that:

A person may see and evaluate similar events in one way in one set of circumstances and in quite a different way in another set of circumstances; and the contrast of circumstances which determine such a change may be either internal (for example, a shift of mood) or external (that which is approved and valued in war may be regarded with horror in time of peace).[27a]

Transmission

Transmission is the third process needed for the sharing of information. It refers to the actual expression of information from the sender to the receiver. Theoretically there are numerous others to whom one is capable of sending information, thus an appropriate channel is needed for the message. For example, if a person wished to make his or her feelings regarding a foreign government's treatment of a particular situation known, the telephone could be an appropriate channel if both parties spoke the same language and had telephone connections. If a nurse wanted to inform a hospitalized client that diagnostic tests had been canceled, the intercom might be an appropriate channel if the client could hear. In many circumstances there are not channels, or the channels available are not adequate for message transmission.

PATTERNS OF COMMUNICATION

The concept of pattern organization is relevant not only to the study of our characteristic mode of behavioral response but also to the study of our characteristic mode of communication response, because communication is a form of behavior.

Relating pattern

Travelbee[32] has outlined a communication pattern that is essential for the fulfillment of nursing goals. Called *relating*, this pattern is:

An experience, or series of experiences, characterized by meaningful dialogue between two people . . . wherein each experiences openness, closeness, and understanding of the other. . . . Relating is characterized by purposeful, reciprocal communication. What is discussed is relevant, and appropriate.[32]

To use primarily the relating pattern, a nurse must have high self-esteem or a feeling of adequacy, competency, and trust in her ability to assist another. She must also have a knowledge of her areas of weakness, the ability to reveal those weaknesses when necessary, and recognition of resources available to compensate for the weaknesses. Because the relating pattern is reciprocal, both participants must be willing to share meaningful dialogue. A skilled nurse may be able to assist a client in using a relating pattern, but this is not always possible. Relating requires an awareness of the self, an awareness of another, and the ability to share. It is a goal, although it is not always attainable.

In an exploratory research study conducted by Ramos,[22] nurses were asked to describe their closest professional relationship. Ramos identified a pattern of relating that she labeled as level III bonds. Level III bonds were similar to the relating pattern of Travelbee. The nurses who described level III bonds "were professionally energized by having experienced them."[22] Nurses stated that in the presence of these bonds they believed that the best possible nursing care occurred. In a personal experience described by Mackay,[17] a similar type of relating pattern was described, creating a special sense of "connecting" to another person.

Peterson et al.[20] conducted research to identify the factors that determine supportive encounters between nurses and nurse administrators. They identified a pattern of communication that they named rhetorical design logic. This pattern of communication was similar to Travelbee's relating. To create supportive messages the speaker often redefined a situation and tried to promote the receiver's self-esteem. Messages attempted to create interpersonal harmony.

Defensive communication patterns

The relating pattern of communication occurs within a supportive environment in which the client can communicate freely. In contrast, other environments can produce defensive communication patterns that attempt to protect the individual from a perceived threat. Defensive communication requires an appreciable amount of energy and tends to produce defensive postures in the listener, thus it is a circular reaction. Communication that is primarily defensive tends to be inefficient and distorted. Gibb[11] outlined six behaviors that can produce defensive communication patterns: evaluative speech, controlling speech, strategic speech, neutrality in speech, superiority, and certainty.

Judgmental or accusing speech is termed *evaluative* and leads to defensive behavior by the listener. In contrast, nonjudgmental statements are labeled *descriptive communication* and help to promote a supportive environment in which relating can occur. *Controlling speech* tends to evoke resistance and produce defensive patterns; the implied message in all controlling behavior is that the listener is in some way inadequate. The opposite behavior is problem oriented, where the speaker tries to engage the listener in a mutual attempt to define and solve a problem. Such communication is permissive, allowing the clients to define and set their own goals.

Strategic speech produces defensive communication patterns. It is characterized by several indefinite motivations. Strategic speech includes deliberate assumptions of innocence and natural simplicity in

the listener. In actuality most listeners are able to pick up when someone is trying to use a "gimmick" on them, regardless of the end goal. In contrast, spontaneous behavior promotes a relating pattern. This is behavior in which the sender is seen as having an uncomplicated motivation rather than hidden goals.

Neutrality of speech indicates to the listener a lack of concern rather than a nonjudgmental attitude. It is characterized by speech with low affect and little caring or warmth. In contrast, empathic behavior facilitates a relating pattern of communication.

Whenever a speaker communicates a feeling of *superiority*, the listener may respond with a defensive communication pattern. The opposite behavior is equality, which characterizes the relating pattern. *Certainty* can also evoke a defensive communication pattern in the listener. To be able to relate, the nurse must demonstrate a degree of provisionalism, or a willingness to experiment with behavior, attitudes, and ideas. A person with provisionalism appears to be searching for information rather than debating issues. Most of the following communication patterns are reflective of some type of nonsupportive environment.

Satir[30] outlined four communication patterns that occur in reaction to stress and impending damage to one's self-esteem: placating, blaming, computing, and distracting. They are used to conceal a feeling of weakness—a weakness that one's self-esteem is vulnerable and may be decreased. All are double-level messages; therefore the verbal and nonverbal communications are incongruent.

The *placating pattern* is characterized by verbal agreement with any message received. The purpose is to prevent anger. Many of what hospital staff commonly refer to as "good patients" are really placaters. For example, Mr. I. always takes his medicine. If he is told to void, he does. If he is told to sleep, he does. If he is told he is cured, he is. The incongruency is that while the verbal is saying "Yes, I agree," the body is saying, "I am helpless and totally dependent on you. You are responsible for me. Take care of me."

The *blaming pattern* is the opposite of the placating one; the verbal communication disagrees with any message received. To prevent damage to his self-esteem, the blamer tries to establish himself as strong and invulnerable to attack. The characteristic "bad patient" in the hospital situation often uses this communication pattern. Mr. T. accuses the nurses of being lazy, the physicians of being greedy, and the technicians of being incompetent. By getting someone to obey his demands and orders, he attempts to increase his own self-worth. While the words say "You are wrong," the body communicates that the blamer is the boss even though feelings of loneliness and unworthiness are present.

The *computing pattern* attempts to protect the self by denying the presence of a threat and to prove self-worth by an onslaught of intellectual statements. A common example is the very "competent" physician or nurse who when asked a question by a client or colleague replies with a lengthy, theoretic dissertation on the subject that rarely answers the original question. In the computing pattern the verbal message consists of six-syllable words while the nonverbal message is "I'm very vulnerable."

The *distracting pattern* attempts to ignore threats to the self with irrelevant communication. The purpose is to ignore the threat long enough in the hope that it will disappear. For example, a nurse asks Mr. H. about his sexual relationships, and Mr. H. starts discussing the inflationary spiral, juvenile delinquency, and police corruption, then finishes with his own plan for world peace. The verbal message of the distractor is irrelevant to the sender; the nonverbal message is "No one cares" (Table 4-3).

Meyers[19] has reported that irrelevant or distracting communication by nurses increases the client's tension. It prohibits the client from "cognitively structuring" or giving meaning to the situation. In fact, not having verbal communication is more effective than having irrelevant communication.

Games as communication patterns

Another way to examine communication patterns is based on transactional analysis. Games are communication patterns that are designed to bring about relief from the "I'm not OK" position—a way to alleviate feelings of low self-esteem. Games represent a form of interaction for people who cannot tolerate withdrawal and at the same time are not able to maintain a mutual relationship without exploitation.[4]

Rather than attempt a review of transactional analysis, we will explore only one part of this theory—games. Games are characterized by their repetitive nature, ulterior motives or psychologic payoffs, and devious methods for attempting to increase self-esteem.[4] Berne has outlined an extensive list of games, which he has admitted is by no means inclusive. Probably one of the best known, and the one the nurse encounters most, is "Why Don't You . . . Yes, But" (WDYB).[3] This game involves one person asking another or a group for solutions to a problem; however, every solution presented is negated by this person until the helper(s) are silent. The aim is to obtain reassurance that "I'm not such a bad person. (I'm really OK.)" Instead of asking directly for the reassurance or stroke, the player of WDYB maneuvers the helper into a frustrated silence, thus demonstrating the player's one-upmanship. On the surface the interaction appears like two adults problem solving, but the player is in reality using his child to show what a bad parent the other is. Stated another way, the player tries to increase his own self-esteem by pointing out the frailties of another.

TABLE 4-3   Satir's defensive communication

PATTERN	BEHAVIOR	VERBAL MESSAGE	NONVERBAL MESSAGE
Placating	Agreement with any message	"I agree."	"I am helpless. You are responsible for me."
Blaming	Disagreement with any message	"You are wrong."	"I am the boss, but lonely and unworthy."
Computing	Intellectualization	Six-syllable words	"I am in control but not really."
Distracting	Irrelevant messages	Anything not related to previous messages	"No one cares."

Many of the client's recurrent behaviors or communication patterns can be analyzed in terms of a game. This framework is useful in identifying patterns, speculating probable causes for what is observed, and most important, planning alternative ways to respond and thus stopping the unhealthy games.

Interactional patterns

Still another approach is suggested by Bernal and Baker,[2] who examine couple communication in terms of five interactional patterns that progress from concrete to abstract. In level one communication patterns the focus is the issue. It may be finances, a vacation, in-laws, physical illness, or the like. Level two communication patterns are characterized by content regarding the individual, "often including mutual accusations and blaming." The actions of one member are considered as reactions to the behavior of the other member. "It's you or it's I" is the communication pattern of level two. This type of communication pattern is often found in couples who are experiencing marital difficulties. Level three communication patterns are described as transactional. The focus is on the actual pattern of relating. "It's you and I" is the communication pattern in level three. Level four communication patterns are termed *relational.* The concrete issue is no longer the focus, but rather what the issue says about the relationship. "It's us" is the communication pattern in level four. Level five patterns are contextual in nature, and Bernal and Baker state that contextual communication patterns focus on a "discussion of growth in its (the relationship's) context and life goals." This is often the type of communication that occurs in a therapy situation. The authors state that communication patterns one and two represent linear causal thinking, whereas the higher levels represent an acknowledgement of the process of relationship development.

Communication patterns used in the nurse-client relationship have also been identified. Gibb and O'Brien[10] conducted a study of the communication between nurses and elderly clients during morning care. They recorded 1 hour of morning conversations with clients, and transcripts of these conversations were analyzed to establish categories or patterns of communication. Two patterns or

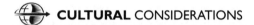 **CULTURAL** CONSIDERATIONS

Cultural background also affects communication patterns used by individuals. For instance, Winkler and Doherty[35] studied communication patterns in American and Israeli couples. They found that Israeli couples used more verbally aggressive communication patterns but were less physically violent during marital conflict than were American couples. These authors contend that communication style is highly dependent on cultural factors. The Israeli aggressive communication patterns did not correlate with levels of marital satisfaction. In contrast, American couples who use calm, reasonable communication patterns tend to have high levels of marital satisfaction. This relationship did not hold for Israeli couples.

styles of communication while providing morning care were identified. They were named *dissection* and *journey,* and they varied partly as a result of the physical activity engaged in by the nurse. The journey style was associated with a more personally engaging social interaction that appeared to be mutually beneficial to the nurse and client. The dissection style appeared to constrain the way the nurse interacted and was identified as a more formal style of relating. In the dissection style the focus was on the task, with several tasks being performed at the same time. Also, the routine was less predictable.

Communication patterns are not only affected by culture but also by the needs of the participants. Bollinger[5] contends that couples tend to communicate based on unspoken expectations, many of which are unconscious. When these unspoken expectations are not met, the long-term quality of the relationship is affected. One example of an unspoken expectation is dependency, in which one participant needs to be taken care of within the relationship. In this case one partner uses parent communication patterns and the other, the dependent partner, uses a child's patterns. This relationship can be satisfactory as long as the unspoken needs do not change and continue to be met. However, if perhaps the parent communication patterns change to adult, the partner may not be able to tolerate this shift, and discord results.

In conclusion, the concept of pattern organization, an individual's usual way of responding to stimuli, is also relevant in studying an individual's characteristic style of communication. An individual tends to respond in a similar way to similar stimuli. This section presents various ways to classify or categorize characteristic communication responses, none of which is exclusive. The cultural background, needs, and the individual's perception of the self and situation all influence his use of various communication patterns. Individuals do not use one communication pattern exclusively. Over time and in various situations, needs change, perceptions of the self change, and communication patterns change as well.

FACTORS AFFECTING THE COMMUNICATION PROCESS

Throughout the previous discussion of communication, factors affecting the communication process (i.e., the influence of cultural background and the level of language development) were mentioned. In general there are five broad factors that influence the communication process: pattern organization, relationship, purpose, content of message, and time.

Pattern organization

Pattern organization refers to the uniqueness of each human being, the sum total of those characteristics that make each self different from any other self. It includes many facets previously discussed, such as the past experiences of the individual, the culture of the individual, perceptions, developmental level, and communication patterns used. For example, if Ms. M., a pediatric nurse specialist, desired to prepare her client Jimmy for a tonsillectomy, she would need to consider her own pattern organization and that of the client to plan effective communication. The communication used would depend on Jimmy's age, past experience with hospitalization and surgery, perception of the experience, self-concept, communication patterns, and many other specific variables. In addition, Ms. M. would need to examine her own perceptions and feelings regarding hospitalization and surgery, communication patterns, level of language development, and so on. From this assessment of her own and the client's individual pattern organizations, Ms. M. would be aware of potential strengths and weaknesses that could facilitate or hinder their communication. For example, the nurse would recognize a potential problem if she was aware that she per-ceived the tonsillectomy as a minor procedure whereas the client perceived it as a major event. If the nurse did not have this awareness, the incongruency in the nurse's and the client's perceptions could hinder effective communication. A thorough assessment of pattern organization would also assist the nurse in planning the words she would use, such as how simple or complex the explanation of the surgical procedure and the hospital routine should be, and how often she would need to repeat or reinforce the message.

Relationship

The second general factor affecting the communication is the *relationship* between the sender and receiver. Consider the variations in communication between a parent and child, a teacher and student, casual acquaintances, and a husband and wife. If the nurse has developed a relationship with a client who is admitted to the hospital for a tonsillectomy, her communication to prepare the client for surgery and hospitalization is different from that of a nurse who has met a client for the first time.

Purpose

The third factor that influences communication is the *purpose* or reason for the communication. Compare the following interactions:

INTERACTION 1.
A: Hello.
B: Hi.
A: How are you?
B: Fine. Thank you. And you?
A: Fine, also. Take care. See you later.
B: You, too. Bye.

INTERACTION 2.
A: Hello. How are you today?
B: My back still hurts.
A: Your back hurts?
B: Yes, every time....
A: And the medication. Does that seem to help?
B: Only for a while....
A: In what positions are you more comfortable....
B: Lying flat....
A: I'll see about having the medication changed....
B: Bye.

The first interaction depicts what Berne[3] has termed the *American greeting ritual*. The purpose is only to acknowledge the presence of another. In the second interaction A's purpose is to assess B's pain and the action of the medication administered. In the first interaction B could not answer A's initial question of "How are you?" with the reply "My back still hurts," because the purpose of the communication is only to acknowledge the presence of another. If B had responded, "My back still hurts," A could have continued with the same purpose by responding, "Well, take care. See you later." Or A could have followed B's lead and changed the purpose of the interaction by responding with "Your back still hurts?" Therefore the purpose of the interaction, whether it is stated or unstated, influences the communication of the participants.

Content

The fourth factor affecting communication is the *content or message* being sent—how the participants plan to accomplish the purpose. This includes choice of words, sentence structure, tone of voice, volume, pitch, congruency of verbal and nonverbal levels, and metacommunication. In addition, the medium used, such as the telephone, personal contact, the written word, and so on, is considered.

Time

The fifth general factor affecting communication is *time*. This includes the location or setting of the interaction. Is the room noisy and crowded or hot and humid? It also involves what has preceded the interaction and what is to follow. Is the client on his way to surgery, or has the client's son been arrested for shoplifting?

Ley and Spelman[16] have reviewed research on communication with clients in a hospital setting. One important fact they found is that within the hospital setting clients forget over one third of what they are told. They believe that both high- and low-anxiety levels facilitate forgetting, as does lack of comprehension.

SUMMARY

Communication serves as an interpersonal function in the establishment, maintenance, and termination of the nurse-client relationship. From communica-

tion behaviors it is possible to define the type and nature of the interpersonal relationship used as the vehicle for nursing intervention. Through this relationship the nursing process of assessment, planning, nursing diagnosis, implementation, and evaluation occurs. In nursing the function of communication is to assist the client in obtaining or maintaining a high level of wellness.

People communicate on two levels: verbal and nonverbal. Verbal communication is the spoken word, and nonverbal communication includes all other forms of human interaction, such as touch, gestures, and facial expression. It is mandatory that the verbal message be congruent with the nonverbal message.

The communication process is composed of five functional components: sender, message, receiver, feedback, and context. In addition to these functional components there are three operations necessary for communication: perception, evaluation, and transmission. Together, these functional components and operations make up the necessary ingredients for human communication.

Because communication represents a form of behavior and consistently recurring behaviors are patterns, there are also communication patterns. Various patterns of communication are described. One that is essential in nursing is relating. By relating, people show that they are secure in their own worth and are able to reach out and help others. The other patterns tend to defend the self from a threat, whether real or imagined. Patterns in couple communication are also discussed.

In summary, numerous factors can affect the communication process. These potential influences are classified into five broad categories: pattern organization, relationship between the sender and receiver, purpose of the communication, content or message, and time.

DISCUSSION QUESTIONS

1. Give examples of how people communicate affection and displeasure in infancy, childhood, adolescence, and adulthood.

2. Compare the greeting ritual of two dogs with that of two humans casually meeting on the street.

3. Using only nonverbal communication, attempt to tell another person where you would like to go to dinner and what you would like to order.

4. Visit an ethnic neighborhood or restaurant and observe cultural differences. Be aware of grammar, syntax, use of the body, and facial expressions.

5. Identify your own favored mode of representation—auditory, visual, or kinesthetic. Attempt to mirror another person who uses a different mode of representation. Discuss how this feels and the problems encountered in changing to a different representational system.

6. Observe your own family and identify the communication patterns that they are using.

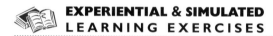

EXPERIENTIAL & SIMULATED LEARNING EXERCISES

1. Verbal and nonverbal communication number 1

PURPOSE: To identify the importance of understanding both verbal and nonverbal communication.

PROCEDURE: Assign half the students in a class to watch a familiar television situation comedy without sound. The other half of the class is assigned to watch the same show with sound. The students should be instructed to record what they are watching. In the next class period divide the students into small groups of four to eight students, composed of half who watched picture only and half who watched picture and sound. Each group should select a recorder to keep notes on the group discussion. Class time should be allotted so that half of the scheduled time, at least 15 to 20 minutes, can be spent in small group discussion and half the time spent listening and responding to the individual group recorders.

DISCUSSION: The students should be instructed to discuss what they saw, particularly differences in perception when nonverbal communication is not validated with verbal communication and also double-level messages.

2. Verbal and nonverbal communication number 2

PURPOSE: To understand the importance of congruent verbal and nonverbal communication.

PROCEDURE: Write each of the following situations on a separate slip of paper. Distribute them folded to the students and ask them *not* to open it until it is their turn. In turn, ask each student to read the situation and critique it for the congruency or incongruency (mixed messages, hidden meanings) of the communication. Then ask the group for additional comments. Each student should get a turn.

1. A student falls asleep during a lecture and later approaches the teacher with compliments concerning the content of audiovisual material.

2. A father, inspecting his son's report card, frowns and says, "I'm pleased with your grades. Three A's are fine, but what about the C?"

3. A student nurse has just finished explaining to a clinic physician the interdependent expanded role of nurses, then hesitantly examines a patient's heart and breath sounds and is unable to explain what was heard.

4. A husband comes home and writes I LOVE YOU in large letters in the dust on the coffee table.

5. A nurse enters a patient's room and begins fiddling with the IV. While adjusting the drip she says, "Any problems, Mrs. Jones?"

6. A client has come to the clinic because she discovered a lump on her breast. As she tells you this, you notice she is smoking, swinging her leg, and avoiding eye contact. You ask her, "Are you anxious about all this?" and she changes the subject.

7. Your long-term client has arrived 10 minutes late. She explains that she had trouble cashing her check at the bank and asks you to sit down. You remain standing and say "If you'd rather not participate in this relationship, I'd really understand."

DISCUSSION: Should take place after each situation is read, focusing on the areas described above.

3. Pantomine of feelings

PURPOSE: To promote increased awareness of the variety of ways a feeling may be communicated.

PROCEDURE: Prepare a list of different feelings such as anger, joy, love, fear, friendship, or hate. Write each feeling on a small card. Replicate each card approximately three times. Instruct the students to select three cards each and to conceal their choices. Then each student is to communicate one of the selected feelings to the group *nonverbally,* and the group is to identify which feeling is being communicated. Each group member successively presents a feeling. After all have presented, group discussion is held. Large groups may be subdivided to facilitate this exercise. Videotaping of the exercise can also promote discussion.

DISCUSSION: Allow group members to describe their perceptions of:

1. How they presented the feelings.
2. How they perceived others were reacting.
3. How the other students did react.
4. How different students attempted to communicate the same feelings.

4. Perception

PURPOSE: To identify differences in perception and how various factors influence the perceptual process.

PROCEDURE: Allow students to choose a controversial current event of interest. Ask them to identify various characters who are involved in this issue. For example, if the issue selected is abortion, the participants may include a pro-life advocate, a pro-abortion advocate, a pro-choice advocate, a pregnant teenager who wants an abortion, a Catholic priest, a counselor from Planned Parenthood, a prenatal clinic nurse, and so on. Ask several students to take the role of each of the identified characters and discuss the issue according to their role.

DISCUSSION: A group discussion should follow that includes each character's perception of the situation. Focus on the individual's selection of stimuli and interpretation of those stimuli. Discuss how needs, values, beliefs, and self-concept are related to the perceptual process.

5. Congruent communication

PURPOSE: To identify specific examples of congruent and incongruent communication and to explore the role of verbal, nonverbal, and metacommunication in congruent or incongruent communication.

PROCEDURE: Ask the students to watch a particular dramatic television series, then ask them to identify as many specific examples of congruent and incongruent communication as possible. Remind them to focus on the verbal, nonverbal, and metacommunication involved in each example.

DISCUSSION: Ask students to share their particular examples. In each example they need to include the verbal, nonverbal, and metacommunication on which their classification of congruent or incongruent communication was based. Discuss who formed the same conclusions. If there were differences, why?

REFERENCES

1. Argyle M: *Bodily communication,* ed 2, New York, 1988, Methuen.
2. Bernal G, Baker J: Toward a metacommunicational framework of couple interactions, *Fam Process* 18:293, 1979.
3. Berne E: *Games people play: the psychology of human relationships,* New York, 1964, Grove Press.
4. Berne E: *What do you say after you say hello: the psychology of human destiny,* New York, 1972, Grove Press.
5. Bollinger RA: Unspoken marital contracts, *Med Asp Hum Sex* 17:74, 1983.
6. Burnard P: The language of experiential learning, *J Adv Nurs* 16:873, 1991.
7. Clark JM: *Verbal communication in nursing.* In Faulkner A, editor: *Recent advances in nursing communication,* vol 7, New York, 1984, Churchill Livingstone.
8. Culley L: A critique of multiculturalism in health care: the challenge for nurse education, *J Adv Nurs* 23:564, 1996.
8a. Duldt BW, Griffin K, Patton B: *Interpersonal communication in nursing,* Philadelphia, 1984, FA Davis.
9. Feyereisen P, de Lannoy J: *Gestures and speech: psychological investigations,* New York, 1991, Cambridge University Press.
10. Gibb H, O'Brien B: Jokes and reassurance are not enough: ways in which nurses relate through conversation with elderly clients, *J Adv Nurs* 15:1389, 1990.
11. Gibb JR: Defensive communication, *J Nurs Admin* 12:14, 1982.
12. Ginsburg H, Opper S: *Piaget's theory of intellectual development: an introduction,* ed 2, Englewood Cliffs, NJ, 1979, Prentice-Hall.
13. Hamachek D: *Encounters with the self,* New York, 1971, Holt, Rinehart & Winston.
14. Janzen S: Taxonomy for development of perceptual skills, *J Nurs Educ* 19:33, 1980.
15. Knowles RD: Building rapport through neurolinguistic programming, *Am J Nurs* 83:1011, 1983.
16. Ley P, Spelman M: *Communication with the patient,* St Louis, 1967, Warren H Green.
17. Mackay L: Just chatting, *Nurs Times* 87:31, 1991.
18. Meyers A, Meyers G: Discussion of papers on nonverbal communication, *Comp Group Stud* 3:487, 1972.
19. Meyers M: The effect of types of communication on patients' reaction to stress, *Nurs Res* 13:131, 1964.
20. Peterson L et al: Communicating with staff nurses: support or hostility? *Nurs Manage* 26:36, 1995.
21. Piaget J: *The language and thought of a child,* Atlantic Highlands, NJ, 1969, Humanities Press.
22. Ramos MC: The nurse-patient relationship: theme and variations, *J Adv Nurs* 17:496, 1992.
23. Reimer T, Brink P, Saunders J: Cultural assessment: content and process, *Nursing Outlook* 32:78, 1984.
24. Riley LR: *Psychology of language development: a primer,* Lewiston, NJ, 1987, CJ Hogrefe.
25. Rime B, Schiaratura L: *Gesture and speech.* In Feldman RS, Rime B, editors: *Fundamentals of nonverbal behavior,* New York, 1991, Cambridge University Press.

26. Rothenburger RL: Transcultural nursing: overcoming obstacles to effective communication, *AORN* 51:1349, 1990.

27. Ruesch J: *Disturbed communication: the clinical assessment of normal and pathological communicative behavior,* New York, 1972, WW Norton.

27a. Ruesch J, Bateson G: *Communication: the social matrix of psychiatry,* ed 2, New York, 1968, WW Norton.

28. Ruesch J, Kees W: *Nonverbal communication,* Los Angeles, 1956, University of California Press.

29. Satir V: *Conjoint family therapy: a guide to theory and technique,* ed 3, Palo Alto, Calif, 1983, Science and Behavior Books.

30. Satir V: *Peoplemaking,* Palo Alto, Calif, 1972, Science and Behavior Books.

31. Speigel J, Machotka P: *Messages of the body,* ed 2, New York, 1982, Irvington Publishers.

32. Travelbee J: *Intervention in psychiatric nursing: process in the one-to-one relationship,* ed 2, Philadelphia, 1979, FA Davis.

33. Trevarthen C: Communication and cooperation in early infancy: a description of primary intersubjectivity. In Bollowa M, editor: *Before speech: the beginning of interpersonal communication,* New York, 1979, Cambridge University Press.

34. Wilkens H: Transcultural nursing: a selective review of the literature, 1985-1991, *J Adv Nurs* 18:602, 1993.

35. Winkler I, Doherty WJ: Communication styles and marital satisfaction in Israeli and American couples, *Fam Process* 22:221, 1983.

36. Wood BS: *Children and communication: verbal and nonverbal language development* , ed 2, Englewood Cliffs, NJ, 1981, Prentice-Hall.

Suggested Readings

Argyle M: *Bodily communication,* ed 2, New York, 1988, Methuen.

This is an excellent and comprehensive textbook on non-verbal communication, both the theory and research. It includes information on cultural and personality variations, and reexamines the functions of nonverbal language. Argyle has separate chapters for various types of nonverbal communication, such as facial expressions, gazes, gestures, posture, touch, appearance, and social skills.

Berne E: *Games people play,* New York, 1964, Grove Press.

This interesting text discusses transactional analysis and lists a number of specific "games." It is particularly useful after reading the text to try to develop ways to therapeutically terminate particular games. Available in paperback.

Brockopp DY: What is NLP? *Am J Nurs* 83:1012, 1983.

This introduction to neurolinguistic programming gives specific examples of the nurse mirroring the information-processing modality used by the client.

Davis A: The skills of communication, *Am J Nurs* 63:40, 1963.

A classic discussion of Reusch's theory of communication as a framework for communication skills, which includes a discussion on evaluation of communication and an application of Ruesch's theory to nursing practice.

Janzen S: Taxonomy for development of perceptual skills, *J Nurs Educ* 19:133, 1980.

A method for teaching students perceptual skills is described. A model for a communication process that focuses on an individual's field of experience is outlined.

Martin JAM: *Voice, speech and language in the child: development and disorder,* New York, 1981, Springer-Verlag.

An interesting textbook that incorporates scientific and clinical information. The first half discusses the development of communication in the newborn and young child. The second focuses on the causes and treatment of specific communication disorders.

Meyers M: The effect of types of communication on patient's reaction to stress, *Nurs Res* 13:126, 1964.

This study demonstrates the impact of the nurse's communication style. The results reinforce the negative impact of the distracting pattern of communication.

Shanks SJ, editor: *Nursing and the management of pediatric communication disorders,* San Diego, 1983, College Hill Press.

This text includes several interesting chapters, especially one on a conversational approach to language-delayed children. It provides a framework for identifying problems and guidelines for potential solutions regardless of the cause. There is also an excellent chapter on augmentative communication methods.

Weiss CE, Lillywhite HS: *Communicative disorders: prevention and early intervention,* ed 2, St Louis, 1981, Mosby.

This is an excellent source book on the development of communication. It includes ways to screen for communication disorders, as well as assessment programs for speech and hearing. The text includes a number of valuable charts from the development of language to signs of speech problems.

Is there anyone out there, anyone at all?
Is there anyone out there, hear my call.
Please wake me from this horrible slumber.
I feel so lost, just another number.
Some statistic in some useless book.
Someone hear me! Turn and look!

Alex Cohen
Hear My Call

LEARNING OBJECTIVES

After studying this chapter, the student should be able to:

- Differentiate between therapeutic and nontherapeutic communication.
- Identify ways to improve one's own communication skills.
- Plan alternative communication channels when the verbal channel is missing or inadequate.
- Compare and contrast structured and unstructured communication.
- Analyze ways in which interorganizational and intraorganizational communication can affect the nurse-client relationship.
- Evaluate specific interactions on their effectiveness, appropriateness, adequacy, and efficiency.

Chapter 4 provides theoretic information regarding the communication process. The focus of this chapter is the application of theory in the development of therapeutic communication skills. Therapeutic communication facilitates the formation of a working nurse-client relationship and fulfills the purpose of the nursing process. The factors that hinder nurse-client communication are explored, and specific forms of nurse-client communication are discussed. These include structured communication and organizational communication. Finally, this chapter explores the acquisition of communication skills in nursing education programs.

THERAPEUTIC COMMUNICATION TECHNIQUES

Communication in nursing can be broadly classified as either therapeutic or nontherapeutic. Therapeutic communication facilitates the formation of a working nurse-client relationship and fulfills the purposes of the nursing process. It allows for adequate and accurate data collection—the objective compilation of appropriate facts. Planning, intervention, and evaluation are performed with the client, not to or for the client, when therapeutic communication is used. Therefore therapeutic communication permits and encourages a mutuality or sharing throughout the nurse-client relationship.

Nontherapeutic communication, in contrast, hinders relationship formation. It prevents the client from becoming a mutual partner within the relationship, and it relegates him to the role of an object—a passive recipient of nursing care.

To facilitate the development of therapeutic communication skills specific techniques can be used. In addition to using these methods or procedures, the nurse must recognize the principles underlying her behavior and be able to evaluate how comfortable she is in using certain techniques. The use of therapeutic communication techniques does not guarantee therapeutic communication. Because of the many factors involved in human relationships, it is impossible to say that any particular method or procedure guarantees a relating pattern. All factors affecting the relationship must be considered.

Listening

Listening is probably the most effective therapeutic communication technique available. Although it is usually considered a passive process of receiving information, therapeutic listening is actually an active process that requires the nurse's complete attention and a great deal of energy. Kron[39] has outlined various levels of listening. The lowest level is isolation, which implies an absence of evaluation of the messages received; the highest is introspection. In contrast to the isolation type of listening, introspection involves actively examining one's reactions to messages received and the influence of these messages on behavior. Therapeutic listening is similar to introspection. The nonverbal message the client receives by the nurse's listening behavior is "You are a person of worth. I am interested in you as a unique person."

Van Dersal[62] suggests that while listening the nurse should keep three key questions in mind:
1. What does the speaker mean?
2. How does the speaker know?
3. What is being left out?

Because words can have various meanings, the nurse must attempt to determine what the client's words mean to that individual. The 500 most-used words in the English language have 14,000 meanings. The second question alerts the nurse to listen for the reasons behind the information given. By identifying the source, the nurse will hopefully be better able to understand the client's message. For instance, if a pregnant client states that she was told she would not be able to breastfeed her infant, to find out who told her would be important in understanding this client's message.

The third question is also important in determining what the client is saying. Important facts may be left to the deduction of the listener. It is often falsely assumed that one understands what has been said even though some information has only been alluded to rather than stated.

In addition, Van Dersal lists a number of general rules for therapeutic listening. One is to relax while listening. Straining makes it more difficult to comprehend what is being experienced. Another general rule is to be patient and nonjudgmental in allowing the speaker to finish without interruptions. The final general rule concerns symbols of authority. Van Dersal contends that if an individual is intimidated by rank or other external symbols,

listening is hampered; on the other hand, if an individual does not possess external trappings of status, this does not mean that what they say is not valid. It is necessary to hear what the individual is saying and to evaluate the statements independent of external criteria.

Garvin and Kennedy[25] reviewed all nurse-client communication research from 1980 to 1989. They concluded that when the nurse focuses on the client, the desired outcome is achieved. Also, the availability of the nurse was considered to be the most-supportive nursing behavior. Their review supported the need for active listening, with its focus on the message of the client, and the therapeutic value of the nurse's physical presence even in silence.

Silence

Many times a client finds it impossible to put thoughts into words. The nurse can use periods of *silence* to nonverbally communicate her interest in the client. Often the client may feel compelled to produce verbal material to keep the nurse interested. By telling the client verbally and, more important, nonverbally that he does not have to talk, that she is willing to just sit with him, the nurse can increase the client's sense of self-worth. The message the nurse is trying to send is "You are a person of worth. I am willing to follow your lead. When you are ready to talk, I will be here. Words are not the only form of communication." Congruency of verbal and nonverbal levels of communication is particularly important. During periods of silence the nurse should be aware of her own nonverbal communication. Verbally telling the client that it is not necessary that he talk and then nonverbally communicating the opposite message by gazing around the room, squirming in a chair, or busying oneself with some available task such as filling out forms sends the client a double-level message.

Short silences often give the client an opportunity to arrange his thoughts. It is also a valuable time for the nurse to examine the nonverbal communication of the client and herself. Although the appropriate use of silence has great therapeutic value, it often provokes anxiety in the nurse and client, particularly if it continues over a period of time. Discussion of the feelings and manifestations of this anxiety can be a valuable experience for both the nurse and client.

Establishing guidelines

Establishing guidelines is a therapeutic technique that should be used at the beginning of each nurse-client interaction. It includes an introduction of the nurse and a statement of the purpose. This is not only a basic courtesy but a statement of the individuality and worth of the client. In addition, it helps the client to know what is expected. Any limitations, such as time or confidentiality, should be included. Essentially this technique is similar to contract formation, which is discussed in Chapter 7. It is also a form of assertive communication. Assertive communication is defined by Clark[12] as "setting goals, acting on these goals in a clear and consistent manner, and taking responsibility for the consequences of those actions." Assertiveness is authentic communication, truthful and open, that conveys to the client the nurse's expectation of the client and what the client can expect from the nurse. Assertiveness includes not only authenticity but mutuality, as discussed in Chapter 7.

Although a nurse may have met with a specific client numerous times in the past, it is still essential to state the purpose of the current meeting. This may serve as a reminder of past meetings and past goals as well as to focus on the task planned for the current meeting. An example of a nurse's introductory statement that restates a past goal but also gives the option to the client to begin is:

We had decided to use this hour to discuss _____ when you left last week. Would you like to begin there or at another point?

It is possible that goals set at the last meeting may not be appropriate for this meeting. For instance, Nurse A has been seeing Mr. R. in the medical clinic during his last two visits. Mr. R. is a 67-year-old man living alone who was recently diagnosed as having diabetes. At his last clinic appointment the nurse and client mutually agreed to spend this time planning a diabetic diet using the foods that Mr. R. likes to prepare. However, at the start of this meeting Mr. R. complained of symptoms indicative of insulin shock. Instead of discussing diet as planned, the nurse started with a discussion of the causes, symptoms, and treatment of insulin shock, which was more pertinent to the needs of the client.

Giving the client broad openings

In this discussion of establishing guidelines another therapeutic technique has been indirectly mentioned. These are examples of the therapeutic technique of giving the client *broad openings:*
1. What would you like to discuss?
2. What are you thinking about?
3. How have things been going?
4. For what reasons did you come to the clinic today?

These place the emphasis on the client's needs. What does this client want to do with this time? In essence the nurse is placing the responsibility with the client for direction in the interaction. The message is "I believe that you are capable of helping yourself. I will facilitate that process."

Not only can the nurse use this technique in allowing the client to choose topics, but broad, open-ended comments throughout the interaction continue to focus on the direction the client desires. Examples are statements such as "And then what happened?" or "Yes, go on." In addition to allowing the client to focus on material that he feels is most relevant, broad, open-ended comments are also encouragements to the client to continue. They are statements that tell the client that the nurse is listening.

Reducing distance

Reducing distance is essentially a nonverbal therapeutic communication technique that refers to the actual diminishing of physical space between the nurse and client. Sitting behind a desk or across the room creates distance between the nurse and client. Physical distance makes it more difficult for the nurse to hear what the client is saying, and it gives the client a negative nonverbal message of noninvolvement. By removing physical obstacles and moving closer to the client, the nurse is able to hear better and focus more easily on the nonverbal messages of the client rather than on unrelated stimuli in the environment. In addition, by moving closer the nurse gives the nonverbal message of involvement; "I want to get to know you" and "I want to hear what you have to say" are messages that can be communicated by removing physical distance.

Acknowledgment

Acknowledgment is the recognition given to a person for his contribution to a communication.[24] Without acknowledgment communication often sounds like a command. Statements that basically say "I am listening," "I hear you," "I am trying to understand you," or "I want your input" are all examples of acknowledgment. The message is that the client is a valued participant within the relationship. The therapeutic communication techniques of restating, reflecting, seeking clarification, and consensual validation also acknowledge the client's participation within the relationship. The following communication demonstrates the absence of acknowledgment:

NURSE: You cannot gain any more weight.
CLIENT: But I've tried all kinds of diets and nothing works.
NURSE: You are going to have to find a way. You can't gain any more weight.

In this interaction the nurse does not acknowledge the client's communication. Essentially the nurse is saying "I am giving you an order that you must obey" and "I am an authority figure." Compare this interaction with the following that includes acknowledgment:

NURSE: Ms. C., I would like to discuss your weight with you when you have time.
CLIENT: I don't have to pick up my child for another 30 minutes. Can we talk now?
NURSE: That will be fine. Let's see if there is an empty office.
CLIENT: OK.
NURSE: Ms. C., please look at your weight chart. In the last 8 weeks you have gained 20 pounds.
CLIENT: I didn't think it was that much. What can I do about it?
NURSE: Perhaps we can work together to find a solution. I know you are concerned about your health.

In this interaction the nurse acknowledges the client's role in the communication by asking when the client will have time to discuss her weight, offering to work with the client on a mutually identified problem, and recognizing the client's concern for her own health.

Failing to give acknowledgment requires less time. It happens every time some written material is handed to a client with the only communication being "Here read this" or an order like "You're N.P.O. after midnight" is given to a client. Although time is saved, communication is hindered.

Restating

Restating is simply repeating to the client what the nurse believes is the main thought or idea that the client has expressed. It is another way of saying, "I am listening to you." Restating also asks the client to validate the nurse's interpretation of the message ("Is that what you meant to say?") The following is an example of this technique:

CLIENT: I can't hear anything in this ear. I can't remember how long it has been since I could hear out of this ear. When I was a child, just a little kid, about 5 or 6, my father got real angry with my mother and me. I remember him hitting me a couple of times and throwing me against the wall. I guess that was the last time I heard anything in this ear.
NURSE: You haven't been able to hear anything in your left ear since your father hit you as a child.
CLIENT: Yeah, that's right. I guess he busted my eardrum or something like that . . .

Reflecting

Reflecting is directing back to the client the client's own ideas, feelings, questions, or content. The nurse is attempting to communicate to the client that his ideas, feelings, and so on are the ones that are important, not those of the nurse or others. Reflecting also attempts to help the client recognize ideas and feelings as being part of his self-system.

Berne's game "Yes, but" is a good example of how reflecting can be used by the nurse.[4a] The protagonist in "Yes, but" asks for advice ("What can I do about this problem?"). When suggestions are given, the response is "Yes, I could do that, but. . . ." To focus on the ideas and feelings of the client, the receiver of the message "What can I do?" can reflect back the question "What do you think would be helpful?" The reflecting technique enables the client to explore his own ideas and feelings regarding the situation. The listener then takes on the role of facilitator rather than that of advice giver.

The following situation demonstrates the nurse's use of reflection to help the client recognize her feelings:

Ms. K. has come to the OB-GYN clinic for a 6-week check-up following a spontaneous abortion. She is complaining of generalized fatigue, headache, and anorexia. Ms. K. has been married for 3 years. She and her husband have no children. This was her second spontaneous abortion in a 6-month period.

CLIENT: I've gone back to work now, but things aren't right at home. I'm not really myself, yet. I'm just so tired most of the time. Usually when I get home from work, I just collapse. I don't even bother with dinner. If I try to do anything like ironing or cleaning, I get a headache. It's as though all my energy had been drained. I don't think I lost much blood. Maybe vitamins would help.
NURSE: You seem to feel emotionally and physically drained by the loss of your baby?

In this interaction the nurse attempts to help the client get in touch with her feelings. Although the client discusses physical complaints and seems to be looking for a physical cause, blood loss, the nurse verbalizes the feelings of loss that she interprets from this message. After the client recognizes this feeling as part of her self, she may be able to examine her behaviors in relation to her feelings.

Clarification

Seeking *clarification* is an attempt to understand the message of the sender through feedback asking for additional information. Some examples of the clarifying technique are "I'm not sure that I understand that," "Would you go over that again?" and "I'm still somewhat confused." With these statements the nurse is communicating to the client that she is listening, she wants to understand the message, but she needs help in understanding the message. The nurse or sender can also clarify her own messages with statements such as "Maybe I didn't make that clear. I'll go over that again," or "I meant this rather than that." In the following example the feedback the sender receives is not congruent with the message sent; clarification is necessary:

NURSE: Take one of these tablets after each meal.
CLIENT: How many do I take each day?

NURSE: You should take three of these a day. They should be taken after you eat.

In this interaction the nurse presumes that the client eats three meals a day. From the feedback received the nurse recognizes the need to clarify the original message.

Consensual validation

Seeking *consensual validation* is similar to the therapeutic technique of clarifying. However, clarification refers to the broad overall meaning of the message, whereas consensual validation usually applies to an accord in the meaning of specific words. The following interaction demonstrates the use of seeking consensual validation:

CLIENT: My son lives so far away, and he is so busy. He never comes to visit.
NURSE: Do you mean that your son has *never* come to visit you here?
CLIENT: No … not *never* never. He only comes on holidays like Christmas and my birthday. Probably because he feels guilty.

In this example the nurse is seeking consensual validation for the term *never*. She is asking for shared denotative and connotative meaning for the words they are using.

Focusing

The therapeutic technique of *focusing* attempts to help the client expand on and develop a topic of importance. It is often useful in working with clients who use the distracting pattern of communication. The following is an example of focusing:

NURSE: You feel frustrated by your wife's lack of sexual interest in you.
CLIENT: Perhaps frustrated is not a good word. The political situation, with so much graft and corruption, frustrates me. I told my son that he should change his major to political science. …
NURSE: It seems that your relationship with your wife is a point worth examining more closely.

In this interaction the nurse is attempting to deliver the message "This seems to be a problem area for you." By directing the conversation toward a topic of importance, the nurse is asking, "Are you ready to discuss this?" If the client avoids the topic again, this may represent increased anxiety and an inability to focus on the subject. The nurse should not persist in trying to develop the topic but should be alert for its reemergence at a later time. Areas of concern to a client tend to reappear throughout interactions. Examining interactions for general topics and themes is often useful in determining issues of importance. For example, when Mr. G. discusses the topics of his sexual relationship with his wife, his inability to handle his sons' acting-out behavior, and his general apathy toward home life, the underlying theme of his topics is "What is my role in the family since my wife has returned to work?"

Summarizing and planning

Toward the conclusion of an interview with a client or after the discussion of a significant area, it is often useful to *summarize* with the client the main points of the discussion. A statement such as "During the hour we have discussed . . ." is an example of the summarizing technique. Summarizing serves to help the client separate the relevant from the irrelevant and gives a sense of closure to the interaction. It can also act as a review in a health-teaching situation or as a method to verify the amount of information that the client has absorbed, areas of weakness, what the client considers salient, or all of these. From the summary it is often possible to *plan* areas for future interactions or actions that the client will take in the future by saying, for example, "Next week we will discuss . . ." or "It may be a good idea to go over your diet again next week after you have tried to use it for a week." Table 5-1 summarizes the therapeutic communication techniques described in this chapter.

NONTHERAPEUTIC COMMUNICATION TECHNIQUES

In general, the use of nontherapeutic communication techniques hinders effective communication and the establishment of a helping nurse-client relationship. It is important to recognize not only the presence of nontherapeutic techniques but also to examine the function that they serve to the self.

Nontherapeutic communication techniques can be broadly grouped into two types: nontherapeutic techniques of omission and nontherapeutic techniques of commission. The former represent the nurse's failure to perform; the latter represent the nurse's performance in an undesirable form. Often when individuals hear that the client should be allowed to take the lead or that restating and reflecting are valuable communication tools, they begin to envision the nurse as an almost passive observer who occasionally makes open-ended comments or restates what the client has just said. The nontherapeutic techniques of omission point out the fallacy of this misconception.

Nontherapeutic techniques of omission

Just as listening is the most important therapeutic technique that a nurse uses, the nontherapeutic technique that is most devastating to relationship formation is *failure to listen*. Failure to listen represents an inability to place the needs of the self secondary to the needs of the client. Because the higher level of listening—introspection—requires the nurse's active participation in the communication process, any factors that decrease the energy available for the interaction also decrease the ability to listen. Failure to listen gives the client the message "You are not of value," or "I am bored; you must entertain me." To prevent internal and external factors from hindering her ability to listen, it is necessary for the nurse to first be aware of their presence and then to determine their function for the self.

Failure to probe is a nontherapeutic communication technique that, like failure to listen, represents an omission of the nurse. Fritz et al.[22] define a *probe* as any discourse that both the client and nurse use to increase the depth of mutual understanding and to generate for the nurse a richer appreciation of the client's perspective. Failure to probe can be discussed in terms of failure to use the therapeutic communication techniques of seeking clarification and consensual validation.

Kesler[37] has listed various examples of failures to probe: eliciting vague descriptions, getting inadequate answers, following standard forms too closely, and not exploring the client's interpretation. All of these nontherapeutic techniques represent forms of inadequate or incomplete data collection.

When the client has stated that she has been having pain in her breasts associated with breast-

TABLE 5-1   Summary of therapeutic communication techniques

TECHNIQUE	DEFINITION	THERAPEUTIC VALUE
Listening	An active process of receiving information and examining one's reaction to the messages received	Nonverbally communicates to client nurse's interest in client
Silence	Periods of no verbal communication among participants	Nonverbally communicates nurse's acceptance of client
Establishing guidelines	Statements regarding roles, purpose, and limitations for a particular interaction	Helps client to know what is expected of him
Open-ended comments	General comments asking the client to determine the direction the interaction should take	Allows client to decide what material is most relevant and encourages him to continue
Reducing distance	Diminishing physical space between the nurse and client	Nonverbally communicates that nurse wants to be involved with client
Acknowledgment	Recognition given to a client for contribution to an interaction	Demonstrates the importance of the client's role within the relationship
Restating	Repeating to the client what the nurse believes is the main thought or idea expressed	Asks for validation of nurse's interpretation of the message
Reflecting	Directing back to the client his ideas, feelings, questions, or content	Attempts to show client the importance of his own ideas, feelings, and interpretations
Seeking clarification	Asking for additional inputs to understand the message received	Demonstrates nurse's desire to understand client's communication
Seeking consensual validation	Attempts to reach a mutual denotative and connotative meaning of specific words	Demonstrates nurse's desire to understand client's communication
Focusing	Questions or statements to help the client develop or expand an idea	Directs conversation toward topics of importance
Summarizing	Statement of main areas discussed during interaction	Helps client to separate relevant from irrelevant material; serves as a review and closing for the interaction
Planning	Mutual decision making regarding the goals, direction, and so on of future interactions	Reiterates client's role within relationship

feeding, the following is an example of *eliciting vague descriptions*. The nurse may begin by making a broad, open-ended statement such as "Tell me about the discomfort." The client responds, "It just seems to hurt at times when the baby nurses. I think I should wean her." Additional data are needed to determine what is happening to this client. Information is lacking regarding the type of pain (burning, throbbing, stinging), the duration of the pain (throughout the feeding, initially, when the milk lets down), and so on. To stop data collection to make recommendations at this point is not warranted.

Inadequate answers, like vague descriptions, represent incomplete data collection. In the preceding

example when the nurse asked the client when the breast pain began, assume the client responded "It's been going on for a while, on and off." To clarify the information the nurse can then use close-ended, specific questions, questions that can be answered with a simple yes or no:

NURSE: When you were here for the baby's 2-week checkup, were you experiencing the pain?
CLIENT: No, it was a few days after that, because I can remember thinking something was wrong but I had just seen the doctor and he said everything was fine.

By changing from nondirect to direct questioning, the nurse is able to fill in information gaps. If the nurse had stopped with the client's initial statement regarding duration, the data collection would have been incomplete. The nurse's first question had elicited an inadequate answer, but by relating time to specific past occurrences the nurse was able to collect more complete data.

Failure to explore the client's interpretations represents another form of inadequate data collection. When the client states that her breasts "hurt," the nurse needs to explore what "hurt" means to this client. Some possible interpretations of this discomfort could be that this pain is a danger signal that something is wrong, that this pain is so severe that it makes nursing unpleasant, and so on. What the nurse needs to find out is how this client at this time is interpreting these body messages.

In this example, failure to probe could lead to incorrect conclusions being drawn. The nurse could quickly react to the client's second statement regarding cessation of nursing and start to instruct the client on weaning and the use of formula. A quite different conclusion would be reached if the nurse first gets the client to describe fully what she is experiencing, to answer questions completely about the type and duration of the discomfort, and finally explores the client's interpretation of what she is feeling. Following this format the nurse obtains a complete picture of what the client is experiencing and draws conclusions based on a complete assessment. In this particular example a complete assessment showed that the client was interpreting the let-down reflex as breast pain when the breasts were very full. In the afternoon and early evening when the breasts were less full, the same sensations were not experienced. When the nurse explained the let-down reflex and related it to what the client was feeling, the client was then able to read these body sensations as an indication that her milk was flowing. Instead of experiencing sensations of fullness and tingling as pain, the client interpreted them more accurately as a temporary discomfort caused by the pressure of the milk moving down to the nipple area, indicating that all was going well.

Following standard forms too closely is an additional nontherapeutic communication technique of omission. Most health care facilities have data collection forms of various types to assist in information gathering. Probably most familiar are the standard checklist-type forms used by private physicians and dentists that list a series of health problems requiring the client to check yes or no. Although much valuable information can be gained in a brief period by using these forms, much valuable information is also lost. Whenever standard forms are followed too closely, the possibility of inadequate data collection is increased. For instance, when the client answers that his mother, father, and brother died of heart attacks and he is complaining of chest pain, there is no standard question to explore this client's interpretation of chest pain and how it may or may not be related to his well-being. When the nurse uses any standard form too closely, data collection is actually hampered. Such usage relegates the client to the role of object from which information is obtained. The communication follows a question-and-answer format in which the nurse is in control, deciding what information is important. Stated differently, this situation places the nurse in the role of a parent, deciding and declaring, while the client is in the role of a child, listening and obeying. Although this may be the fastest way to gather needed information, it is not congruent with the reality of the situation. In reality it is expected that the client will return home and carry on adult roles. An example may help clarify this dilemma:

Mr. A. comes to the clinic complaining of headaches. The nurse follows a standard form, collecting data in a question-and-answer format. Mr. A. is examined, diagnosed as having hypertension, and given a prescription. The nurse gives Mr. A. standard instructions regarding medication, diet, and a return appointment.

It is expected that Mr. A. will go home and take his medication, follow his diet, and return to the clinic in 1 month. Whether Mr. A. will comply with his regimen depends on a variety of factors. The expectations require the client to assume an adult role; however, during his contact with the health care system he is placed in a child role. This child role fosters dependency and prevents mutuality in goal setting, thereby hampering goal accomplishment.

Parroting is a nontherapeutic communication technique discussed by Bradley and Edinberg.[6] They define parroting as the continual repetition of the client's phrases as an attempt to reflect or paraphrase. Restating and reflecting were previously discussed as examples of therapeutic communication techniques; parroting represents the extreme use of these techniques. Comedians have often portrayed talk therapists as nonentities nodding their heads and repeating back what has just been said. Novices in the field of therapeutic communication often latch on to these stereotyped "listener/facilitator" roles and fail to see the total interaction rather than the isolated techniques.

The following is an example of how parroting gives the opposite message of reflecting and restating:

CLIENT: I have such a headache today.
NURSE: You have such a headache.
CLIENT: My head is just throbbing, throbbing.
NURSE: Your head is throbbing.
CLIENT: I can hardly focus my eyes the headache is so bad.
NURSE: You can hardly focus your eyes.
CLIENT: I don't like when you repeat everything I say.
NURSE: You don't like it when I repeat everything you say.

Parroting is another way of telling the client "I'm not listening to you."

Nontherapeutic techniques of commission

The second broad category of nontherapeutic communication techniques is nontherapeutic techniques of commission. These are characterized by the nurse performing undesirable behaviors as opposed to the previous techniques in which the nurse failed to perform desirable behaviors.

Being judgmental involves a number of responses that essentially tell the client that to be accepted "You must think as I think." Judgmental statements include such responses as "That's good," "That's bad," "You shouldn't do that," and "You should do…." They tend to place the nurse's values, beliefs, and perceptions above those of the client. All approving or disapproving statements imply that the nurse has the right to pass judgment on the client's behavior. They make the relationship conditional, that is, "I will help you only if you do as I say." In general they negate the self-worth of the client. The message is "You need me. You are not capable of helping yourself." Seeking to make the client dependent on the helper, they place the client in a role that is subservient to the helper.

Brown and Keller[9] have proposed that anxiety generates a judgmental attitude. Those who have achieved self-acceptance do not need to judge others. Making judgmental statements often represents a fear of others and decreased intimacy with them, which has been learned from significant others in one's life who have similarly sat in judgment and made arbitrary demands. Some specific judgmental nontherapeutic techniques are reassuring, rejecting, defending, and giving advice.

Reassuring statements, such as "Everything will be fine," attempt to do magic with words. Sullivan[58] has stated that such verbalisms reassure the helper rather than the client. They negate the feelings of the client and block the client's communication regarding them.

Rejecting statements, such as "I don't want to discuss that," are another way that the nurse refuses to discuss feelings or topical areas with the client. In addition to having communication rejected, the client often feels rejected. Rejecting statements are usually made to defend the self from increased anxiety or to keep from revealing an area of personal weakness. The Clinical Example shows how rejecting is used to defend the self:

CLINICAL EXAMPLE

*M*s. *K. was a student nurse assigned to work with a geriatric client during a 10-week course to develop communication skills. Throughout their first five meetings, the client, Ms. Z., discussed only her problems with food intake and elimination. By the sixth meeting the student was frustrated by their relationship. Ms. Z. continued to repeat the same messages—the food was too starchy, and she was always constipated. During the sixth visit the student told Ms. Z. that she did not want to talk about the client's intake and output anymore. She wanted to discuss other areas of interest to the client. The client's behavior changed dramatically after this visit. She missed appointments with the student. She constantly forgot the student's name. There were long periods of silence, and the client manifested many signs of anxiety. For example, her rocking in her chair increased, and she refused to meet the student in a quiet place but insisted on meeting in the central lobby where the client talked to everyone but the student.*

Although there were numerous other problems within the relationship, the student's rejection of what the client considered important represented rejection of the self for his client. Feeling rejected as a person, the client became increasingly anxious within the relationship. The student's inability to handle what the client considered important represented her own feelings of anxiety and incompetence.

Defending is a nontherapeutic technique that attempts to protect someone or something. It prevents the client from expressing opinions or feelings. If a client states that the clinic staff is incompetent or looking for experimental subjects and the nurse defends her colleagues by saying, "I've worked here for 5 years, and I know that the staff is very qualified and dedicated," she is rejecting the client's opinions. Probably the most threatening attacks are those that are directed toward the self. Often hostile comments regarding colleagues or institutions are interpreted by the nurse as also being directed toward her. Defending statements deliver the message "You do not have the right to complain or express an opinion."

Giving advice, like other judgmental techniques, implies that the client has an inferior status and a basic inability to direct the self. Giving advice differs from supplying the client with information. Giving information supplements the client's knowledge with additional facts from which the client can make a decision. However, giving advice takes away from the client's decision-making powers.

Stereotyped responses are nontherapeutic in that they negate the uniqueness of the client. Examples include platitudes, clichés, and other trite expressions that are virtually meaningless. The following interaction demonstrates how stereotyped responses prevent meaningful communication:

NURSE: How are you today?
CLIENT: Miserable. I wish I were dead.
NURSE: Everybody has bad days.

The nurse's stereotyped response that "Everybody has bad days" negates the significance of the client's message. The nurse is essentially telling the client that he is meaningless. The message is "I don't have time for you."

In addition to meaningless expressions, stereotyped responses also refer to classifying groups of people together and treating them as though they were the same. When the nurse assumes that all alcoholics are similar or all depressed adolescents have the same needs, she is preventing a relationship with the client beyond that of nurse and client's diagnosis. It is certainly true that there are similarities among clients diagnosed alcoholic, but there are also unique, individual differences. To date, although many have tried, no one has been able to formulate a personality pattern unique to alcoholics. Gross' book *The Brain Watchers*[26] powerfully depicts the futile attempts to develop personality profiles for selected groups. It is the obsession with being able to predict the behavior of another that forces the stereotyping of individuals into groups.

Changing topics is a nontherapeutic technique that puts the nurse in charge of material discussed. It essentially says to the client, "We will talk about what I consider important." Changing topics is often used to protect the self from anxiety-laden areas. It can also result from failing to listen to what the client is saying or from believing that the client is not capable of helping himself and, therefore, that the helper should determine the areas that are significant.

Patronizing is a style of communication that involves verbal, nonverbal, and metacommunication. The message to the client is that "you are on a lower level than me." It is represented by a tone of voice that is often "too sweet," singsong, or of a higher pitch. Other nonverbal communications that are indicative of patronizing are standing over a seated client and lack of eye contact with the client. Verbal communication includes the use of the word *we* instead of *you* or *I* and the use of baby talk. Bradley and Edinberg[6] contend that patronizing the client can result in decreased self-esteem, increased dependence, or anger in the client. Patronizing communication says that this relationship is not symmetric, not based on equality, but rather is complementary and based on unequality, with one partner assuming a superior position.

Table 5-2 summarizes the nontherapeutic communication techniques described in this chapter.

BARRIERS TO COMMUNICATION

Therapeutic communication is not simply the use of therapeutic communication techniques and the

TABLE 5-2   **Summary of nontherapeutic communication techniques**

TECHNIQUE	DEFINITION	THERAPEUTIC THREAT
Failure to listen	Not receiving client's intended message	Places needs of nurse above those of client
Failure to probe	Inadequate data collection represented by eliciting vague descriptions, getting inadequate answers, following standard forms too closely, and not exploring client's interpretation	Inadequate database on which to make decisions; client care not individualized
Parroting	Continual repetition of client's phrases	The metacommunication is "I am not listening" or "I am not a competent communicator"
Being judgmental	Approving or disapproving statements	Implies that nurse has the right to pass judgment; promotes a dependency relationship
Reassuring	Attempts to do magic with words	Negates fears, feelings, and other communications of client
Rejecting	Refusing to discuss topics with client	Client may feel that not only communication but also the self was rejected
Defending	Attempts to protect someone or something from negative feedback	Negates client's right to express an opinion
Giving advice	Telling client what nurse thinks should be done	Negates the worth of client as a mutual partner in decision making
Stereotyped responses	Use of trite, meaningless verbal expressions	Negates the significance of client's communication
Changing topics	Nurse directing the interaction into areas of self-interest rather than following lead of client	Nonverbally communicates that the nurse is in charge of deciding what will be discussed; possible to miss important topics for individual client
Patronizing	Style of communication that displays a condescending attitude toward the client	Implies that the nurse-client relationship is not based on equality; places the nurse in a "superior" position

avoidance of nontherapeutic techniques. As discussed in Chapter 4, numerous factors affect the communication process. In this section barriers, or factors that hinder therapeutic communication, are explored.

Parry[49] outlined seven general barriers to human communication—obstacles to understanding the message of another and to forming relationships. These barriers are limitation of the receiver's capacity, distraction, unstated assumptions, incompatibility of schemas, intrusion of unconscious or partly conscious mechanisms, confused presentation, and absence of communication facilities.

Limitation of the receiver's capacity is a barrier to communication because of an individual's basic inability to hear, see, and comprehend all stimuli. Therefore if the sender is talking too fast, overusing audiovisual aids, or presenting too many ideas, the receiver goes into system overload. The receiver is unable to understand all of the information presented. This knowledge of the receiver's capacity is particularly relevant in planning health teaching. For example, if the nurse wants to teach a client methods of contraception, it is important to remember not to overload the client with facts so that she forgets the information or remembers only distorted information. Being able to pick out important facts, repeating important ideas, and asking for feedback to see if these ideas have been received as intended is more important than presenting everything one knows about contraception.

Distraction is another important barrier to communication that is often avoidable. Distractions, or noise, are both external and internal to the system. External noise includes environmental distractions, such as a hot and humid room, a crowded waiting room, traffic, or other competing auditory stimuli that prevent the receiver from concentrating on the message of the sender. If at all possible, it is best to interview a client in a quiet, private, comfortable area to decrease the harmful effects of environmental noise.

Internal noise includes any stimuli within the system that hinder communication, such as anxiety, low self-esteem, hunger, or fatigue. Decreasing internal noise is often more difficult, because the sender is often unaware of its presence. At times nonverbal communication is indicative of internal noise; for example, fidgeting in a chair or continuously twisting a strand of hair may represent increased anxiety. Also, double-level communication patterns are often an attempt to mask feelings of low self-esteem. Although ideal conditions are not always available, the sender needs to be aware of the harmful effects of internal and external distractions.

"The commonest source of everyday misunderstanding originates in the speaker or writer making an assumption which he thinks [is] unnecessary to render explicit."[49] If the nurse teaching contraception assumes that the client knows the denotative meanings of the terms *uterus, vagina,* and *diaphragm* or of the phrases *coitus interruptus, regular menstrual cycle,* and *hormonal blood levels,* this is making unstated assumptions. *Unstated assumptions* also imply that words have the same connotative meaning for both the sender and receiver. To seek shared meaning for each word used in communicating is impractical. However, the nurse needs to remember that critical words should have an agreed-on meaning and that a thorough assessment of the client to decrease the effect of unstated assumptions would include educational level and cultural background.

Incompatibility of schemas is the fourth general barrier to communication. Schemas are similar to pattern organizations. They are defined as "persistent, deep rooted and well organized classifications of ways of perceiving, thinking and behaving."[49] They are termed *incompatible* when irreconcilable accounts are deduced from identical data.

CRITICAL THINKING *Question* ....

Ballinger[3] described factors that can impede effective communication. She related a personal experience, a time when she was called to the health center to see a Somali client and her daughter. Both were visibly upset. After finding a small private room, Ballinger called the language service to find an interpreter. He was male. The client would not discuss her problems at home with a male. In what other cultures may it be considered inappropriate for a female to discuss personal problems with a male?

....

Ms. G. is a devout Catholic who believes that birth control is immoral. The nurse working in the OB-GYN clinic has liberal views on birth control, abortion, and sexuality in general. Ms. G. has six children. She has been advised that her hypertension and aortic valve disease make it medically inadvisable for her to have any more children. Ms. G. agrees that she is chronically tired and cannot financially afford a seventh child. The nurse sees family planning as the responsibility of Ms. G. and her husband. Ms. G. believes that for her to intervene in "fate" would be wrong; the responsibility of family planning rests with someone else.

The schemas of the nurse and Ms. G. are incompatible.

The fifth general barrier to communication is the *influence of unconscious and partly conscious mechanisms.* This includes all of the methods that the human mind employs to select and distort material received so that it is congruent with the self-concept of the receiver. (See Chapter 9 for a further exploration of unconscious mechanisms.) An example is the client who considers himself to be in the best of health. He talks about how he never goes to a doctor, how he has not had a cold in his life, and how his body is in excellent condition for a 50-year-old man. Although he has had stomach pains for years, he attributes this to poor-quality food or cooking. Finally he is rushed to the hospital with massive intestinal bleeding. What has prevented this client from recognizing his need for health care? His self-concept is based on the premise that he is physically incapable of needing health care, thus any messages from his own body, such as stomach pain, or from the environment, such as his wife telling him to see a doctor, are ignored and distorted.

Nurses can also be influenced by partly conscious or unconscious mechanisms. This is often seen when nurses allow personal biases to influence their interactions. There are clients that a nurse may instinctively like. Usually they are people reflective of the nurse's self-ideal; it is not difficult to be warm, empathic, and genuinely interested in such clients. However, there are also clients that a nurse will instinctively dislike. They may represent parts of the self that are also disliked or manifest characteristics that the nurse was taught were undesirable. When the nurse allows personal biases to interfere with a nurse-client relationship, communication can be affected in many ways. Often the result is reaching conclusions not based on facts, similar to the client's behavior in the preceding example. A further example would be Ms. A., who complains of headache and chronic fatigue, but the nurse has decided that Ms. A. is a hypochondriac. Rather than gathering more information on this client's complaints, the nurse groups them all under the personal-bias category of hypochondria.

The idea of *confused presentation* as a barrier to communication is self-explanatory. If the sender overuses complex grammatic constructions, jumps from topic to topic, and lacks general organization of thoughts, this will hinder message transmission to the receiver. The distracting pattern of communication is a good example of confused presentation.

Smith[56] discusses specificity as a component of therapeutic communication. Smith defines specificity as "being detailed and clear in the content of our speech. It means being concrete so that our communication is focused and logical." Specificity is the opposite of a confused presentation.

The last barrier to communication discussed by Parry[49] is the *absence of channels*. If there are no means available to bring potential senders and receivers together, or if the methods available are not appropriate, there is a block to communication. The English-speaking nurse who is attempting to take a history from a client who does not speak English encounters an absence of appropriate channels. Although she may be able to communicate concern and similar feelings nonverbally, data collection is severely limited by the lack of a common language.

According to Braverman,[7] a potential barrier to communication is the client's emotional state and behavior. Negative client emotions and behaviors that may hinder therapeutic communication include anger, anxiety, depression, manipulation, and seductiveness. Anger may be expressed directly or indirectly. Direct manifestations include verbal or physical expression; indirect manifestations may include refusing treatment, sabotaging treatment, or uncooperative behavior. The client's anger may result from the hospitalization experience itself or from feelings regarding lack of control or frustration. Anger could also result from family- and work-related difficulties, especially the financial strain of any illness. Communication that may be beneficial when working with the angry client includes speaking calmly, firmly, and reassuringly to the client; allowing the client to vent anger in a nondestructive manner; and allowing the client the opportunity to express feelings. Braverman recommends that if a client is out of control, it is best not to confront or touch the client. Rather, the nurse should allow the client to have sufficient physical space so that he does not feel threatened. Braverman also recommends that nurses should get help in managing an angry client whenever they feel threatened.

Anxiety is another emotion that can hinder therapeutic nurse-client communication. Indicators of anxiety can include rapid speech, restlessness, inattention, irritability, hypervigilance, increased startle response, increased muscle tension, increased heart rate, diaphoresis, and dry mouth. Anxiety can be caused by an illness or be a result of the hospital experience. A lack of information or a lack of a feeling of control may also cause increased anxiety. To decrease the client's level of anxiety, the nurse can give information in a reassuring and structured manner. Braverman suggests that communication with the anxious client should be simple, concise, and unhurried.

The depressed client is often suffering from depression related to illness. Depression is commonly associated with many physical illnesses, and it has been associated with various medications. Behaviors that may reflect depression include sleep disturbances, lack of appetite, weight loss or weight gain, nausea and vomiting, lack of interest in sexual activity, preoccupation with body functions, withdrawal, poor

Barriers to Communication

Limitation of receiver's capacity
Distraction
Unstated assumptions
Incompatibility of schemas
Influence of unconscious or partly conscious mechanisms
Confused presentation
Absence of channels
Client's emotional state—anger, anxiety, depression
Client's manipulative behavior
Client's seductive behavior

eye contact, lack of spontaneity, slowed speech and movement, and difficulty concentrating. Open-ended questions may result in little information from the client. Often the nurse needs to provide the client with more structured questions and give the client added time to answer. Braverman suggests that the nurse avoid empty clichés in an attempt to "cheer up" the client; rather, the nurse should express an awareness of the client's feelings and an acceptance of them.

Manipulative behaviors may also hinder communication. Expressions of these behaviors may include lying, excessive flattery, playing staff members against each other, helplessness, intimidation, and suicidal gestures. Manipulative behaviors can result from poor and inadequate coping skills or be a pattern of behavior. Braverman recommends that the nurse use communication that provides structure and sets limits when working with manipulative clients.

Finally, Braverman discusses seductive behavior as a barrier to communication. Like manipulative behavior, seductive behavior is a way of coping with a situation or a pattern of behavior. Examples may include idealizing, flattering, attachment behavior, flirtations, sexual innuendos, or overt sexual behavior. Communication that is helpful is firm and limit setting. Braverman suggests that the ignoring of concealed seductive behavior is often beneficial.

SPECIAL COMMUNICATION PROBLEMS

Throughout this discussion on communication, the focus has been on the nurse-client relationship in which a verbal channel of communication is available and is used. However, there are nurse-client interactions that demand special skills and ingenuity on the part of the nurse, because the verbal channel of communication is not present or adequate. Some examples are the client who does not speak the same language as the nurse, the aphasic client, the sensory-impaired client, the noncommunicative client, and the child. When confronted with clients such as these, the importance of nonverbal communication is magnified.

Lack of common language

Nurse-client interactions in which a common language is not present pose special problems for the nurse. Interpreters are often used to overcome this barrier to communication. Kay et al.[33] have listed a number of problems in the use of translators. Primarily there are cognitive differences between medical personnel trained in a special science and the public. These authors contend that "in the absence of shared ideas, simple translation will not work." In addition, language changes, idioms, and folk ideas regarding diseases and medicine affect word meanings, making translation difficult. Even if the nurse or interpreter speaks the same language as the client, there are regional differences within language. For instance, Spanish spoken in the Southwest is quite different from Puerto Rican Spanish.

To overcome these obstacles special care needs to be taken in the training of interpreters; they must be aware of regional dialects and folk medicine practices. At the same time the nurse needs to avoid the use of medical terms and be attuned to all nonverbal communication. This awareness of nonverbals should include a consideration of cultural and background factors that influence nonverbal messages. Brosnan[8] has recommended that whenever possible, the nurse should make attempts to use the language of the client. No matter how limited, such attempts tend to make the client more comfortable in a strange situation and give a message of caring, "I want to communicate with you."

Sherman[54] outlines a number of nursing strategies that can be implemented when there is not a common language between the nurse and client. She recommends assessing the cultural background of the client. She also recommends assessing the amount of common language spoken by the client, the client's family members, and the nurse, as well as the amount of common language that can be read. There is often a discrepancy between what can be read and what can be spoken in nonnative languages. Sherman believes that it is important to identify nonverbal behaviors that can be used to communicate, along with a list of basic words and simple sentences. She encourages the nurse to learn a few words in the client's native language. In addition, the nurse should seek out information about the client's culture. Culture often affects the client's perception of illness and adherence to a treatment plan.

The aphasic client

The aphasic client presents another special communication problem for the nurse. Again, when the verbal level of communication is not present, the nonverbal level is accentuated, playing an even more important role in the nurse-client relationship. Therefore the nurse must become more aware of the nonverbal messages of both self and client. The use of writing pads, signs, and signal systems can be arranged to facilitate message transmission.

Mast[43] discussed a number of nonoral, alternative communication systems. The first is a communication board. This can be any size, shape, or form, from notebooks to easels, consisting of prewritten messages to alphabet letters. A second alternative system is mechanical devices. An example is a clock-face communicator with messages placed at intervals around the clock face. The clock hand scans the messages, and the client can stop the hand when the desired message is reached. Mast discussed other similar mechanical devices that are available through various medical supply companies. Local rehabilitation units should have information regarding what mechanical aids are commercially available in their area. A third type of nonoral system discussed by Mast consists of finger spelling and sign-language systems. "There are numerous recognized sign language systems . . . selection of a signing system will depend on the situation, need and particular patient."[43] Finger spelling is used primarily by the deaf and is a system in which each alphabet letter has a corresponding hand configuration. The last nonoral communication system is gesturing. As discussed previously in the section on sign nonverbal communication, there are universal

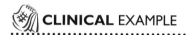

CLINICAL EXAMPLE

Mr. P. was a 65-year-old client who was aphasic after a severe stroke that left the right side of his body almost completely paralyzed. Because Mr. P. was righthanded, he could not write out his needs. With the client the nurse prepared a list of daily needs (e.g., drink, television on and off, and so on) that the client frequently needed assistance in performing. The client gestured his approval or disapproval regarding their addition to his list. The list was then attached to the siderail so that Mr. P.'s left hand could point to what he needed. Numbers were added for those things most frequently requested. By raising the appropriate number of fingers, Mr. P. could make his requests known. Later, Mr. P. used a large, lightweight writing pad, with the assistance of the nurse, to communicate messages.

gestures, such as placing the index finger to the lips to mean quiet.

The Clinical Example shows how one nurse attempted to deal with the special communication problems of an aphasic client. Ingenuity is the key factor.

Such attempts by the nurse help clients maintain some degree of control over their environment. They also help maintain the client's self-esteem while communicating a caring attitude by the nurse.

The sensory-impaired client

Problems in relationship formation and communication can develop whenever a client is handicapped by an illness that affects the senses, perceptions, or cognitive skills, which are the essence of the communication process. One example is the elderly confused client. Sensory impairment can take the form of hearing loss, decreased visual acuity, decreased olfactory acuity, or decreased cognitive acuity. Williams[63] suggests communication guidelines to identify some of the common communication difficulties and to provide the nurse with specific actions and behaviors.

The first guidelines are to approach the client in a confident and friendly manner and to achieve a successful introduction. Clients with sensory impairment may not see or hear the nurse approach. It is important to make sure that the client knows that the nurse is present to avoid startling or frightening the client. Williams suggests that the nurse's introduction should include her full name to permit the client to choose whether to call the nurse by first or last name. Williams also cautions against speaking to the client as if he were a child, even the regressed elderly client, because this fails to show respect for him as a person and also does not facilitate an adult-to-adult interaction.

Another guideline discussed by Williams is to encourage the client's active involvement in the communication process. To facilitate the client's involvement the nurse needs to be aware of the physical and cognitive impairments that could lead to problems. For example, the nurse needs to check that hearing or visual aids are working and being used appropriately.

Chovaz[11] discusses her own traumatic hearing loss and ways to help keep communication channels open. Four primary methods are used to communicate by the hearing impaired: sign, lip-reading, hearing aid, and reading and writing notes. Clients may use one method or any combination of methods to communicate. Nursing assessment should include the identification of the client's preferred method of communication.

Elderly clients also usually require increased time to respond; they often need extra time to process the nurse's statement and formulate a response. Williams also states that it is easier for elderly clients to discuss their past lives and experiences.

Braverman[7] states that clients with cognitive impairment may manifest any of the following behaviors: intermittent confusion, forgetfulness, inability to attend, drowsiness, lethargy, and emotional lability. There are many causes of cognitive impairment, including chronic brain syndrome, metabolic changes, cerebral tumors, drug or alcohol use, and sleep deprivation. Braverman contends that the nurse needs to focus on the nonverbal communication of the client. The client's nonverbal communication can provide the nurse with needed information, such as the client's ability to groom, motor coordination, orientation, attention span, and state of consciousness.

The noncommunicative client

The noncommunicative client also presents a special challenge to the nurse. Because it is impossible not to communicate, this is really a misnomer and refers to the client who refuses, for whatever reasons, to verbally communicate with the nurse. Often extremely depressed or very angry clients will refuse to speak. The angry client often fears a loss of control, and the depressed client may not have the energy available to speak. The nurse's physical presence and ability to allow the client to choose not to speak communicate the nurse's acceptance of the individual. The following Clinical Examples demonstrate methods that the nurse can use in dealing with a noncommunicative client:

CLINICAL EXAMPLE

Ms. J. recently had a radical mastectomy for a breast carcinoma. She refused to have visitors and to speak with any of the staff beyond simple yes and no statements. Mr. T., the nurse assigned to the client, included 15 minutes each day to "talk with the client about her surgery, cancer, feelings, etc." Each day Mr. T. announced his purpose. The client would turn on the television and stare blankly ahead, and then Mr. T. would reiterate that he would return the next day for 15 minutes. By the fourth day the client smiled when Mr. T. entered. Mr. T. commented on the television news show, but the client failed to respond.

On the fifth day Mr. T. entered and made his usual announcement of purpose and duration, and the client started to cry. When he got up to get her a tissue, she said, "Please don't go." For the rest of the time he held her hand in silence.

By the sixth day when Mr. T. entered, the client was smiling and the television was not turned on.

MR. T.: I'd like to come and sit with you for a while. If you like we can talk. I'll stay for 15 minutes.

CLIENT: Today I'd like to talk.

By the time of discharge Ms. J. had discussed her feelings of hopelessness with the nurse and her feeling that someone cared, which was communicated by the nurse's quiet periods of waiting. She stated that she was so sad she couldn't talk and was afraid that crying would make others uncomfortable. Mr. T.'s acceptance of the silence and her tears demonstrated his acceptance of the client. On this base of acceptance it was possible to build a therapeutic relationship.

In a similar situation a student nurse was assigned to care for a young male client who had bilateral leg amputations following a car accident.

In this vignette (see box below) the nurse could not tolerate silence and refused to meet the client on his terms. By constantly attempting to get the client to verbally communicate, the nurse gave a negative message, "I will not accept your decision." This was an angry, silent client. Instead of accepting his current method of dealing with his loss, the nurse kept trying to "help" him express his feelings. Although the nurse's intentions were legitimate, the methodology focused on the needs of the nurse rather than on those of the client.

The nurse should not feel helpless or useless with noncommunicative clients, but rather should realize that a wealth of nonverbal messages pass between them. The nurse should take this opportunity to focus on the nonverbal communication that both participants are using.

🕮 CLINICAL EXAMPLE

. . . .

Mr. D. *refused to speak with the nurse beyond yes and no statements regarding his needs and physical care. Initially it was suggested that the nurse set aside a portion of the day to sit quietly with Mr. D. The nurse responded negatively to the suggestion but eventually said she would try this approach. Although the nurse stated to the client that she would stay with him for a designated period of time each day and he could talk if he wanted to, she found herself continually asking questions in an attempt to find some area of mutual interest. Mr. D. would respond with quick yes or no replies and usually ask the nurse to leave. Next, the nurse attempted to involve the client in activities—usually card or board games—which he would refuse. For 4 days the nurse persistently tried to engage Mr. D. in some type of verbal interaction. Finally, on the fifth day the nurse arrived with a war-type game that she had brought from home.*

NURSE: I brought this game from home. I thought you might enjoy playing it.

The nurse proceeded to set up the game and explain the rules. Mr. D. glared at the game, then at the nurse, and then swept the game to the floor never speaking a word. The nurse literally ran from the room.

. . . .

The child

The final example of special communication problems concerns nurse-client interactions with children. Chapter 2 and the material on language development presented in Chapter 4 give some indication of the special needs of this client population. Knight[38] contends that children represent a segment of the population most in need of a communication channel. Because children tend to believe everything told to them, they also represent a segment of the population most vulnerable to the absence of appropriate communication channels.

There are two principal ways that nurses can facilitate communication with children. Primarily nurses need (1) knowledge about child development, and (2) expertise in the use of alternative communication channels. They need to be able to recognize developmental needs and to be aware of stages of development and the progression of these stages. As in all of the nurse-client interactions discussed in this section, nurses need an increased awareness of all nonverbal messages when working with children.

In infancy a basic developmental task is the establishment of trust. A hospitalized infant will need continuity of care—preferably the same nurse each shift—to foster the development of trust. Communication during infancy is primarily nonverbal. The infant senses the concern of the nurse through holding, touching, and other physical demonstrations of caring. Throughout childhood, and particularly in infancy, the parents' interpretations and reactions are very important, because parent and child are still emotionally bound. Parents who are anxious and frightened need to be supported and helped to express their feelings. The nurse needs to explain to parents how parental feelings are transferred to the child. Perhaps at no other time is the statement so true as during childhood that the nurse cares not only for the client (child) but for the entire family.

As the child begins to comprehend verbal messages (which is earlier than the child can verbalize) the nurse begins to communicate more verbal messages to the child. The intellectual development of the child and the characteristics of certain developmental periods are important to the nurse who works with children. For example, there are age-related differences in questioning that should influence the nurse's response to children. The 3-year-old child is usually seeking information when asking why. In contrast, the 4-year-old asks multitudinous questions related to why and how, often only to make conversation. Although the 5-year-old asks fewer questions concerning what, who, and when, the questions are more relevant and are asked because the child really wants an answer. The nurse needs to be aware of these differences and to be able to give brief and accurate answers that are appropriate to the intellectual level of the particular child.

In facilitating communication through the use of alternative communication channels, play and the therapeutic use of play are often recommended in working with children, because their verbal and cognitive skills are limited. Through the child's play the nurse can determine the child's fears and concerns, as well as individual strengths and weaknesses. Play also offers the child a constructive, alternative way to express feelings. Dramatic play can be an excellent therapeutic tool, because the child can act out with dolls, puppets, or self the situations that are being encountered. Art can also be a useful play method; as mentioned in Chapter 3, it can be used to assess body image and also as a means to communicate to the nurse what the child cannot verbalize. After the age of 5 years children usually have sufficient fine muscle control to use crayons and pencils to produce what they want, but even younger children can use art as an expresssive tool. Stollack[57] discusses the establishment of a program to train nursing students in the use of free play. The Clinical Example demonstrates how play can be used with children.

Elmassian[16] reports on the therapeutic use of play in a situation where the child initially refused to participate. The child was a paraplegic who was able to use her upper extremities. When she was scheduled to have sutures removed, she became hysterical and screamed violently when anyone attempted to explain the procedure. She refused to participate in any type of play therapy, and the time for preparing her was short. The nurse decided to "play out" the child's feelings for her. The nurse drew two pictures. The first was of a sad girl in traction with stitches. The nurse told a story about how the little girl was afraid, how it was normal for the little girl to be afraid of something that may hurt, and how the nurse might also be afraid if she were in the same situation. The second picture was that of a smiling girl with her stitches gone. Elmas-

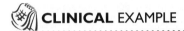

CLINICAL EXAMPLE

A *5-year-old boy was brought to the clinic because of insomnia. The nurse asked the 5-year-old if he would draw her a picture of his family doing what they usually do. After he was finished the nurse asked him to tell her who the individuals in the picture were and what they were doing. The two large figures in the drawing were identified as his parents. They were fighting with each other. The other figure was his 11-year-old brother. He wasn't doing anything. When the nurse asked about the lines drawn over the brother figure, he said that he had tied him up. The child had not included himself in the drawing. When asked where he was, he said his brother had locked him in a closet. The child's drawing of his family was an accurate description of his family as he perceived it. His parents were separated, and the mother often used the 11-year-old as a baby sitter for the younger child. When the younger brother would not listen, the 11-year-old locked him in a closet. The family was referred to a child psychiatric nurse for counseling.*

sian reports that the child stopped crying and was able to verbalize that the story was about her.

Elmassian outlines four basic steps in dealing with conflicts based on the work of Stollack. The first is to identify the feelings or needs that the child is expressing. This is followed by a message of acceptance of those feelings or needs as valid experiences, but this does not necessarily mean an acceptance of the actual behaviors of the child. In the previous example the nurse accepted the little girl's fear, although hysterical crying and screaming behaviors were not acceptable. The third step is an *I* statement of how the nurse thinks and feels about the child's needs and feelings (e.g., a statement such as, "I would feel the same way."). The last step is offering alternative behaviors to the child that are more appropriate for the present and future situations. In the example the nurse offered alternatives, such as medication to help the child relax in the present and talking or drawing how she might feel in future frightening situations.

In summary, to facilitate communication with the child the nurse needs background knowledge regarding normal growth and development. For instance, the nurse needs to be able to determine that a colossal imagination with startling fabrications, surprising fears (like fears of dust and feathers), and "I won't" responses are typical behaviors for a 4-year-old, but in a 7-year-old they are cause for concern because they are no longer appropriate. Readings and lectures, as well as actual experiences with children at different levels, can assist the nurse in acquiring this knowledge. In addition, nurses working with children need to develop alternative means of communicating, such as free play. As in all situations where the verbal level of communication is inadequate or inappropriate, the nurse will need a heightened awareness of the nonverbal messages of self and client.

STRUCTURED COMMUNICATION

Some of the definitions of communication presented in this chapter identify the purpose of communication as the transfer of information. This purpose is particularly appropriate when discussing structured forms of communication. Structured communication refers to definite, planned content that the nurse wants to transfer to another person or group. Three types of structured communication are discussed in this section: health education, oral reports, and written reports.

The type of communication previously discussed usually involves an unstructured format. The nurse meets with a client, and although specific goals and actions are planned before this meeting, the focus is on the needs of the client at that particular point in time. The nurse allows present needs to take precedence over any previously planned goals. For instance, Mr. A. is scheduled for an operation in the morning. The nurse and client mutually planned a time to discuss postoperative exercises; however, when the nurse enters the room, Mr. A. appears preoccupied. He gazes out the window and tells the nurse that he is too tired and not interested in learning exercises at this time. The nurse explores Mr. A.'s feelings, and their discussion centers on surgical risks and the client's fear of dying. The nurse is meeting the needs identified by the client at this particular point in time. Although this interaction did not meet the goals mutually defined by the nurse and client a few hours before, the communication was more appropriate based on the client's current needs.

Structured communication does not involve the same degree of flexibility. There is specified content or a particular message that the nurse wants to send. This does not mean that structured communication must be rigid; it may involve some specific content along with an opportunity for further communication based on the particular needs of the listeners. Unstructured communication is usually found in a one-to-one relationship or a small group where the needs identified are similar. In contrast, structured communication with its preplanned content is often associated with groups of clients, such as group health education sessions or preplanned staff interactions like case presentations in the form of oral and written reports.

Health education

Health education is one form of structured communication, and this topic is discussed fully in Chapter 10. Essentially, there are two formats for health education: formal and informal. Formal health education refers to the presentation of structured, planned, and scheduled content. The advantages of formal health teaching are twofold. First, most of the methodologies discussed allow more time for staff to spend in other activities; second, content is standardized, which is important when considering the large number of medical personnel who have client contact. When there are a multitude of teachers potentially covering the same content, client confusion can result. Although many teachers are not inherently wrong and may have certain advantages, a standardized content format should produce less client confusion, because all personnel are working from the same knowledge base. Differences in emphasis and modes of reinforcement will still exist. However, differences in what is essential content hopefully will be worked out in the development or choosing of a standardized content format.[21,23] For instance, Nurse A believes that a newborn should be nursed with the mother seated in a chair with a pillow across her lap, but Nurse B believes that a side-lying position is more advantageous. In the production of a sound-slide presentation, Nurses A and B discuss their differences and decide either to present both methods to each mother as equal alternatives or to enumerate the situations in which one position is superior to another. In either case the new mother is presented with a unified approach.

Informal teaching refers to all unscheduled nurse-client communication. It can be equated with giving the client information. Schweer and Dayani[52] believe that although informal teaching is the most common type of health education, it is often not pursued. In nurses' daily contacts with clients there are innumerable opportunities for health education. Owing to a variety of factors, such as lack of time, increased technologic responsibilities, and lack of preparation and teaching skills, many of these opportunities for client teaching are not used to their fullest.

The major difference between formal and informal health education is scheduling. Informal health education is not previously scheduled and is unplanned to that extent. Informal health teaching can involve either structured or unstructured communication. For example, Nurse M. brings Ms. Y. her baby from the nursery, and the mother wants to know about bathing the baby. Nurse M. informs her of a class in bathing and general care of the newborn in the nursery at one o'clock, but Ms. Y. cannot attend. The nurse arranges for the class in Ms. Y.'s room that morning. The bathing and general infant care communication is structured but unscheduled.

Oral reports

Oral reports are another form of structured communication. Lesikar[42] states, "In its broadest sense, an oral report is any presentation of factual information using the spoken word." The oral report varies widely in its degree of formality. At one extreme it includes the routine and informal reporting situations that occur among all medical personnel. An example is the team leader giving information to a team member about the clients assigned for that particular shift. At the other extreme are the highly formal presentations that take place in nursing, such as an oral report on a preliminary hospital study at a nursing conference. Change of shift reports, case conferences, and classroom reports made by students are all examples of oral reporting that are common in nursing. There are many similarities between oral reports and health teaching; in both the speaker is trying to get a particular factual message across to the listener. Health education can be discussed in terms of a nurse giving health information to other nurses or other medical personnel, but oral reports are usually defined in terms of medical personnel presenting information to other medical personnel. Many of the same principles involved in planning health education are also appropriate in planning oral reports. For instance, the first step in planning an oral report is the assessment of the listeners' characteristics: Is this an oral report for nursing assistants? A case presentation to other registered nurses? What is the educational background of the listeners? What is their past experience with this topic? What are the needs of this particular group in reference to this topic?

A second consideration in planning an oral report is preparation. As the degree of formality of the report increases, the need for preparation also increases. Preparation involves thorough knowledge of the content to be covered. In addition, it involves choosing visual aids, planning the order of the content, and most of all, practice in delivering the report. The speaker should test all material in advance to prepare for possible contingencies. Visual aids should be used to help clarify confusing points or to stress important points in the oral presentation. Part of preparing the presentation is to arrange the visual aids so that they are available when needed. Planning also involves making sure that equipment, such as projectors, is in working order and that the audience will be able to see the visuals unencumbered by obstacles, such as structural posts or the speaker. The speaker should look at visual aids only when it is appropriate for the listener to look at them.

The third aspect of oral reporting is measuring and responding to feedback from the listeners. No report should be so rigidly structured that the needs of the listeners are lost in the speaker's need to present the content.

Lesikar[42] lists a number of personal characteristics of the speaker that facilitate oral reports, and these characteristics are outlined in the box. The

Characteristics of an Effective Public Speaker

1. Produces an image that gives the listener confidence
2. Is sincere
3. Is thorough yet concise
4. Is friendly
5. Is aware of nonverbal messages, such as those conveyed by posture and gestures
6. Varies pitch, speed, and volume

From Lesikar R: *Business communication: theory and application*, ed 3, Chicago, 1976, Richard D Irwin.

first is confidence. If speakers have confidence in themselves, their knowledge of the subject matter, and their ability to transfer information to the listeners, they tend to produce an image that gives the listener confidence in the speaker. In addition to knowledge of the subject matter, Lesikar suggests that physical appearance and speaking in a strong, clear voice also tend to give the listener confidence in the speaker. A second personal characteristic that facilitates oral reporting is sincerity. Listeners tend not to believe the message if the speaker is not sincere. "Rarely is pretense of sincerity successful." A third personal characteristic is thoroughness. Presentations that cover a subject in a complete manner are usually better received than those that are scant and hurried. However, it is necessary to balance thoroughness with conciseness, because it is possible to lose listeners in a sea of information. A fourth personal characteristic is friendliness. People are more receptive to friendly speakers, and like sincerity, speakers rarely can fabricate friendliness successfully.

Nonverbal communication also affects the speaker's ability to transmit a message. Some of these nonverbals include posture, walking, gestures, and facial expressions. In addition, voice characteristics such as pitch, speed, and volume affect the success of oral presentations. The pitch of voice in an oral report needs to vary. Speaking in a monotone is usually a habit and can be reversed. The speed of presentation should also vary, and complex information should be delivered at a slower rate than is simple, straightforward information. Pauses are useful in oral reporting to emphasize particular points and to give the listener a chance to process information received. Speakers should never fill in pauses with meaningless sounds, such as "uh"s, which distract from the presentation. The volume of the voice needs to be loud enough to be heard, and by varying volume, pitch, and speed, the speaker can effectively emphasize various points in the presentation.

Leech[41] outlines a number of communication distractors that speakers should avoid in oral presentations; these are summarized in the box at right. The first is speaking in language that the audience does not understand. He suggests explaining all ambiguous terms and avoiding the use of unclear

phrases. Many times, whether a phrase or word is unclear is determined by the characteristics of the listener. When discussing operating room policy with a group of nurses, the term *O.R.* is appropriate; however, when teaching a prenatal class to young mothers, the acronym *O.R.* might be confusing. Leech describes an advanced form of obfuscation that comes from the German method of noun stacking, the combination of small words to produce large words. An example provided by Leech is a U.S. Air Force Bulletin asking all supervisors to report for a "merit pay appraisal system research field test training session."

Other examples of word groups that block understanding of the spoken word are buzzwords (paradigm; quality circles, or Q.C.'s), empty words (unique, really), inflated words (ineffaceable, quiddity), or indirect words ("attitude adjustment hour" instead of "coffee break"). In most instances the use of clear terminology makes the message more comprehensible to the listener.

A second common distractor discussed by Leech is the improper use of the English language. Incorrect speech patterns tend to distract the listener from the intended message. Common problem areas include grammatic flaws such as double negatives and verb confusion. For instance, "The drug company didn't never publish the adverse reactions." What is the speaker trying to say? Or, "The focus of the following studies were." Also included as common distractors are basic pronunciation flaws, such as adding extra consonants and erroneously sounding silent letters. Leech suggests that the time to correct language usage is not during an oral presentation. To speak correctly during an oral

Common Distractors to Avoid in Public Speaking

Distractor
  1. Use of unclear or ambiguous terms
  2. Incorrect use of the English language

Examples
  Buzzwords, empty words, inflated words
  Grammatic flaws, pronunciation flaws

From Leech T: *How to prepare, stage and deliver winning presentations,* New York, 1982, American Management Association.

presentation, when anxiety is increased and attention needs to be focused on content and audience feedback, one must practice correct speech patterns at all times.

In summary, oral reports rely on the speaker's ability to orally transmit a message, usually to a group of people, clients, or peers. The ability to present oral reports is a skill that needs to be practiced. Preparation is an important key to successful oral reports.

Written reports

Written reports are the third type of structured communication, and these are any written communication of factual information. Fiesta[19] contends that clear and effective written communication among health professionals is one deterrent to client dissatisfaction, client injury, and possible litigation. Nurses use written communication in many areas. Some of the most common examples are staff evaluation, case reports, nurse's notes, and care plans.

There are a number of differences between oral and written reports. Written reports have the advantage of visual cues. These cues show the reader the structure of the message through sentence construction, paragraph formation, and punctuation. In written reports the reader has control of the presentation. The reader can reread any confusing sections and control the pace of the message. This is not possible with oral reports. Therefore oral reports must be easier to comprehend. Written reports demand a higher degree of accuracy than do oral reports in terms of grammar, punctuation, and sentence structure, because written reports are permanent and subject to a high degree of scrutiny by their readers.

The following are general guidelines in the preparation of a written report:

1. Define and state the problem or reason for the written communication This is one of the most important aspects of preparing a written report. Commonly the writer operates under a false premise regarding what is actually expected. There are numerous examples in which the writer failed at this initial step. The result may be a comprehensive and well-written report; however, the basic problem identified is erroneous. For example, Nurse A is asked to report on the nursing care of mentally handicapped clients in the general hospital. Nurse A writes a detailed and comprehensive report on the mentally handicapped, including the nomenclature used, characteristics of various subgroups, and learning objectives for skills of daily living. Nurse A has not accurately identified the problem, which is how general hospital nurses need to change their patterns of care to provide for the special needs of this kind of population. The definition of the problem is the most important step in writing a written report.

2. Organize thoughts on the topic Organization of thoughts involves thinking about the problem and what needs to be said regarding it. This step is primarily a mental exercise, consisting of the reshuffling of ideas and attempts to make sense out of personal thoughts on the topic. The product of this mental exercise is the written outline. In many cases this may simply be short notations jotted down during the workday before writing nurses' notes. In the case of a formal written report the outline may represent an elaborate detailing of the content to be included.

3. Write the report Clarity, continuity, and unity are the three key factors in writing an effective report. Continuity and unity refer to how the ideas within the report are held together: Is there a central point? Are the secondary points related to this central idea? Does the message flow? Are the expectations of the reader being met? When continuity and unity are not present, the written report is often said to "miss the point." This is because the central idea is not adequately addressed. To present a continuous and unified message it is often suggested that a deductive reasoning format be used. When this format is used, the writer starts with the conclusion reached and then shows the reader various data supporting the conclusion that has been drawn rather than a reverse procedure of specifics to general information.

4. Read and edit The final step in any written communication is to read and edit what has been written. Often it is advantageous to have another person perform the editing. After working with material for an extended period of time, content that may seem clear to the writer may be confusing to another.

Daily nursing documentation is often in the form of narrative nurses' notes and requires planning and organization, as previously discussed. It consumes a considerable amount of nursing time, but recent advances in computer technology may assist in decreasing the amount of time spent documenting nursing care. Miller and Pastorino[45] advocate the use of a flow sheet to standardize routine elements of observation and care given. A checklist format saves considerable time over the usual narrative notes, and it can also increase legibility and accuracy. The authors report a 40% to 50% decrease in charting time using the check sheet rather than narrative notes.

In summary, the three forms of structured communication discussed—health education, oral reports, and written reports—require two key factors. They are preparation, which includes not only knowledge of the subject matter but also knowledge of the characteristics and needs of the listener, and practice.

ORGANIZATIONAL COMMUNICATION

The focal relationship within this text is that of the nurse and client. In many cases the term *client* includes family and significant others in addition to the identified client. The concept of context as a functional component of the communication process has already been discussed. The term *context* refers not only to the physical setting but also to the time dimension and the pattern organization of the participants. In addition, there is a broader view of context, as the focal nurse-client communication process takes its place within a network of other communication channels. Some of these other channels directly affect the nurse-client communication process; others affect it only indirectly. For example, Nurse A works in a prenatal clinic. In addition to the focal relationship with a specific Client B, Nurse A's communication is influenced by communication with various other groups. Figure 5-1 divides the other communication lines into those occurring within the organization where Nurse A and Client B are interacting and those that are external to the organization. Intraorganizational communication that can influence the nurse-client interaction includes other clinic personnel. For instance, the physician who examines Client B gives information to Nurse A and possible suggestions for health education. Other nurses in the clinic may also affect this one-to-one relationship. Clinic administration is another intraorganizational group that can influence the nurse-client relationship; for example,

the administration may decide that all prenatal clients with specified characteristics should have sonograms performed. Other clinic groups are listed as the third type of intraorganizational communication that can affect nurse-client communication. For example, Client B is also being followed by the medical clinic for hypertension, and the medical, low-sodium diet must be incorporated into client B's prenatal diet.

Various organizations external to the clinic can also influence the focal nurse-client communication process. Some of those listed are community groups, the local hospital, the media, and lawmakers. In this example Client B is attending prenatal childbirth classes in the community. Some of the questions that the client asks the nurse are based on these experiences in the childbirth classes. The local hospital may also influence the nurse-client communication process, such as by their policies and procedures. In this example the hospital requires that anyone who plans to be in labor and delivery with the mother attend certain courses, tour the labor and delivery unit, and have the physician's prior approval recorded. The media is also listed as an external organization. In this specific example Client B has seen a documentary on local television in which siblings are present during labor and delivery, and Client B discusses this with the nurse.

In Fig. 5-1 only the communication lines between the nurse-client relationship and the other organizations are included. In actuality these groups can all affect each other. For instance, community groups such as Lamaze Childbirth Preparation have communication with local hospitals, the media, and other community resources. This communication can be direct or indirect. As an example, perhaps some of the Lamaze instructors have seen the local television documentary on labor and delivery (indirect communication). They know of only one area hospital that has a policy to include siblings, and they decide to contact other area hospitals to see if they have a definite policy regarding siblings in labor and delivery (direct communication).

Administrative communication

A number of recent articles discuss communication among various groups within an organization. Communication skills for administrative personnel

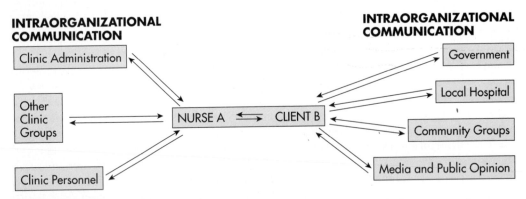

INTRAORGANIZATIONAL COMMUNICATION

INTRAORGANIZATIONAL COMMUNICATION

Fig. 5-1 Two categories of organization communication affecting the focal nurse-client communication process.

are often emphasized. According to Lancaster,[40] administration should be designed so that communication can occur in both an upward and downward direction. Communication that goes from administration to personnel functions to give direction and coordinate activities and is considered downward; it often takes the form of job instructions, policies, procedures, and rules. Lancaster believes that downward communication creates the greatest dissatisfaction among employees and offers suggestions to prevent some of this dissatisfaction. She encourages clear messages and informing personnel that a directive is to be issued before its actual distribution. Upward communication refers to communication from personnel to administration and is necessary for sound decision making by administration; it often takes the form of group meetings, suggestion boxes, task forces, and open forums. Lancaster believes that upward channels of communication give employees a sense of recognition and importance. If an organization does not supply appropriate upward channels of communication, it often develops underground channels that tend to be less productive. When underground channels carry the same message as official channels, the communication is complemented and the underground channel should be fostered. When the message is not the same, the false message needs to be quickly refuted by a statement of the truth. This statement should not include a repetition of the false rumor, because it is possible that some members of the organization may not have heard it originally. Lancaster states that the presence

of rumors and their content is a good indication of the feeling tone of the participants.

O'Brien[48] questioned staff nurses regarding their opinion of how administrators should communicate. She found honesty to be a primary positive characteristic that nurses want in administrative personnel. Concrete examples of honesty include making promises that one intends to keep, not showing favoritism, taking an unpopular but needed stand, and not stating half-truths to alleviate pressure on the self. Some of the other characteristics that the nurses valued in administrative personnel were directness coupled with tact, listening with follow-through, giving reasons for policies made, and respect for the individuality of the person.

In general, administrators need to use the therapeutic communication skills discussed regarding the nurse-client relationship in their nurse-administrator contacts. The rigid, rejecting, and judgmental techniques that are detrimental to a nurse-client relationship have the same effect on a nurse-supervisor relationship. The administrator should want all employees to feel that they are valued and respected individuals. If an administrator dictates a policy change as an order without discussion and input from personnel, the message communicated is that "You are not important. You are not a person of worth. You are not knowledgeable." If on the other hand an administrator asks personnel for input, listens, tries to understand their position, and plans a policy change mutually with them, the message is also clear that "You are respected."

CRITICAL THINKING *Question* ....

Which of the following represents assertive communication? Which are examples of aggressive communication? What are the reasons for your choice?

1. "The schedule can't be changed. It's your fault for not requesting the days off."
2. "I can't do that now. I'll have time after 2 o'clock."
3. "It's not possible to see that number of clients."
4. "Can't you do anything right!"
5. "I want you to take Mr. K. to x-ray now."

Bara and Rugg[4] believe that assertive communication is a core skill for good leadership. Assertive communication demonstrates responsibility and accountability. Assertive communication is not aggressive communication because it is not blaming another; it is an expression of a personal view of another's behavior.

Using quality circles is one method to improve communication between administrators and personnel.[28] Quality circles are part of the Japanese model of participative management. They are basically meetings between personnel and administration scheduled to discuss specific issues that affect both. They serve to improve communication.

Kepler[36] believes that the classic functions of management, planning, organizing, directing, and controlling need to be broadened to include understanding and communication. Through understanding management recognizes that individuals have various needs, perceptions, and goals. Through communication these differences are recognized and aligned to the basic goals of the organization.

Horizontal communication

Another form of intraorganizational communication is communication among comparable units or groups within the organization. In the initial example there was communication between the prenatal clinic and the medical clinic. Lancaster[40] refers to this as horizontal communication. It is necessary for organizing and coordinating activities. Horizontal communication becomes more important as the interdependence among groups increases, such as if one area begins a task and another completes it. Some examples of hor-

izontal communication are committees, conferences, and task forces that can all generate a team spirit if the communication is kept active and honest.

Phippen[50] contends that horizontal communication needs to be done through recognized information sources from one organizational unit to another to be most effective. He believes that interpersonal communication is not as effective. For example, if the operating room personnel want to arrange an assessment program on the surgical units, it is more effective for the designated operating room spokesperson to contact the designated surgical unit spokesperson to arrange this than for an operating room nurse to speak with a surgical floor nurse. Phippen also points out that the designated entry-exit point for organizational information may not be the supervisor or head nurse for that particular unit. It could be the secretary or unit manager. Therefore it is necessary to assess each unit to see where the information enters and exits the unit. The goal of communication among subunits is the interdependence, not the autonomy, of each unit. Some of the same factors that are important in nurse-client communication are also important here, especially individual and group perceptions and their experience base.

Staff communication

The third type of intraorganizational communication is staff communication. Many studies indicate that nurses spend more time talking with other health care personnel than with clients.[1] Part of this communication among health care personnel is about clients. In the initial example Nurse A received information from Client B's physician. Allen[1] studied communication on a psychiatric day unit for 11 weeks. She found that most of the communication among staff was not about client care; rather, its focus was social contact and the personal or professional needs of the staff. This included "the needs of stimulation and social support, for role affirmation, and the defense of 'professional' definitions of their work." Allen concludes that although a great deal of time was spent in meeting staff needs, the communication was ultimately effective. She did not believe that alternative communication patterns would have the same degree of effectiveness, because without such communication there would be a greater amount of staff turnover, which would be counterproductive to the efficiency of the staff team.

Bourhis et al.[5] studied the communication of doctors, nurses, and clients in a hospital setting. Convergence was described when one or both participants attempted to use the speech patterns of another. Participants were asked to complete a questionnaire regarding nurse, client, and doctor use of everyday language and medical language. According to the findings, doctors thought that they used everyday language with clients, but nurses and clients did not perceive them as using everyday language. The role of the nurse was described as a mediator between the everyday language of the client and the medical language of the doctor. All of the groups believed that clients should be spoken to in everyday language and that the use of medical language was seen as a cause for decreased understanding.

A study by Nowell[47] examined communication between unit managers and nurses in four midwestern hospitals. The result of the self-report questionnaires showed that both groups were satisfied with the accuracy and completeness of the communication. Problem areas were not caused by lack of communication but by basic disagreements regarding roles, duties, responsibilities, power, and status. Nowell suggested work sessions to reach compromises on the areas of disagreement. This is an important point in communication at all levels. If Client X does not think he is overweight, there is nothing the nurse can do, regardless of the communication skills available. The nurse can only recognize the basic difference in opinion and perhaps try to change the client's perception or reach some compromise.

Government

The second major category of communication that affects the nurse-client relationship is interorganizational communication. Government is the first external organization listed in Fig. 5-1. This includes lawmakers, courts, and government agencies in general. They affect nurse-client communication by passing laws or determining, for example, what programs will receive funding. As in communication with administrators, this type of communication is most effective when it operates in two directions, so that lawmakers and government agencies are not

only giving directions to medical organizations but are also receiving input regarding what programs are most needed or how a limited budget can be spent most effectively. By joining and actively participating in local and national nursing organizations, the individual nurse can unite with others who have similar concerns, thus increasing their input regarding the direction of health care. An example of how government affects the primary nurse-client relationship is the area of abortion. When abortion is defined as illegal, it is no longer an option to explore with a pregnant client who does not want a baby. Nurses need to make their voices heard on issues affecting their relationships with clients.

Another way in which government affects the nurse-client relationship is through communication regarding what is considered legal or illegal practice. Some recent court decisions regarding nursing and communication demonstrate the need to document and ensure that a message is received. These decisions can directly or indirectly affect nurse-client communication. The *Regan Report on Nursing Law*[51] published a court decision holding a physician negligent in failing to communicate to staff nurses that a hospitalized orthopedic client had suicidal tendencies in the past. The nurses did not provide special precautions, and the client committed suicide. The client's chart is the appropriate place for formal communication between physicians and nurses in the case of every hospitalized client. Although the physician noted in the progress notes that the client should have 24-hour attendance, no special precautions were ordered. Verbal communication is often lost in a busy day, and all important communication needs to be documented to avoid legal battles and to ensure the client's rights.

Cushing[13] reports a similar case in which the nurse documented in writing on the client's chart the critical condition of the client but failed to ensure verbally that the information was received. Therefore the nurse was still liable for the harm that the client suffered. In this particular situation the client needed immediate attention of a physician. Cushing cautions that failure to communicate, or even a delay in communication, can lead to liability. When the nurse is unable to obtain the attending physician, Cushing states that documenting that the attending physician was paged five times without a reply does not absolve the nurse of responsibility.

Medical organizations

The second external organization that can influence nurse-client communication is the local hospital or other medical organizations. The communication between the nurse-client unit and the external medical organization would be an example of horizontal communication, because the systems are relatively equal and interdependent. It is similar to the communication between the nurse and clinic personnel in that the same language is spoken. The perspective is different, however, so this is a possible problem area. Another similarity between the two is the effectiveness of communicating through designated spokespersons rather than on an interpersonal level.

Community groups

The third form of interorganizational communication that affects the nurse-client interaction is communication between nurse-client and community groups. The term *community groups* refers to those groups that are directly related to the particular nurse-client interaction. In the initial example groups such as childbirth education groups and breastfeeding support groups would be directly related to the nurse-client unit in the prenatal clinic. In the postpartum period the mother may want information on weight loss or exercise groups in the community. The nurse has the responsibility to know about community resources available to the client, their philosophies, and how they function. In addition, the nurse needs to take an active role in supplying inputs to these various community groups. In addition to medical organizations there are other community groups that can also affect the nurse-client relationship. Some examples are places of employment, churches, and schools.

Differences in objectives, language, and expectations can create communication problems, and Michal[44] discusses communication problems between medical organizations and the schools. He suggests the combining of objectives to represent both disciplines. The primary objective in the school is to learn. The primary objective in nursing and medicine is to become healthy. Michal's combined objective is to help the child cope with life. Another suggestion to decrease communication problems is to clarify expectations and develop an awareness of the limitations in each discipline. Language differences can be minimized by avoiding foreign terminology and jargon. Michal recommends joint training sessions, team approaches to difficult students, and finally, school health conferences as methods to facilitate intraorganizational communication.

Media and public opinion

The fourth external organization that affects the focal nurse-client interaction is the media and public opinion. The term *media* is used as both a reflection and a maker of public opinion. Kalisch and Kalisch[31] conducted a study using a nationwide clipping service in 1978. They reviewed 3098 articles about nursing that appeared in the print media during that year. The researchers concluded that the quantity and quality of news about clinical nursing varied by specialty area. The majority of these articles were about community-health nurses, but the articles portrayed a stagnant image of nurses in this field. In contrast, psychiatric nurses had the lowest number of articles, but the articles portrayed a progressive role. The authors believe that through media, citizens can be informed and their opinion of nurses influenced. This function of media is particularly important for individuals who have no direct experiences with nurses in a particular field. The current image projected in the media is often that of a sympathetic caregiver. Although this is a positive image, nurses need to go beyond that and depict themselves as knowledgeable and accountable health care providers whose primary responsibility is the promotion of the client's health.

Kalisch and Kalisch[31] recommended ways to increase news coverage of nursing and to show the critical role that nurses play in health care. They suggested trend stories about clinical nursing. They also encouraged stories explaining longrange developments as well as daily events, such as a story on the changing role of the nurse. Their most important recommendation was for nurses to develop relationships with the media to inform the public of what they are doing, because public opinion is such a critical force in politics and organizational units. For example, if the nurse knows that child neglect and abuse is a problem in a particular area and that more funding is needed for this problem, working with the media to show what nursing is currently doing regarding this situation and what still needs to be done is important in influencing public opinion and gaining support.

Assessment of organizational communication

Components of organizational communication are directly related to job satisfaction. They are:

1. A positive communication atmosphere
2. Positive communication between staff nurses and supervisors
3. Feedback on job performance

Farley[17] outlines a method to assess the communication system of an organization by asking members to complete survey questionnaires. There are six aspects of the formal communication system that should be assessed, which are outlined in Table 5-3.

Farley cautions that when assessing communication, the staff must be aware of the purpose of the assessment and what will be done with the information collected to encourage staff participation. One aspect of assessment outlined in Table 5-3 is accessibility of information. The staff needs to know where to obtain information that is needed to do their jobs. Another aspect of accessibility is related to the ease of obtaining needed information.

Another area to assess is the availability of communication channels in the organization. The primary concern is the degree of congruence between the formal and informal communication systems as well as links in the formal channel. Survey questions would include items to determine how often and from whom organizational communication is received. Organizations have both explicit and implicit communication rules. When communication rules, both explicit and implicit, are observed, dissonance is reduced and stability is maintained. A third area to assess is the clarity of messages, both written and verbal. Concise, clear messages are more likely to be heard or read and remembered than are long, cumbersome messages. If messages are assessed by staff as being unclear, it is important to know precisely why they are difficult to understand.

Farley also recommends assessing the span of control or the number of people for whom a supervisor is directly responsible. There are advantages and disadvantages to both large and small spans of control; either can have communication problems. Assessment questions should reflect the staffs subjective feelings of satisfaction with the current span of control. Large spans are advocated when staffs are composed primarily of professionals reflecting autonomy.

A fifth area of assessment is flow control and communication load. "Flow control refers to the ability of managers to regulate the dissemination of a message to other employees. Communication load refers to the amount of information received by an

TABLE 5-3   Assessment of communication in organization

AREA	ASSESSMENT QUESTIONS
Accessibility of information	I have the information I need to do my job. I know where to obtain the information I need to do my job.
Availability of communication channels	I receive information about my job from _____. How often?
Clarity of messages	The communications I receive are clear and understandable. If not, why are they hard to understand?
Span of control	I am satisfied with the type of messages I received about my job. I am satisfied with the frequency of messages I receive.
Communication load	I receive sufficient information about things that are happening in the organization.
Communicator effectiveness	Administrators effectively communicate with employees. Administrators in this organization are good listeners.

Modified from Farley MJ: Assessing communication in orgranizations, *JONA* 19:27, 1989.

individual within a specified period of time."[17] There needs to be a balance between the amount of communication conveyed to the staff and the needs of the staff for information. When flow control is too low, the staff receives too much irrelevant information, which results in a communication overload.

The final area of assessment discussed by Farley is communication effectiveness. This refers to the individual's ability to accurately encode and decode information. It is highly dependent on the communicator's ability to actively listen. "Communicator effectiveness occurs when the outcome of a message can be accurately predicted and when recipients of messages feel satisfied with the communication."[17] Interpersonal competence has been shown to be one of the best predictors of organizational success. Assessment involves the staff's perception and feelings of satisfaction with current interpersonal communication.

Kennedy and Garvin[35] assessed the effectiveness of interpersonal (doctor-nurse) communication. The research results showed that 87% of the interactions were confirming. Confirming responses recognize the other person, are relevant, and are a direct response to another or express acceptance of another. Confirmation is a process of recognizing and endorsing another and contributes to the staff's perception of a positive communication atmosphere.

In summary, the term *context* was initially introduced to describe the physical setting, pattern organization, and fourth dimension of time in which nurse-client communication occurs. This term is expanded to include interorganizational and intraorganizational communication channels that can directly and indirectly influence the focal nurse-client communication process. Interorganizational and intraorganizational communication channels were discussed only in terms of their possible effect on nurse-client communications. In actuality these interorganizations and intraorganizations have the possibility of influencing each other, as well as the focal nurse-client relationship.

ACQUISITION OF COMMUNICATION SKILLS

The acquisition of communication skills is a topic of concern to all nursing educators. Eastwood[15]

found that communication skills were perceived by 80% of the nurses surveyed to be of at least equal importance to practical skills.

Although the findings of other studies indicated that students can learn communication skills, retention of skills was not demonstrated. Harrison et al.[27] examined the acquisition of communication skills in a sample of nursing students.

All students in one nursing school were the subjects. Subjects were asked to sort 100 statements into one of nine categories ranging from least characteristic to most characteristic. The statements described aspects of interpersonal communication. "Generally, students seemed to make gains in acquiring the therapeutic norms of sympathetic and egalitarian treatment of clients, and they perceived improvement in their verbal and nonverbal expressiveness."[27] On the negative side, older students perceived themselves as being less likely to listen carefully and more likely to disagree, interrupt, and criticize. Although the therapeutic communication skills can be learned, use of some of the skills declined over time.

Various methods are used to foster the development of therapeutic communication skills. Severtson[53] outlined a seminar course format to provide students with a "safe and supportive environment" to try out new communication strategies.

The learning activities at the end of each chapter of this book were formulated to assist in the development of the skills previously discussed. Regardless of the methods used, however, there are basic premises on which the development of communication skills depends.

Understanding the communication process

The individual needs to have an understanding of what therapeutic communication actually is— some definition of the process and the factors that affect the process. More specifically, the individual needs to be able to describe concrete behaviors associated with therapeutic communication. Theoretic discussions often are devoid of concrete representations; for instance, the nursing term *support* was used for years without an adequate description of behaviors reflective of support. Therapeutic communication can suffer in the same way unless it is defined concretely and behaviorally.

Self-assessment

The development of therapeutic communication skills involves self-assessment and self-growth. Just as it is necessary to have behavioral goals to know what the desired outcome is, it is also necessary to have an accurate assessment of the starting point. This necessitates the ability to look at the self critically in comparison with stated goals and to assess strengths and weaknesses.

Methods of skill acquisition

The third factor in the acquisition of therapeutic skills is the one most often discussed and that follows logically from the others. It is the ways or means of moving from the starting point to the desired end point. The reading of theoretic material on communication and various processes of skill acquisition is certainly not to be negated; however, as in the acquisition of any skill, some type of actual practice is necessary. The standard format for therapeutic communication skill acquisition typically consists of some reading, discussion, or lecture, followed by practice and then some form of assessment by self, others, or both. Keller[34] describes one program to help baccalaureate students develop communication skills. In this program first-semester nursing students interview hospitalized clients to assess their general health. In addition to this standard format other methodologies have been used, specifically role playing and videotaping. In the standard format the actual practice is left unsupervised. The nurse meets with the client and returns with information on what transpired. What has happened with the client is often clouded by the perceptions of the nurse, and there is a heavy reliance on the memory of the nurse. Even if videotapes or audiotapes are used, the nurse is not able to make changes in what has already been done. When nurses are given the opportunity to try out new skills in a controlled environment, practice with them, discuss them, and then make another attempt, the avenues for learning are increased. Role playing and videotaping offer these opportunities for exploration. The values of videotaping the role playing of various nurse-client interactions have been discussed in the literature.[10,29] Expense is listed as one of the major disadvantages. Role playing

alone, without video playbacks, gives the nurse an opportunity to try out skills; however, it is devoid of the feedback received when nurses see themselves in action.

Even if it is not practical to videotape all role playing of nurse-client interactions, a single videotaping session may be beneficial. Nontherapeutic verbalizations, mannerisms, facial expressions, and gestures that a nurse is unaware of may be evident during a single taping session. When similar nontherapeutic techniques are brought out by other nurses during role playing situations, the response tends to be more negative, accompanied by defending or explaining. However, often when the nurse is confronted with a playback of actual behaviors, no comment is necessary. Behavioral changes tend to be more rapid, because the need for change comes from within the individual. Hence videotaping, even when limited in use, can serve as an excellent learning and self-assessment tool.

Student-teacher relationship

There is a fourth factor in the acquisition of communication skills: the relationship between the student nurse and the nurse instructor. Karns and Schwab[32] reviewed literature on student-teacher communication and found that therapeutic communication skills are rarely applied in interactions with students. According to the authors there are several reasons why this situation exists. First, some teachers believe that good relationships with students lead to decreased student motivation and performance. Second, excellence in teaching is not rewarded, and third, the use of therapeutic communication techniques requires time and effort or increased involvement. Karns and Schwab contend that the characteristics of empathy, congruence (honesty), and positive regard (respect) that are so important in a therapeutic relationship actually enhance student learning. When the authors asked junior nursing students to list teacher behaviors that promote a positive relationship, 93% identified behaviors reflecting empathy, 65% identified behaviors indicating congruence, and 81% identified behaviors demonstrating positive regard. The students also listed instructor availability and teaching ability as behaviors promoting a positive relationship.

Fishel and Johnson[20] discuss another method to improve student-teacher communication. According to them, clinical supervision of students should include the nurse supervisor from the unit where the student is working. The authors state that diadic communication about triadic concerns can create problems. In some cases the student aligns with the nursing supervisor against the instructor or with the instructor against the nursing supervisor. This can be a problem, especially when the student is functioning below an acceptable level in the instructor's or the supervisor's opinion. The phases in the three-way conference parallel the phases in a therapeutic relationship. It serves not only to decrease conflict in the clinical area but also to increase the student's feeling of security. Obviously, it is necessary that the educator and supervisor have a good relationship, with a thorough understanding of the instructional goals and objectives and the defined role of the nurse.

Therapeutic communication skills need to be used by the instructor as a role model in relationships with students. They are not skills that are used exclusively in contacts with clients. The three-way conference is a good method for demonstrating to the student the practical use of a therapeutic relationship and communication skills. The focus is on a positive discussion of how the student can grow within the assigned clinical experience. During the conference the processes of evaluation, review, and feedback are used. Fishel and Johnson suggest the three-way conference in all areas where students are assigned to practice therapeutic communication skills. An additional benefit in using the three-way conference is decreased conflict between real work situations and academia. This conflict tends to increase with the educational preparation of the student; baccalaureate students demonstrate the greatest role stress.

Factors that handicap skill acquisition

Fielding and Llewelyn[18] warned that although there is evidence that communication training is needed and welcome, implementation of training programs without consideration of a number of critical issues can lead to partial or complete failure.

One of the major critical issues to be considered is whether the individual or the organization truly wants to improve communication. Since the days of Florence Nightingale, nursing leaders have called for improved communication skills. However, communication continues to be "one of the most demanding and difficult aspects of a nurse's job, and one which is frequently avoided or done badly although being central to the quality of patient care."[18]

Naish[46] believes that the environment must be supportive of nurse-client communication. Even though research has shown that time spent communicating with clients is cost-effective and improves the quality of care, evidence shows that communication time is often deleted first when an attempt is made to reduce costs.

According to Fielding and Llewelyn, several principal factors can handicap the effectiveness of communication training. First, administrative nursing tasks are often valued more than client interaction. Often the nurses who spend time communicating with clients are nursing students and nursing assistants rather than more senior nurses. A second factor is failing to understand that poor communication exists for a reason and actually serves a purpose. Clear communication can increase conflict or lead to confrontations and other unacceptable consequences. According to these authors, individuals in positions of authority may feel that they have more control if communication is kept "fuzzy." A third factor is cultural values, and Fielding and Llewelyn contend that there is a deep-seated cultural suspicion of communication, which is expressed in proverbs such as *Silence is golden* and *Actions speak louder than words.* Cultural values that are anticommunication would explain the continued need to improve communication skills.

CRITICAL THINKING *Question* ....

Jarrett and Payne[30] reviewed the literature on nurse-client communication. They concluded that researchers have neglected the role of the client in nurse-client communication. Do you agree? Why should this be an issue of concern? What should be the focus in research on nurse-client communication?

EVALUATION OF NURSE-CLIENT COMMUNICATION

In the assessment and evaluation of nurse-client communication three important questions need to be answered:

1. Who are the participants?
2. What are they saying?
3. Is their purpose being accomplished?

Some of the information necessary to answer these questions has been previously discussed in this chapter.

Who are the participants?

The importance of self-knowledge has been previously stated. This includes knowledge about strengths, weaknesses, and habitual ways of responding. In addition, the nurse needs knowledge about the client. A complete nursing assessment of the client will produce a more accurate description of the participants. However, the nurse and client are not isolated entities. Part of defining the participants is examining the context of the communication. Where is it occurring? What is the relationship between the participants, and at what time—defined broadly as earlier in this chapter—is it occurring?

What are they saying?

Essentially, this question asks for the meaning of the verbal and nonverbal messages of the participants. To attach meaning to their messages a number of factors that can influence communication must be considered. These include imitation, culture, and pattern organization. On the verbal level the importance of idioms and denotative and connotative meanings, as well as the difficulty in finding words to express thoughts and ideas, were discussed previously in this chapter. Therefore to answer the question, "What are they saying?" it is necessary to consider both the verbal and nonverbal levels of communication together with the host of factors that can affect specific meaning. In addition, the metacommunication of participants needs to be considered, as well as the congruency among all levels of communication and the patterns of communication used.

Is their purpose being accomplished?

The importance of having specific behavioral goals has been previously stated. When nurses evaluate

their own communication, it is done in terms of nursing goals. There are five criteria that can assist the nurse in evaluating communication: effectiveness, appropriateness, adequacy, efficiency, and flexibility.

Effectiveness is the overall general criterion. It determines how successful the communication is in meeting the goals of the interaction. Because it is often impossible to tell how effective a given interaction is in the present, the other four criteria can be used to predict effectiveness. If communication is appropriate, adequate, efficient, and flexible, it will usually be effective; the opposite is also true.

To determine effectiveness it is necessary to have preplanned behavioral goals against which to measure the behavioral outcomes of the interaction. If the nurse's goal is to teach Ms. P. about iron deficiency anemia and dietary treatment for it, specific client behaviors are needed that are indicative of accomplishing this goal. Examples of specific client behaviors are Ms. P. defining iron deficiency anemia, listing foods high in iron, planning a weekly menu using foods high in iron, eating foods high in iron three times a week, and so on.

The goal of the interaction may be more general; for example, it may be to establish a therapeutic nurse-client relationship. However, specific client behaviors are still needed to measure success. What are the behaviors indicative of a therapeutic nurse-client relationship that the nurse could use? Trust, discussed in Chapter 6, is one of the concepts associated with a working relationship. However, to say that the client will trust the nurse is still not sufficient. Specific client behaviors such as sharing confidential material are needed. Therefore measuring the effectiveness of communication requires a well-defined purpose and client behaviors that reflect the purpose or goal.

Thobaben[59] discusses specific concrete evaluation questions that can be used to determine whether a therapeutic relationship has been established. Some examples of the questions are: Is the time frame of the relationship explained? Is the client included when the goals are changed or met? Are the client's expectations clarified? The case study and care plans in Chapter 12 also show how to measure effectiveness with client behaviors.

A common problem in evaluating effectiveness is subjectivity—determining effectiveness based on feelings without considering behaviors. The following interaction demonstrates the potential error in subjective evaluation:

MS. G.: Mr. X., I am expecting an important telephone call from Mr. P., the social worker. I'm going to be in a staff meeting in room 3C until 1 o'clock. If Mr. P. calls, will you please tell him that I will call him back after 1 and ask him for a phone number where I can reach him this afternoon?

MR. X.: (Smiling) Certainly.

MS. G.: Thank you.

Ms. G. left this interaction feeling that her communication had been effective. Mr. X. had said he would take a message if the social worker called. At 1 o'clock Ms. G. returned to the office to ask Mr. X. if the social worker had called and where she might reach him.

MS. G.: Did Mr. P. call?

MR. X.: Yes, a while ago, but when I couldn't find you on the floor, I transferred the call to the page operator. She said she thought you had left for the day.

MS. G.: But I was in the staff meeting. . . .

If Ms. G.'s communication had been effective, as her subjective evaluation believed it was, Mr. X.'s behavior would have been quite different. He would have asked Mr. P. for a number where Ms. G. could reach him after 1 o'clock. Thus based on the behavioral outcome, the communication was not effective.

As stated previously, many times the behaviors to measure effectiveness are not apparent for hours, weeks, or sometimes years after the interaction. Therefore the nurse needs to examine appropriateness, adequacy, efficiency, and flexibility to predict the possible success or failure of the interaction.

Appropriateness refers to the relevancy of the communication in meeting the desired outcomes. It also takes into account the uniqueness of the participants and the context or time of the interaction. In the example of Ms. G., was the communication relevant to her goal of having a message delivered and taken by Mr. X.? Ms. G. did not include any unrelated facts in her communication; however, she did fail to respond to the fact that Mr. X. was talking on the phone while she was delivering her message and that he had been extremely busy all day because his co-worker was ill. Although Ms. G.'s communication

was appropriate to her goal, there is no evidence that this goal was shared by Mr. X. Because Mr. X. was busy it may have been more appropriate to write out the information in addition to telling it to him, thus leaving him with object, nonverbal communication to reinforce the verbal communication. Another possibility would have been to wait until Mr. X. had finished with his current task before asking him to take a message. Trying to arrive at a shared purpose for the communication would have also increased appropriateness. In retrospect, Ms. G.'s communication was appropriate to her goal but not to the receiver or the time.

Adequacy refers to the amount of communication used to reach the desired goal. Is there sufficient communication to accomplish the purpose? Has sufficient feedback been received, acknowledged, and accurately interpreted? Ms. G. told Mr. X. everything she expected him to do—to ask the social worker for a phone number where she could call him after 1 o'clock. (If she had only said, "Mr. X., I am expecting an important phone call from Mr. P. I'm going to be in a staff meeting in room 3C until 1 o'clock," and then later returned, expecting a telephone number to return Mr. P.'s call, the communication would have been inadequate.) In the area of feedback, however, the communication was inadequate. Ms. G. interpreted Mr. X.'s "Certainly" to mean "I have received and understood your message." She was making an unstated assumption. She needed additional feedback to validate her assumption that the message was received and accurately interpreted.

Efficient communication uses direct and simple language. Instructions are clear and agreed on. It uses the smallest amount of energy. Efficient communication is direct communication.[14] Ms. G.'s communication meets the criteria of efficiency. The following example demonstrates inefficient communication:

WIFE: Did you like the beef stew?

HUSBAND: It was OK; maybe less potatoes next time and a beef gravy instead of tomato sauce.

What the husband in this interaction wants to say is "I hate stew. Don't make it again." The communication is not efficient. It is not direct. He only implies his dislike and hopes or expects his wife to receive this covert message. He is wasting energy by trying to subtly communicate his true message. Inefficient communication often is incongruent on the verbal and nonverbal levels. For example, while the husband is verbally saying that he likes stew, his nonverbal communication, eating half of what he normally eats for dinner, is delivering the opposite message.

The last criterion for successful communication is *flexibility*. This refers to control versus permissiveness within the interaction.[14] Rigid approaches (exaggerated control) are not flexible. A good example of a rigid approach is the overuse of a history form or any type of interview format that is systematically adhered to by the nurse. The following interview demonstrates exaggerated control in communication:

NURSE: Have you ever had a venereal disease? Gonorrhea? Syphilis?
CLIENT: No.
NURSE: How many children do you have?
CLIENT: None.
NURSE: What type of birth control …?

Exaggerated control prevents the nurse from knowing the client as a unique person. The interaction becomes computerized, and the client is relegated to the role of an object. On the other hand, exaggerated permissiveness is often interpreted by the client as lack of interest or incompetency. When the nurse offers nothing of herself (no direction, thoughts, perceptions, or so on), the client feels as if he is speaking into a tape recorder.

The original question in evaluation asked whether the purpose of the participants was being accomplished; however, all of the preceding has referred to nursing goals. In the best situations the goals of nurse and client would be identical and mutually determined. There are, however, many instances in which the nurse and client do not have similar, or even compatible, goals. These situations can occur even when the client states goals similar to those of the nurse, as in the following instance:

Nurse J. enters Mr. P.'s room to provide routine morning care. Mr. P. states that he does not want any breakfast and does not feel like getting out of bed to take a shower. To regain his strength after surgery Mr. P. needs to eat, and he needs the activity that would accompany a shower.

What is the goal of Mr. P.'s communication? To be able to answer the question "Is their purpose being accomplished?" the nurse needs to identify Mr. P.'s goal. In this situation Mr. P.'s communication does not seem effective if his general goal is to recuperate quickly or to be discharged from the hospital.

Sloboda[55] contends that to understand the communication of a client, the nurse must analyze the client's self-concept, perceptions, and reactions to stress and loss. Although the client's communication may not seem to be effective in meeting the general goal of wellness—presupposed for all clients—it may be meeting some more pressing goal for this particular client at this point in time.

When a client is scheduled for any type of major surgery, the nurse expects some degree of apprehension. In the previous example Mr. P. told the nurses that his surgery didn't matter because he was old and useless anyway. His later refusal to eat and lack of daily physical care fit into the same pattern, indicative of his low self-concept. Such clients, who often are labeled as either depressed or uncooperative, are communicating quite effectively the message that they are worthless.

Just as the self-concept can influence communication, client's perceptions have an effect on their goals and resultant messages. Ms. X. perceived her stay in the hospital as a vacation from her job and three small children at home. Ms. X. was on a restricted diet, but the nurses constantly found the remains of forbidden foods in Ms. X.'s room. When confronted, she dismissed the situation as unimportant. Her goal was to extend her hospital stay as long as possible. Her communication was effective based on her perception of the situation.

The client's reaction to stress as discussed in Chapter 8 can also help the nurse to evaluate the client's communication. When the client's stress increases, the communication may function to decrease the stress state. For instance, Ms. T. came to the clinic for a routine physical. When she was told that she had a lump in her breast and needed surgery, she smiled and said nothing. She failed to make a return appointment and left as cheerfully as she had entered. The client's communication would not be considered effective in meeting a general goal of wellness. However, at that point in time the client was completely overwhelmed and communicated effectively the message "This is more than I can handle."

Reactions to loss can also help the nurse analyze the client's communication. Loss refers not only to death but also to loss of body parts and functions, independence, skills, or any type of physical, emotional, or intellectual loss whether real or perceived. Mr. Y. had recently had a stroke. When the nurse came into the room to assist him in eating breakfast, Mr. Y. told the nurse that breakfast was ruined by the nurse putting sugar in his tea, and he ordered the nurse to leave. The client's verbal abuse communicated effectively his anger resulting from a loss of independence, although by not allowing the nurse to help him eat, he was not meeting a general goal of wellness.

By examining clients' communication in terms of the individual goals, it is obvious that many times even if clients do have a general goal of wellness, other needs and goals at a particular time may be more important. They may need to deal with increased stress or a loss, or their communication may be influenced by self-esteem and perceptions that at this time may be more important than the general goal of wellness.

The preceding analysis is based on the effectiveness of the communication process in accomplishing behavioral goals with a client. Approaching evaluation from another direction, Topf[60] has listed eight areas of communication, each containing ineffective and effective behaviors. The nurse can use this list to check those behaviors that are found in each client interaction to determine areas of weakness and

Criteria for Evaluating Nurse-Client Communication

1. Effectiveness
   Does this communication meet the goals of the interaction?
2. Appropriateness
   Is this communication relevant to the stated goals?
3. Adequacy
   Is there sufficient communication and feedback to meet the stated goals?
4. Efficiency
   Does this communication use the minimum amount of energy necessary to meet the goals?
5. Flexibility
   Is there an appropriate balance between control and permissiveness in the interaction?

strength. The eight areas outlined by Topf are initiating the interaction, questioning, listening, observation, problem solving, interpretation of the interaction, evaluation of the interaction, and recording of the interaction. According to Topf, behaviors that are useful in evaluating the interaction include identifying not only the nurse's strengths but also weaknesses, examining not only the nurse's role within the interaction but also that of the client, formulating goals for the client, and formulating goals to improve the skills of the nurse. Chapter 12 gives further examples of analyzing the nurse-client communication using these effective behaviors.

SUMMARY

Communication that fosters mutuality in the nurse-client relationship is therapeutic. One of the most important therapeutic communication techniques is listening. Numerous other therapeutic techniques are also important in the course of the helping relationship. In contrast, communication that hinders relationship formation is nontherapeutic. It is important to examine the function that nontherapeutic communication serves in the relationship.

When the verbal channels of communication are unavailable or inadequate, the nurse needs to rely more on the nonverbal messages of self and client. Special communication problems, characterized by the inadequacy of normal communications channels, are presented by the client who does not speak the same language, the aphasic client, the sensory impaired client, the noncommunicative client, and the child client.

Structured communication is a special form of communication. It is defined in terms of definite, planned content that the nurse wants to transfer to another person or group. Three forms of structured communication are included in this chapter: health education, oral reports, and written reports.

Although the nurse-client communication is the focus, it does not occur in a vacuum. There are many interorganizational and intraorganizational communication channels that can influence the nurse and client. They can have both a direct and an indirect effect on the focal nurse-client relationship.

In the development of communication skills, four basic premises are outlined. They are the need for behavioral outcomes reflective of therapeutic communication, self-assessment, methodologies useful in the acquisition of communication skills, and the instructor-student relationship.

Last in the process of communication is evaluation of the nurse-client interaction. Using all of the information presented regarding why and how communication occurs, an attempt is made to critically analyze communication to assess areas of weakness and strength. Three important questions need to be answered:

1. Who are the participants?
2. What are they saying?
3. Is their purpose being accomplished?

The importance of communication in nursing, as in any helping profession, cannot be overly stressed. It is only through open and honest communication that participants can share their inner feelings and thoughts. It is only through communication that relationships are born and human beings are able to help their fellow human beings.

DISCUSSION QUESTIONS

1. Analyze a recent interaction and identify therapeutic and nontherapeutic techniques used. Identify those that you use the most and those that you feel most comfortable using. Explore your own feelings regarding specific techniques that you constantly use and those that you tend to avoid.

2. Analyze a recent process recording, selecting general factors that enhanced or hindered the communication.

3. Plan alternative communication channels to use with an uncommunicative client and a client who speaks only a foreign language.

4. Outline five behaviors indicative of various feelings in children of different age groups. Read about or observe children in these age groups and try to identify other behaviors not originally included that are representative of the same feelings.

5. Make a list of the positive and negative features of both structured and unstructured communication. For each negative characteristic try to identify nursing actions that would minimize or remove this negative characteristic.

6. Take a written report and plan the changes that would be necessary for it to be used as an oral report.

7. Compare and contrast the writing style of an author in a research journal, a newspaper article, and a popular novel.

8. Describe the interorganizational and intraorganizational communication patterns that can affect your communication with a specific client. Discuss how the included organizations can affect each other.

9. Develop a survey to assess communication in a familiar organization.

10. Identify one current nursing event that you believe deserves media attention. How would you proceed to obtain media coverage? Write the story.

11. Identify current legislation that affects nursing that you believe needs to be changed. Discuss ways of changing this law.

12. Identify three ways to improve your own communication.

EXPERIENTIAL & SIMULATED LEARNING EXERCISES

1. Validating

PURPOSE: To check to be sure of a clear understanding of another person's ideas, information, or suggestions.

PROCEDURE: Ask two students to volunteer to role play a short dialogue. Each student should only read his own part. They should *not* know the description of the other student's role.

SITUATION I

Student 1: He or she has seen student 2 cheating on an examination. He or she decided to talk to student 2 about it but wants to do it tactfully.

Student 2: He or she knows student 1 wants to talk about a fellow classmate cheating on examinations.

SITUATION II

Student 1: The student should play the role of a college football player who has come to talk to his coach. He talks about a fellow student on the team who has a drug problem. He is really talking about himself but doesn't want to admit it.

Student 2: The student should play the role of the college football coach who is talking to one of his players but is really preoccupied with practice, team schedules, and so on.

DISCUSSION: After a short role-playing period (5 to 10 minutes) ask the group to critique the actors for validation. After a thorough group discussion ask for two more student volunteers to role play either the same situation or the unused situation, making a conscious effort to validate. Following the second role play ask the group to discuss the ways in which the interaction changed when the participants were actively engaged in validation.

DISCUSSION: Allow group members to describe their perceptions of:

1. How they presented the feelings.
2. How they perceived others were reacting.
3. How the other students did react.
4. How different students attempted to communicate the same feelings.

2. Analysis of communication skills number 1

PURPOSE: To provide experience in the use of communication skills and to use group effort to improve the communication process.

PROCEDURE: Prepare a list of client profiles. For instance, Ms. D. is a 35-year-old female who came to the clinic because of amenorrhea. She has five children, ages 2, 4, 6, 8, and 14. When she was told she was pregnant, she began to cry. In large classes the students can be divided into small groups. Ask for a volunteer to play the role of the client and another to play the role of the nurse. They should read aloud the client profile to the group to set the stage for the interaction. The student playing the role of nurse can be instructed to be as nontherapeutic as possible. Such instructions often decrease the anxiety associated with being expected to perform "right." After the initial role playing the group should make suggestions to improve the nurse's communication, and then the same or different participants can replay the situation with recommendations of the group being interjected as role playing proceeds. This can be repeated until all members of the group have had an opportunity to play nurse or client roles.

DISCUSSION: This is a good activity to videotape when facilities are available. The video playback can be used so that all students can make recommendations for improving the nurse's communication. The students should be encouraged to provide open feedback in a supportive environment with attention given to strengths and weaknesses.

3. Analysis of communication skills number 2

PURPOSE: To identify and analyze the various components of the communication process and to gain an awareness of the effectiveness of communication skills.

PROCEDURE: Select a two- or three-page nurse-client interaction from any source, or write one that incorporates special problems that the majority of students are encountering or fear to encounter. Allow the students to work in small groups with a recorder assigned to critique the interaction. Instruct the students to identify patterns of communication, techniques used, and general factors that enhance or hinder the communication. The students should also be asked to analyze the effectiveness of the communication and to identify ways to improve the communication. The recorders in small groups should report their group's decisions to the total class.

DISCUSSION: Class members should compare the experiences of the various groups and compile a list of effective and noneffective communication techniques. The discussion may also be focused on the interaction that took place within the group.

4. Editing written reports

PURPOSE: To stress the importance of editing written work and to give the student an opportunity to edit a written report.

PROCEDURE: Ask each student to write a brief case presentation (allow only 5 to 10 minutes) and ask them to make as many structural errors as possible. Have the students exchange reports and edit another person's report.

DISCUSSION: Permit editor and author to discuss the written reports with each other to see if they were able to identify all the intended errors.

5. Listening skills

PURPOSE: To develop listening/attending skills

PROCEDURE: Ask the students to number a paper from 1 to 10. Instruct the students that this is a listening task and that each item will be read only one time. At a steady rate read a series of instructions such as those that follow. Make the items as simple or as difficult as needed depending on the listening skills of the students. External distractors, such as loud noises, music, people entering and leaving the room, the speaker turning away from the listeners, and so on, can also be added.

The following is a list of sample instructions:

"Number 1. Draw a square in a circle on line 10 if you have blonde hair.

Number 2. On line 7 draw two sets of parallel lines that intersect.

Number 3. Write the 5th and 25th letters of the alphabet.

Number 4. If line one is blank, draw a circle in a square, if not draw a diamond on line 6.

Number 5. Write three ways to make change for a dime.

Number 6. If you live east of the Mississippi River, write a zero on line 9."

DISCUSSION: The discussion following this exercise should include the nature of listening skills and attention as well as factors that facilitate and hinder listening. Ask the students to develop their own set of instructions to read to their peers.

REFERENCES

1. Allen H: "Voices of concern": a study of verbal communication about patients in a psychiatric day unit, *J Adv Nurs* 6:355, 1981.
2. Reference deleted in proofs.
3. Ballinger P: An attempt to break down barriers, *Nurs Times* 92:29, 1996.
4. Bara M, Rugg M: Assertive communication for effective leadership, *Can Nurse* 85:9, 1989.
4a. Berne E: Games people play: the psychology of human relationships, New York, 1964, Grove Press.
5. Bourhis RY, Roth H, MacQueen G: Communication in the hospital setting: a survey of medical and everyday language use amongst patients, nurses and doctors, *Soc Sci Med* 28:339, 1989.
6. Bradley JC, Edinberg MA: *Communication in the nursing context*, ed 3, Norwalk, Conn, 1990, Appleton and Lange.
7. Braverman BG: Eliciting assessment data from the patient who is difficult to interview, *Nurs Clin North Am* 25:743, 1990.
8. Brosnan S: Communicating with the non-English speaking patient, *J Pract Nurs* 28:16, 1978.
9. Brown C, Keller P: *Monologue to dialogue: an exploration of interpersonal communication*, Englewood Cliffs, NJ, 1973, Prentice-Hall.
10. Carpenter K, Kroth J: Effects of videotaped role playing on nurses' therapeutic communication skills, *J Contin Educ Nurs* 7:47, 1976.
11. Chovaz C: Nursing the hearing impaired patient, *Can Nurse* 85:34, 1989.
12. Clark C: *Assertive skills for nurses*, Wakefield, Mass, 1978, Contemporary.
13. Cushing M: Failure to communicate, *Am J Nurs* 82:1597, 1982.
14. Davis A: The skills of communication, *Am J Nurs* 63:40, 1963.
15. Eastwood CM: The role of communication in nursing—perceptual variations in student/teacher responses in Northern Ireland, *J Adv Nurs* 10:245, 1985.
16. Elmassian BJ: A practical approach to communication with children through play, *MCN* 4:238, 1979.
17. Farley MJ: Assessing communication in organizations, *JONA* 19:27, 1989.
18. Fielding RG, Llewelyn SP: Communication training in nursing may damage your health and enthusiasm: some warnings, *J Adv Nurs* 12:281, 1987.
19. Fiesta J: Assessment and communication, *Nurs Manag* 25:14, 1994.
20. Fishel AH, Johnson GA: The three way conference: nursing student, nursing supervisor and nursing educator, *J Nurs Educ* 20:18, 1981.
21. Friedland GM: Learning behaviors of a preadolescent with diabetes, *Am J Nurs* 76:59, 1976.
22. Fritz PA et al: *Interpersonal communication in nursing: an interactionist approach*, Norwalk, Conn, 1984, Appleton-Century-Crofts.
23. Fulton K: Acknowledgment supports effective communication, *J Nurs Lead Manag* 12:37, 1981.
24. Fulton M et al: Helping diabetics adapt to failing vision, *Am J Nurs* 74:54, 1974.
25. Garvin BJ, Kennedy CW: Interpersonal communication between nurse and patients, *Annu Rev Nurs Res* 8:213, 1990.
26. Gross M: *The brain watchers*, New York, 1962, Random House.
27. Harrison TM, Pistolessi TV, Stephen TD: Assessing nurses' communication: a cross-sectional study, *West J Nurs Res* 11:75, 1989.
28. Hatfield B: Quality circles in nursing, *Hosp Top* 60:40, 1982.
29. Iverson SM: Microcounseling: a model for teaching the skills of interviewing, *J Nurs Educ* 17:12, 1978.
30. Jarrett N, Payne S: A selective review of the literature on nurse-patient communication: has the patient's contribution been neglected? *J Adv Nurs* 22:72, 1995.
31. Kalisch BJ, Kalisch PA: Communicating clinical nursing issues through the newspaper, *Nurs Res* 30:132, 1981.
32. Karns BJ, Schwab TA: Therapeutic communication and clinical instruction, *Nurs Outlook* 30:39, 1982.
33. Kay M et al: *Southwestern medical dictionary*, Tucson, 1977, University of Arizona Press.
34. Keller KL: Curriculum redesign to improve psychosocial assessment skills of first semester baccalaureate nursing students, *J Nurs Educ* 26:81, 1987.
35. Kennedy CW, Garvin BJ: Nurse-physician communication, *Appl Nurs Res* 1:122, 1988.
36. Kepler TL: Mastering the people skills, *J Nurs Adm* 10:15, 1980.
37. Kesler AR: Pitfalls to avoid in interviewing outpatients, *Nursing* 7:70, 1977.

38. Knight I: Communication methods, *Nurs Times* 73:11, 1976.
39. Kron T: *Communication in nursing,* ed 2, Philadelphia, 1972, WB Saunders.
40. Lancaster J: Communication: the anatomy of messages, *Nurs Manag* 14:42, 1983.
41. Leech T: *How to prepare, stage and deliver winning presentations,* New York, 1982, American Management Association.
42. Lesikar R: *Business communication: theory and application,* ed 3, Chicago, 1976, Richard D Irwin.
43. Mast DL: Selecting and implementing supplementary communication systems. In Sharks SJ, editor: *Nursing and the management of adult communication disorders,* San Diego, 1983, College Hill Press.
44. Michal ML: Physicians and educators: how can we better communicate? *J Sch Health* 51:575, 1981.
45. Miller P, Pastorino C: Daily nursing documentation can be quick and thorough, *Nurs Manag* 21:47, 1990.
46. Naish J: The route to effective nurse-patient communication, *Nurs Times* 92:27, 1996.
47. Nowell G: Communication and conflict between unit managers and nurses, *Hosp Top* 60:40, 1982.
48. O'Brien MJ: *Communications and relationships in nursing,* ed 2, St Louis, 1978, Mosby.
49. Parry J: *The psychology of human communication,* New York, 1968, American Elsevier.
50. Phippen ML: Winning through communication, *AORN* 34:1043, 1981.
51. Regan WA, editor: Charting: M.D./R.N. communication errors, *Regan Rep Nurs Law* 20:1, 1979.
52. Schweer SF, Dayani EC: The extended role of professional nursing: patient education, *Int Nurs Rev* 20:174, 1973.
53. Severtsen BM: Therapeutic communication demystified, *J Nurs Educ* 29:190, 1990.
54. Sherman K: *Communication and image in nursing,* Albany, NY, 1994, Delmar.
55. Sloboda S: Understanding patient behavior, *Nursing* 7:74, 1977.
56. Smith S: *Communications in nursing,* ed 2, St Louis, 1992, Mosby.
57. Stollack GE: Learning to communicate with children, *Child Today* 42:12, 1975.
58. Sullivan H: *The psychiatric interview,* New York, 1954, WW Norton.
59. Thobaben M: Evaluation of the therapeutic nurse-patient relationship, *Home Healthcare Nurse* 9:46, 1991.
60. Topf M: A behavior checklist for estimating the development of communication skills, *J Nurs Educ* 8:29, 1969.
61. Reference deleted in proofs.
62. Van Dersal W: How to be a good communicator—and a better nurse, *Nursing* 4:58, 1974.
63. Williams J: Meaningful dialogue, *Nurs Times* 87:52, 1991.

Suggested Readings

Dixon E, Park R: Do patients understand written health information? *Nurs Outlook* 38:278, 1990.

In this article the authors analyze the reading difficulty levels and overall comprehensibility of client-education materials provided in one Midwestern hospital. Their analysis of the reading materials showed the information to be difficult to comprehend not only for the poorly educated but the general public as well.

Grasska MA, McFarland T: Overcoming the language barrier: problems and solutions, *Am J Nurs* 82:1376, 1982.

Intrinsic and extrinsic problems associated with the use of an interpreter are followed by helpful advice from a medical interpreter.

Johnson MH, Zone JB: Concentrating on the process of learning while teaching clearly defined communication skills, *J Nurs Educ* 20:3, 1981.

One method used to make abstract communication skills more concrete is explained, including the objectives and assessment tools used. Also includes a breakdown of communication skills into levels from level 0, nontherapeutic, to level 4, therapeutic intervention.

Rotter DL, Hall JA, Katz NR: Patient-physician communication: descriptive summary of the literature, *Patient Ed Counsel* 12:99, 1988.

This article is a summary of 61 research studies of patient and physician communication. From these studies the authors identify six mutually exclusive categories of communication: information giving, information seeking, social talk, positive talk, negative talk, and partnership building. An appendix describes the specific variables included in each category.

Stetler C: Relationship of perceived empathy to nurses' communication, *Nurs Res* 26:432, 1977.

An exploratory study used 32 registered nurses in a simulated encounter with an ill client-actress. The results of this study favor the possibility that when communication is incongruent, the verbal level plays the weakest role in the client's perception of empathic characteristics of the nurse.

Stollack GE: Learning to communicate with children, *Child Today* 4:12, 1975.

This article discusses the use of free play in working with children. It is a good source for anyone desiring to establish a training program.

Tilden V, Porter K: Manifest and latent content in communication: genesis of an instructional module in psychiatric nursing, *J Nurs Educ* 17:11, 1978.

This article tells how to sensitize students to identify and respond therapeutically to latent content.

Wurzell C: Putting communication skills into practice, *AORN* 33:962, 1981.

A discussion of seven major areas of nonverbal communication that stresses two key elements in communication: listening and understanding.

CHAPTER

6 The Nurse-Client Relationship: Theoretic Concepts

• • • • • • • • • • • • • • •

Now, When I have overcome my fears—of
*   others, of myself, of the*
underlying darkness:
*   at the frontier of the unheard-of.*
*   Here ends the known. But, from a source*
*   beyond it, something fills my being*
*   with its possibilities.*
*   Here desire is purified and made lucid: each*
*   action is preparation for,*
*   each choice an assent to the unknown.*
*   Prevented from the duties of life on the surface*
*   from looking down into the depths,*
*   yet all the while being slowly trained*
*   and molded by them to take the*
*   plunge into the deep whence rises the*
*   fragrance of a forest star, bearing*
*   the-promise of a new affection.*
At the frontier—

Dag Hammarskjöld
Markings*

LEARNING OBJECTIVES

After studying this chapter, the student should be able to:

• Describe the helping relationship.
• Explore her own value system through the application of the values clarification process.
• Identify client behaviors that indicate lack of trust.
• Identify nurse behaviors that are conducive to the development of a trusting relationship.
• Describe the process of empathy.
• Compare and contrast empathy and sympathy.

---

*From Hammarskjöld D: *Markings*. Translated by Sjoberg L, Auden WH, New York, 1964, Alfred A Knopf.

• Assess her own responses to clients according to Kalisch's empathic function scale.
• Analyze the expression of caring in a nurse-client relationship.
• Compare and contrast caring in a professional and a social context.
• Identify the use of touch as a positive nursing intervention.
• Analyze the influence of hope on the helping relationship.
• Discuss the interrelationship between autonomy and mutuality as expressed in the helping relationship.
• Analyze the impact of paternalism on the client's expression of autonomy.
• Describe the advocacy role of the nurse.
• Foster the development of mutuality in the nurse-client relationship.

The interpersonal relationship is the vehicle for the application of the nursing process. From the time the nurse and client first meet and throughout their contacts, progress in relating to each other will be reflected in the degree of accomplishment of the nursing care goals. The nurse must therefore be able to use knowledge of communication theories and of the development of self to facilitate the growth of the helping relationship.

THE HELPING RELATIONSHIP

Rogers has defined the helping relationship as one "in which at least one of the parties has the intent of promoting the growth, development, maturity, improved functioning and improved coping with the life of the other."* These same terms could be used to describe the focus of nursing intervention. In a similar vein, King[18] has noted the importance of interpersonal relationships to the practice of nursing. She views nurse-client relationships as "learning experiences whereby two people interact to face an immediate health problem, to share, if possible, in resolving it and to discover ways to adapt to the situation."

Both of these definitions emphasize positive outcomes of growth, improvement, learning, coping, and adaptation. This should certainly be true for the client while participating actively in health care. The nurse can also benefit from the interpersonal relationship and should continue to grow as a professional and an individual.

The nurse-client relationship

The focus on the nurse-client relationship has occurred as the nursing profession has matured. As nursing theorists have developed philosophies and theories of nursing, the importance of the interpersonal relationship has become apparent. At the same time, as nurses have become more skilled at using the nurse-client relationship to enhance the care they provide, the health care system has been shifting toward shorter episodes of care. This is particularly so in hospitals, where the largest number of nurses have contact with clients. In this context it is important for the nurse to be able to interact effectively with the client. Mastery of interpersonal skills is critical for successfully providing nursing care. Even brief relationships can be meaningful events in a person's life.

The dimensions of the therapeutic relationship have been explored by Truax and Carkhuff.[38] Their research investigated the areas of accurate empathy, nonpossessive warmth, and genuineness, as originally identified by Rogers. They found that these behaviors occur consistently in observations of effective therapists and counselors. Aiken and Aiken[1] have also considered the essential features of positive interpersonal relationships and they give greatest emphasis to the need for "empathic understanding." In addition, they identify dimensions of "positive regard, genuineness and concreteness or specificity of expression." They also mention "appropriate levels of self-disclosure, spontaneity, confidence, intensity, openness, flexibility and commitment" as important but less well-defined components of caring.

Another study focused on the occurrence of exclusion in the nurse-client relationship. Anderson[2] describes this as the opposite of creative, humanistic nursing and as "depersonalization made concrete." When the client is excluded, the client is treated as an object. Exclusion commonly takes place when two or more nurses are caring for a client simultaneously. There is a tendency to relate to the other caregiver. Several nurses noted that it required a conscious effort to direct attention to the client when a peer was present. This information emphasizes the need for the nurse to strive for self-awareness to avoid placing her own needs before those of the client.

Anderson also found that emotional distancing was the primary factor that caused patients to feel excluded.[3] The components of emotional distancing include "facial expression, tone of voice, verbal style, use of silence, use of eyes, and use of touch." Behaviors related to this might be lack of eye contact, talking past the person, content contradictory to the person's own experience, silence, and a negative affect in response to the person.

Knowing the client is essential for participating in a successful nurse-client relationship. Tanner et al.[34] explored the meaning of "knowing" clients for nurses who worked in critical care units. They identified two dimensions of knowing:
1. Knowing the person's typical pattern of responding
2. Knowing the client as a person

They found that knowing the client is the foundation for skilled clinical judgment and allows the nurse to become an advocate for the client. To know a client in this way, the nurse must be involved with the patient in a caring relationship.

Characteristics of the helping relationship

An extremely helpful guide to the characteristics of the helping relationship is the series of questions asked by Carl Rogers:
1. Can I *be* in some way which will be perceived by the other person as trustworthy, as dependable, or consistent in some deep sense?

---

2. Can I be expressive enough as a person that what I am will be communicated unambiguously?

3. Can I let myself experience positive attitudes toward this other person—attitudes of warmth, caring, liking, interest, respect?

4. Can I be strong enough as a person to be separate from the other?

5. Am I secure enough within myself to permit him his separateness?

6. Can I let myself enter fully into the world of his feelings and personal meaning and see these as he does?

7. Can I be acceptant of each facet of a client which he presents to me? Can I receive him as he is? Can I communicate this attitude? Or can I only receive him conditionally, acceptant of some aspects of his feelings and silently or openly disapproving of others?

8. Can I act with sufficient sensitivity in the relationship that my behavior will not be perceived as a threat?

9. Can I free him from the threat of external evaluation?

10. Can I meet this other individual as a person who is in the process of *becoming*, or will I be bound by his past and by my past?*

These questions place the responsibility for the progress of the relationship with the helping person. They involve the need to be open and honest with oneself. In addition, the focus is on the client's needs and response to the relationship. Roger's frame of reference is compatible with that of the nurse-client relationship.

Values clarification

To be able to respond to the questions asked by Rogers the nurse must develop a high level of self-awareness. In addition to the aspects of self-awareness described in Chapter 3, one must be in touch with and act consistently with one's values. An individual's value system represents personal beliefs and attitudes about the worth of anything from a concrete object to an abstract concept. Uustal[40] adds that "values are general guides to

behavior, standards of conduct that one endorses and tries to live up to or maintain." Some values may be identified easily with little conflict; for instance, most nurses would agree that it is important (highly valued) to provide good skin care for a client who is in traction. Other values may lead to high levels of conflict and be difficult for the nurse to describe or, at times, even identify. Such values often include moral and ethical considerations. For example, it requires a great deal of self-examination to analyze one's own values regarding death. One must consider such questions as: Does a person have a right to decide when to die? Is this right affected by the person's age? Is it affected by the person's physical condition? Is it affected by the person's emotional state? There are many more questions that could be asked related to this complex issue, and this is only one of the many issues that must be explored by the nurse to be able to relate to a client openly. The nurse's lack of understanding of her own value system may result in her unknowingly imposing personal values on the client.

The nurse must also be aware of the relationship between perceptions and values. The process of perceiving is based on the person's value system. Therefore others may have different perceptions than ours, because they are founded on different values. For instance, people who base their values on a fundamentalist religious belief may perceive human immunodeficiency virus (HIV) infection as punishment for the sinful behaviors of homosexuality or drug abuse. Others who base their values on scientific findings may perceive HIV as a viral infection resulting from certain high-risk behaviors. The response of a nurse to a patient with HIV infection would depend on one's own value system unless it could be put aside to meet the nursing needs of the patient.

Hawks[14] cautions that nurses need to approach the giving of moral advice with great care. Professional knowledge needs to be clearly separated from personal values and presented as such. People have a tendency to place great faith in any advice given by a professional person. Therefore nurses must be sure that information is accurate and that the person retains responsibility for making his own decisions.

---

*From *On Becoming a Person*, by Carl R Rogers. Copyright © 1961 by Carl R Rogers. Used by permission of Houghton Mifflin Co.

Understanding one's own value system may be achieved by applying the process of values clarification. This process was developed for educators by Raths et al.,[27] later expanded by Simon et al.,[30] and adapted to nursing by Uustal.[40] As described by Raths et al.,[27] the valuing process involves three major activities: *prizing* and *choosing* beliefs and behaviors, and *acting* on beliefs. These are subdivided into seven steps as follows:

- **Prizing:** (1) prizing and cherishing and (2) publicly affirming when appropriate
- **Choosing:** (3) choosing from alternatives, (4) choosing after consideration of consequences, and (5) choosing freely
- **Acting:** (6) acting and (7) acting with a pattern, consistency, and repetition.[27]

In addition to using the values clarification steps for self-understanding, it can also be a useful tool to help clients develop greater self-awareness. It can be particularly useful in helping a client make a difficult decision, as demonstrated in the Clinical Example below.

The nursing student in this situation effectively used values clarification theory. She was aware of the unsettled nature of her own values but did not impose her conflicting feelings on Nancy. She assisted Nancy to identify the beliefs and behaviors that she prized and to list the alternatives available. She then directed Nancy toward completing the process for herself by choosing the best alternative for her and acting on that decision. Ms. P. avoided the temptation to try to influence Nancy toward the decision that she thought was best, even though that had been Nancy's original request.

Knowing and understanding the process of valuing as well as personal use of values clarification by the nurse contribute to critical thinking. To be consistently effective, decisions related to nursing intervention must be based on sound theory. Intuitive or trial-and-error nursing intervention may happen to be effective at times, but consistent therapeutic nursing intervention should be the goal of the professional nurse. This need for a sound theoretic rationale for nursing action is as important in the interpersonal aspects of nursing as it is in physiologic intervention.

In this chapter several basic theoretic concepts related to the nurse-client relationship are considered. An attempt is made to present the viewpoints of several nursing theorists, as well as theorists from other disciplines who have been engaged in examining the various aspects of helping relationships. Concepts explored include trust, empathy, caring, hope, autonomy, and mutuality.

 CLINICAL EXAMPLE

Ms. P., *a senior nursing student, volunteered one evening a week at a church-sponsored teen center in her neighborhood. She was approached by Nancy, a 16-year-old who was an active participant in the center. Nancy asked to talk with Ms. P. alone. She seemed anxious and after several minutes of superficial talk revealed that she had become sexually involved with her boyfriend, David. She was now pregnant and afraid to tell her parents. She wanted to tell David but was concerned that he would reject her. She felt great pressure to decide what to do, because she knew that abortion would be an option for only a limited time. She asked Ms. P. how she should resolve this problem.*

As a nursing student, Ms. P. had been struggling with clarifying her own values about unmarried parents and alternatives to childbirth. She was aware that this was an issue she had not fully resolved for herself yet believed that she needed to help Nancy. She told Nancy that she could understand some of her conflict because of her own difficulty in clarifying her feelings. However, she offered to help her look at the alternatives and her feelings about them. They then analyzed the situation in terms of several important factors, including Nancy's feelings toward herself, the baby, her parents, and David; her present life situation and future goals; and her religious beliefs. They listed and discussed each of Nancy's options related to her pregnancy. No decision was reached by the end of the discussion. However, Nancy told Ms. P. that she understood herself and her alternatives better and had decided that she needed input from her parents and David before making up her own mind about how to proceed.

CONCEPT OF TRUST

2.

The evolution of basic trust has been described by Erikson as an essential element of a successful mother-child relationship and the first task in personality development (see Chapter 2). The relationship between mother and child is in many ways reflected in the relationship between nurse and client. Generally a person is helped through the first experiences with illness by the mother, who responds with comforting and caring actions that help the child cope with discomfort. Nurses use many of these same comforting actions when providing nursing care. An important influence on this behavior by the nurse is the cultural expectation of how a caregiver should behave. The focus of nursing has broadened from the traditional role of providing bedside care to the acutely ill to encompass preventive health care in the community. However, the mothering role has continued to be incorporated into the nursing role. Community health nurses are frequently asked for practical advice and are looked to for comfort in times of crisis.

Reciprocally, the client tends to assume a more childlike or dependent role when receiving health care. Particularly when ill, the individual tends to regress or behave in a manner typical of an earlier developmental stage. This mental mechanism helps the person cope with illness and accept the care that is necessary for health to be regained.

Trust in the nurse-client relationship

If this reciprocal nurse-client relationship is to work effectively, it, like the mother-child relationship must be based on trust. The nurse must therefore become skilled in fostering the development of trust in a relationship.

In the context of the helping relationship, Travelbee[37] has defined *trust* as "the assured belief that other individuals are capable of assisting in times of distress and will probably do so." The quality described by Truax and Carkhuff[38] as *genuineness* is also related to trust in the sense that it describes the person's ability to be authentic and open in a relationship. They describe several levels of genuineness, ranging from a low level, where the helping person is defensive and tries to present a facade, to a high level, characterized by self-congruence, where the helper feels free to be sincere and open in the expression of feelings. They note that the helper is not required to express all feelings to be genuine, but feelings that are expressed should be real. When the client perceives that the helping person is relating genuinely, the client develops a sense of trust that the person will be consistently open and honest.

An attitude of trust is based on past experience. Some people have had experiences that have taught them not to trust. One such person is described in the Clinical Example below.

Johnny had been raised in an environment where there was little reason to trust. He did not have close, stable relationships with his parents, and life offered him little in terms of recreation or creative outlets. The struggles of his parents would not lead him to expect great improvement in the future. When Ms. R. encouraged Johnny to risk seeking help for his

CLINICAL EXAMPLE

Johnny J. was a 14-year-old youth who had always lived in a poor neighborhood. Both of his parents worked long hours to try to provide for their seven children. As a result they had little time or energy for getting to know the children as individuals. The children's guidance and supervision were left to a series of neighbors. Johnny spent most of his time "hanging out" with a gang of older boys in a local park.

Ms. R., a community health nurse, was visiting Ms. G., the neighbor who looked after the J. children. Ms. G. asked her to look at Johnny, who was in bed that day with an upset stomach. Ms. R. noted needle marks in Johnny's arm and signs of drug withdrawal. She spoke with him alone for a few minutes, urging him to accompany her to a drug-abuse center three blocks away. Johnny's response was that he was sure the center would report him to the police, and he refused to accept the nurse's assurances of the trustworthiness of the clinic staff. On her next visit to the G.'s, Ms. R. asked about Johnny. She was told that he had recovered soon after a friend had dropped by to see him and that he was again hanging out in the park.

drug problem, his past experience led him to reject that risk.

Sometimes health professionals encounter clients who are generally trusting people but who have a sense of mistrust directed toward the health care system. This may result from lack of previous experience with health care or traumatic past experiences. It is important to keep in mind that no one is completely trusting in a new situation with a new person. It is necessary to build trust with every new client and family. Past experience only influences the tendency of a person to develop trust in a relationship. It is also necessary to remember that trust is reciprocal, and the nurse also grows to trust the client as the relationship progresses.

Characteristics of the trusting person

Several characteristics of the trusting person have been identified by Thomas.[35] They include a feeling of comfort with growth in self-awareness and an ability to share this awareness with others; acceptance of others as they are without needing to change them; openness to new experiences; long-term consistency between words and actions; and the ability to delay gratification. The person who tends to be distrustful generally shows opposite characteristics. The helping person can use these characteristics to assess the client's ability to trust. These characteristics may also serve as a guideline for self-assessment. A person with a trusting attitude tends to create a sense of trust in others; a trusting attitude by the nurse therefore facilitates growth of trust by the client.

Building a trusting relationship

There are other ways the nurse can enhance the client's ability to trust. Consistency and reliability are both extremely important. It is easy to say to a clinic client, "I'll find out the answer to your question and tell you before you leave today." It is equally easy to become involved with other problems and not notice when that client actually leaves. The client, however, is only aware that the question was unanswered and will hesitate to ask again in the future because of a lack of trust that the nurse really cared. On the other hand, following through on a request from a client has the opposite effect and increases the likelihood that more questions will be asked in the future.

It may seem unnecessary to say that honesty is essential in building trust in the helping relationship. However, it is doubtful that there is a nurse in practice who has not at one time guessed at the answer to a client's question rather than admit a lack of information. The client who later discovers the right answer or gets four different answers from four staff members will not likely trust information received in the future. Similarly, the child who is told that an immunization injection will not hurt (and then it does for several days) will not believe the person who says that the stethoscope is painless. If experiences such as these are repeated, adults and children will develop mistrust of the helping professions. Considerations concerning confidentiality in the helping relationship are also important in establishing and maintaining trust.

The ability to trust is closely related to good communication. Provision of information and an opportunity to share feelings promote a sense of trust. In turn, trust helps the client to share concerns, feelings, and hopes. Without the establishment of trust, the helping relationship will not progress beyond the level of mechanical attention to superficial needs.

CONCEPT OF EMPATHY

The ability of the helping person to empathize with the client gives depth and meaning to the relationship. Empathy has been defined by Kalisch[17] as "the ability to enter into the life of another person, to accurately perceive his current feelings and their meanings." Stotland et al.[33] defined it as "an observer reacting emotionally because he perceives that another is experiencing or about to experience an emotion." Empathy in a helping relationship adds a dimension of real understanding between the participants. LaMonica[19] states that empathy "signifies a central focus and feeling *with* and *in* the client's world. It involves accurate perception of the client's world by the helper, communication of this understanding to the client, and the client's perception of the helper's understanding." Rogers[28] similarly identifies empathy as one of the most important aspects of the helping relationship.

MacKay[22] differentiates between ways to conceptualize empathy. One is *behavioral*, in which the nurse's behaviors while interacting with the client reveal the ability to use empathy (Fig. 6-1). Another

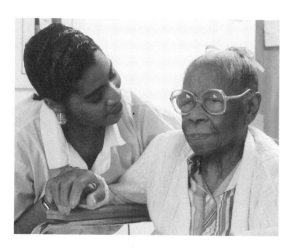

Fig. 6-1 The nurse uses empathy when interacting with the terminally ill client. (From Sorrentino S, Hogan MJ: *Mosby's textbook for long-term care assistants,* ed 2, St Louis, 1994, Mosby.)

is the *personality* perspective, which focuses on the influence of values, attitudes, or personality on one's natural tendency toward empathy.

Truax and Carkhuff[38] include in their definition of empathy the helper's "sensitivity" to current feelings and verbal ability to communicate this understanding in a language that reflects the client's current feelings. It is emphasized that although the helper experiences a real understanding of the client's feelings, these feelings are not shared by the helper. Truax and Carkhuff differentiate between several levels of empathy. At a high level the helping person's communications are congruent with the client's feelings and may even extend awareness of feelings. This level of understanding is communicated verbally and nonverbally; both participants feel that they are in tune with each other. At the lowest level of empathy the helping person does not exhibit awareness of the feelings that the client is trying to express. The helper may try to change the subject or respond to an emotional communication at an intellectual level, and the feeling tone between the participants is one of alienation.

Empathy research

Social scientists have been designing research studies that are intended to explore the link between the experience of empathy and the emergence of helping behavior. It is hypothesized that those who are highly empathic will also be highly motivated to help others. The rationale for this is that the empathic perception of another person's pain will cause the empathizer to try to alleviate that pain.

Gladstein[11] described the problems of designing and carrying out valid and reliable research on empathy. This is because of the complex interaction of verbal and nonverbal behaviors, combined with the client's past experiences and perceptions of the helping person. However, he believes that continued efforts to explore this concept are necessary, including the identification of the various types of empathy. This will facilitate helping professionals to be empathic.

One study that attempts to document empathic behavior and its effect on the helping relationship concludes that high empathic behavior initiated by the counselor did affect the client's self-perception of the level of empathic understanding, depth of self-exploration, and satisfaction with the counseling session.[11] The results of low empathy were more difficult to document. There is a great need for nurses to participate in research related to empathy and its effect on the nurse-client relationship.

Stotland and Mathews[32] studied the behavior of nursing students relative to empathy and helping. During the hospital clinical experience they observed students who had been tested regarding their ability to empathize. They hypothesized that highly empathic students would spend more time with clients, presumably being more helpful to them. The results did not entirely bear out the hypothesis. Early in the semester highly empathic students spent less time with clients than the low empathizers. However, by the end of the semester this tendency had been reversed; the highly empathic students were spending more time with clients. The investigators suggested that it was very uncomfortable for the highly empathic individuals to be with clients when they were insecure in their own abilities to meet the client's needs. Later in the semester they felt more secure in their own nursing abilities and were able to spend more time assisting clients.

Empathy in everyday life

Empathy has been closely related to the experience of anxiety. According to Sullivan, the individual's first experience with anxiety occurs when the mother's anxiety is perceived by the infant. He theorizes that this occurs empathically by means of the mother's nonverbal behavior when she is with the child. This kind of experience is not limited to the relationship between mother and child. It is difficult, if not impossible, to conceal anxiety from others with whom one is in close contact. The nonverbal behaviors of anxiety are readily perceived by others, and frequently uneasiness or discomfort is felt by the observer. This is the empathic experience of anxiety.

Empathy, therefore, is not an alien experience in everyday life. Aside from facilitating sensitivity to the discomfort of others, empathy is a factor in many enjoyable situations. Absorption in a good novel, appreciation of poetry, and the thrill of competition in spectator sports are examples of ways in which empathy can induce pleasure. Close relationships between friends often include long talks with each sharing hopes and fears with the other. The feeling of closeness that comes from sharing is enhanced by empathy.

Sympathy

Sympathy may also be experienced in a relationship between close friends. Whereas empathy implies that a degree of emotional separateness exists between the participants, sympathy implies a kind of fusion with the emotional experience of the other. In the latter instance the needs of the other are seen as one's own. The sympathizer's past experiences and individual responses become entangled with those of the other person. An example may help clarify this distinction:

Susan had been dating Bob for several months and had hoped that they would be married. Bob told her over the phone one evening that he had been seeing another girl and did not plan to date Susan again. Susan turned to her friends Mary and Linda for comfort.

Mary shared her feeling that Bob was typical of all men, selfish and unreliable. She added that she never knew what Susan saw in him anyway. Her suggestion for a way to handle the situation was that Susan should tell Bob exactly what she thought of him.

Linda listened to Susan and encouraged her to cry and express her anger at Bob for rejecting her. She made herself available to Susan but let her take the lead in their conversation. She did not dwell on her own perceptions of Bob but focused her attention on Susan and tried to help her look at her own needs at that time.

In this situation Mary reacted to Susan sympathetically. She probably made herself feel much better, because she expressed some of her own feelings. She assumed that Susan would feel as she did and did not allow Susan to examine her own feelings. Her statement about Bob even indicated that Susan's judgment had been rather poor, because she had become involved with such a loser.

Linda, on the other hand, was empathic. She helped Susan identify her feelings and allowed her to express them. By not placing a value on men, Bob, or Susan and Bob's relationship, she refrained from imposing her own feelings on Susan. By allowing Susan to take the lead, she helped her to confront the situation as she felt able to do so.

Sympathy has a place in human relationships. It can feel good to share the same feelings with another person and feel allied against a common enemy. It also feels good to share feelings of love or enjoyment to the extent that the differentiation between two people is minimized. The point to be made in terms of the helping relationship, however, is that objectivity is lost when feelings are shared sympathetically. If one person is in need, the sympathizer shares that need and may be unable to provide any help in meeting it. The helper has a responsibility to the client to assist in solving the problem. Therefore to identify and clarify alternatives and help the client consider them realistically, the helper must be objective.

Development of empathy

Empathy is a dimension of an interpersonal relationship that evolves as the relationship progresses. It is not an experience that can be approached deliberately. It is not possible to say, "I'm going to empathize with Mr. Jones today." It is more realistic to approach a client with an attitude of openness toward what may be communicated. This is sometimes referred to as "having one's antennas out." Another factor that helps a person be empathic is having had varied life experiences. A person who is open to the unfamiliar is more accepting of interpersonal risks, and empathy can be a risk. Empathic perceptions may be inaccurate. Hopefully the client will feel free to tell the helper when this is so, but it is always uncomfortable to be wrong. Therefore the empathizer should also be a secure person with a well-developed sense of self.

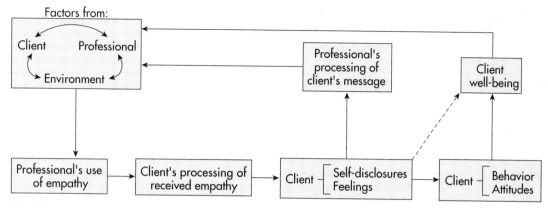

Fig. 6-2 A model of empathy in professional client interaction. (From MacKay RC, Hughes JR, Carver JC: A model of empathy in the helping relationship. In MacKay RC, Hughes JR, Carver JC, editors: *Empathy in the helping relationship,* New York, 1990, Springer.)

Without this there is a great likelihood of the helper being more sympathetic than empathic because of the helper's own need for help. Figure 6-2 presents a model of empathy in the professional-client interaction that was developed by MacKay et al.[23]

CRITICAL THINKING *Question* ....

Is it possible to empathize with someone who is confronting a problem that you have never experienced? Explain.

•••

The empathy process

Ehmann[7] has described a model for the application of the process of empathy (as formulated by Katz) to the nurse-client relationship. There are four steps in the process.

1. **Identification.** The helping person must first be able to comprehend the situation and feelings of the other. This occurs through identification, a psychologic process that allows the helper to "lose consciousness of self and become engrossed in the personality and situation of another person." This involves the relaxation of some degree of self-control so that the other's situation seems real rather than remote.

2. **Incorporation.** Incorporation is a step beyond identification. The experience of the other person is taken into the self of the helper. However, it is still recognized as the other person's experience and not as the helper's own. This step brings the helper closer to the reality of the other's situation.

3. **Reverberation.** The helper next experiences interaction between personal feelings, which are based on past experiences, and the experience identified and incorporated from the other person. This is the step that leads to understanding of the feelings of the other. Ehmann has noted particularly that "if we assume that all human beings possess the same impulses, feelings, and potentialities for experience, we can recognize that it is not necessary to share the very same experience, or share the impulses or feelings of the patient to the same degree."

4. **Detachment.** Finally, the helping person totally returns to his own identity. The results of the first three steps are combined with other objective knowledge about the client. This information is then used as a basis for responding to the client, so that the situation, feelings, and alternative approaches may be clarified.

This process frequently occurs spontaneously and is usually very rapid. It would be difficult to differentiate the phases as they occur, because they tend to overlap. The most important factor to remember is that throughout the process, the empathic person never loses a sense of self. This is the key to successful achievement of the last step, that of stepping back and considering the situation objectively.

A situation in which the nurse might be helpful to the client by responding empathically would be caring for a dying client or the family of a person who is dying. This would be difficult for most nurses, because it would require confronting one's own feelings about death as a very real part of life. Until this had been accomplished to some extent, the danger of reacting with sympathy would be great. In sympathizing the nurse would be trying to cope with personal concerns rather than with those of the client.

Identification and *incorporation* with the dying client would occur at the level of perceiving and accepting feelings related to impending death. However, the nurse who is sensitive to the magnitude of the client's loss will not say, "I know how you must feel," realizing that this is probably not true. Reverberation can be hard to achieve when working with a person who is dying. Although the nurse has probably not actually faced the prospect of her own death, she has most likely experienced losses. Feelings associated with loss play an important part in empathizing with the dying client, because these feelings form the nurse's common frame of reference with the client. In *reverberation* the nurse would be aware of her own feelings about loss and death and would try to relate these to the situation with the client. However, she would not give in to these feelings and become self-absorbed. Instead she would communicate to the client, both verbally and nonverbally, her wish to understand, thus facilitating the client's expression of feelings. This behavior on the part of the nurse would indicate that empathic *detachment* has been achieved.

Nonverbal behaviors that communicate empathy

Empathy is communicated both verbally and nonverbally. Gladstein[11] has identified several nonverbal behaviors that are usually perceived as empathic by a client. These include:

1. Placing oneself so that one is facing the client directly.
2. Maintaining comfortable eye contact. Staring, glancing, and critical looks should be avoided.
3. Leaning forward at about a 45-degree angle but without violating the client's personal space.
4. Smiling in a natural, unexaggerated way.
5. Nodding the head gently in an encouraging way.
6. Keeping the arms in a comfortable position but not crossing them across the chest.
7. Keeping the legs in a comfortable position but not crossing them with the ankle over the knee.

In her discussion of the use of empathy with dying patients and their families, Tyner[39] has added the use of culturally relevant gestures; the use of touch other than that required for physical care (expressive touch); maintaining a calm, quiet demeanor; and speaking in a soft voice. This demonstrates the need to adjust empathic behavior to the situation, as well as the characteristics of the client.

Self-assessment of level of empathy

Because empathy is such an important component of a helping relationship, the nurse may wish to assess her level of functioning in this area. A scale has been developed by Kalisch[17] that categorizes levels of empathic response (Table 6-1). Category 0 represents the lowest level of empathy. At this level the nurse may be totally out of touch with the feelings of the client, even with those feelings that are quite openly expressed. As one progresses through the scale, responses become more accurately attuned to the client's feelings; first to those that are close to the surface and, by category 4, to deeply hidden, indirectly expressed feelings. It is important to note that one should not automatically attach a higher value to a higher-level response. At times a category 2 response may be more appropriate to the setting and the stage of the relationship than one that is representative of category 4. The scale can be most useful when applied to a series of interactions and when used to develop a profile of the nurse's style of relating at a feeling level. To obtain a truly objective assessment, the use of this tool could be incorporated into a supervisory session during which the nurse supervisor could provide input based on observation of the nurse's relationships with clients. When the supervisory process is used in this way the nurse is able to develop greater self-awareness and thus enhance therapeutic effectiveness.

Empathizing with a client and analyzing one's ability to empathize can use a large amount of energy. However, empathy can be a positive experience for both nurse and client, one that brings them

TABLE 6-1   The nurse-patient empathic function scale: a schematic presentation

CATEGORIES OF NURSE EMPATHIC FUNCTIONING	LEVEL OF PATIENT'S FEELINGS	
	CONSPICUOUS CURRENT FEELINGS	HIDDEN CURRENT FEELINGS
0	Ignores	Ignores
1	Communicates an awareness that is accurate at times and inaccurate at other times	Ignores
2	Communicates a complete and accurate awareness of the essence and strength of feeling	Communicates an awareness of the presence of hidden feelings but is not accurate in defining their essence or strength; an effort is being made to understand
3	Same as category 2	Communicates an accurate awareness of the hidden feelings slightly beyond what the patient expresses
4	Same as category 2	Communicates without uncertainty an accurate awareness of the deepest, most hidden feelings

From Kalisch B: What is empathy? *Am J Nurs* 73:1548, 1973.

closer together and enhances the quality of caring in the relationship. Helping a person to share the innermost joys and fears is one of the most rewarding experiences in nursing.

4 CONCEPT OF CARING OR LOVE

The idea of caring is inherent in the purpose of the helping relationship. It is not really conceivable that one can care *for* effectively without caring *about*. However, this is an area where there has been a great deal of uneasiness. Clients question how much nurses really do care about them. This is reflected in statements such as "You're just here because you're paid to do this." Such a comment is usually anger provoking to nurses. One reason for this anger may be that the client is expressing a universal human need: to be loved. The nurse, as a helper, feels a desire to respond to the client's needs; however, this particular need touches an area where the nurse has learned to be wary of too much involvement.

Definitions of caring

Perhaps one reason for this conflict is the prevalent connotation of love in this society. Love, or caring, is generally interpreted in a sexual context. The nurse is apt, therefore, to interpret the client's demand for more caring as a demand for a sexual relationship.

According to standards of professional behavior, however, a sexual relationship between nurse and client is not viewed as appropriate to the helping relationship.

A more precise definition of the concept of love relative to the nurse-client relationship would be that proposed by Hoffman:

I find at the heart of love an unconditional acceptance of the person as he is (even at his most unlovable), together with a vision of what he is capable of becoming.[15]

Hagerman's definition of love in a helping relationship is

a response to others in a manner that expresses awareness and respect for a person as an individual, with knowledge and consideration for his specific needs and eventually mutual sharing with him.[13]

Both of these definitions, related specifically to nursing, are comparable to Erich Fromm's description of mature love as

an active power in man; a power which breaks through the walls which separate man from his fellow men, which unites him with others; love makes him overcome the sense of isolation and separateness, yet it permits him to be himself, to retain his integrity.[9]

Some nursing theorists view caring as a central attribute of nursing practice. Benner and Wrubel[4] state that caring means "being connected and having things matter." Caring helps people determine what is important, what is stressful, and what coping methods they might use. Caring also enables caregivers to feel concern about their clients. Finally, according to Benner and Wrubel, a caring attitude is necessary if help is to be given and received. A nursing action is not likely to be experienced as helpful if caring is absent.

Watson[41] has based her theory of nursing on caring. She has identified 10 "carative factors" (see box below).

Watson views caring as an interpersonal phenomenon. When applied effectively, it fosters growth and promotes health. In a caring relationship people are valued for what they are as well as what they will become. The caring nurse assists the client to develop to his fullest potential and gives him the freedom to choose. Caring focuses on health promotion and is complementary to curing.

The quality that Truax and Carkhuff[38] describe as nonpossessive warmth or unconditional positive regard also is akin to caring in the helping relationship. They have identified the range of this quality from a low level, characterized by a judgmental attitude on the part of the helper who may even express dislike or disapproval of the client or his feelings, to a high level, characterized by warm acceptance of the client's experience with no conditions imposed.

Carative Factors

1. Formation of a humanistic-altruistic system of values.
2. Instillation of faith-hope.
3. Cultivation of sensitivity to one's self and others.
4. Development of a helping-trust relationship.
5. Promotion and acceptance of the expression of positive and negative feelings.
6. Systematic use of the scientific problem-solving method for decision making.
7. Promotion of interpersonal teaching-learning.
8. Provision for a supportive, protective, or corrective mental, physical, sociocultural, and spiritual environment.
9. Assistance with the gratification of human needs.
10. Allowance for existential-phenomenologic forces.

Feeling cared about as an individual helps the client feel secure in a potentially threatening situation. Contacts with health care personnel are usually anxiety provoking for the client. Attitudes of respect and concern can help the client feel less threatened and therefore less anxious. As health care becomes more focused on technology, some worry that technologically competent nurses will be less caring. Locsin[21] points out that proficiency with the technology of health care is itself a demonstration of caring and contributes to the client's feeling of security in a frightening environment. Caring will contribute positively to the growth of trust. It is also difficult to imagine empathy in a relationship if no caring is present.

Development of the ability to care

A client's need for caring from the nurse, and the manner of communicating this need, may indicate the quality of past experiences with being loved and loving. Learning mature love is a developmental process. Most theorists in the psychologic development of the self (including those cited in this book) view a positive, that is, loving, mother-child relationship as essential for successful accomplishment of maturity. In later life corrective experiences through positive interpersonal relationships may help the person who had a negative childhood experience learn to love in a mature way.

Hagerman[13] has identified the developmental process of love between parent and child as follows:
1. Awareness of the child as an individual
2. Respect for the individuality of the child
3. Increased knowledge of the child's need
4. Mutual sharing

Development of the caring relationship

These same steps could be used to trace the development of a caring relationship between nurse and client. The nurse must first become aware of the client as an individual rather than as a diagnosis or a problem. This client must be differentiated from other clients in terms of needs, concerns, strengths, and weaknesses. Awareness of the client as an individual is a beginning, but there must also be respect for the person. Knowing about a person is not meaningful unless this knowledge is put into action. The plan of care must reflect the client's individuality.

Because sincere interest in the client as an individual is communicated actively, the client will become more open and share more of himself. At this point responsibility for planning nursing intervention should be shared by the nurse and client. A mutual experience such as this can have a powerful impact on an individual, adult or child, whose earlier developmental experiences were deficient in demonstrations of love.

Nursing research has revealed the behaviors that clients identify as evidence that the nurse cares for them. Cronin and Harrison[5] found that clients in the coronary care unit believed that professional competence and monitoring of their conditions demonstrated caring. They liked extra, individualized interventions; teaching by the nurse was also viewed favorably. In a study of clients with cancer, Larson[20] reported a marked difference between the nurses' and the clients' perceptions of important nurse caring behaviors. Nurses believed that comforting and trusting behaviors were most important. The clients selected "behaviors that demonstrated being accessible, monitoring, and following through as most caring."

Wolf et al.[44] studied caring behaviors of nurses from the perspectives of clients and nurses. They identified five dimensions of nurse caring:

- Respectful deference to other, which refers to courtesy and regard for others
- Assurance of human presence, which reflects concern for the other's needs and security
- Positive connectedness, which indicates optimistic and constant readiness to help
- Professional knowledge and skill
- Attentiveness to other's experience

These studies represent important contributions to nurses' understanding of ways to communicate caring.

The use of touch

Usually when one thinks about demonstrating love, some sort of physical contact comes to mind. Touch is one of the most universal nonverbal ways of communicating caring. Much of the practice of nursing requires touching the client. "The laying on of hands" is frequently cited as a basic characteristic of nursing, and the use of touch in nursing goes beyond that which is necessary to attend to the client's physical needs. The manner in which the person is touched and the attitude of the nurse who is touching can give a message of caring while physical needs are being met. The use of touch can overcome barriers to verbal communication such as age or language differences. Holding the hand of a woman who does not speak English while she is in labor is much more effective than any effort to communicate with her verbally. Small children also understand the meaning of a gentle touch very readily. The elderly often reach out and touch the person who is caring for them, and comfort to a person who feels sad often means "having a shoulder to cry on." Nurses are in daily contact with a variety of people who are often afraid, lonely, sad, or in pain. Reaching out physically and touching these people is a powerful way to show human concern. This is particularly important when the client is in an unfamiliar environment. The intent to help rather than hurt is much more easily understood when conveyed by a kind touch. Words are subject to endless individual interpretations; touch is much closer to being a universally understood language.

The painful use of touch also takes place in nursing. For instance, giving an injection to a small child must inflict pain. Unfortunately, many children and some adults associate nursing with pain. The establishment of a caring relationship is then very difficult. Perhaps if the nurse who gives an injection to a child would stay for a few minutes and cuddle, the child would be left with a more positive memory. If touch must be used to cause pain for the client, the nurse should make an effort to touch the same client in a caring way.

Weiss[42] has identified the need for nursing research exploring the various dimensions of touch, so nurses can incorporate a scientific theory of the use of touch into their rationale for practice. She describes six tactile symbols that constitute the qualities of touch: duration, location, action (rate of approach), intensity, frequency, and sensation (immediate response of comfort or discomfort). To use touch effectively the nurse needs to understand the nature and meaning to the individual of each of these tactile symbols.

Tommasini[36] identified the intentions of psychiatric nurses who used touch as a nursing intervention. They included "establishing contact with the patient; enhancing communication; communicating caring, interest, and recognition; and providing reassurance and comfort." They also used touch to decrease the client's self-preoccupation. When touch is used with a specific purpose, it communicates the nurse's concern and becomes an effective intervention.

Responses to touching described by nurses and clients in a long-term care setting were described by Routasalo and Isola.[29] They found that both nurses and elderly clients felt positively about being touched. The exception was the perception by some nurses that touching by male clients was sexual, resulting in avoidance of touching by the men. This study demonstrates the reciprocal nature of touching and the pleasure derived by people from both touching and being touched.

Although most nurses are comfortable with touching clients to help them meet their physiologic needs, they seem to be less comfortable with using touch to convey caring. The avoidance of the use of touch for this purpose deprives the nurse of a powerful therapeutic tool.

CRITICAL THINKING *Question* ················

Although there is nursing literature that supports the positive nature of touch between the client and the nurse, this is not always the case. For instance, nurses in the Routasalo and Isola[29] study did not feel comfortable when they perceived that the touches of some male clients were sexually motivated. Responses to touch develop in the context of one's cultural background. Based on your knowledge of cultural attitudes about closeness and personal space, identify nurse-client situations in which touch might be uncomfortable for one of the participants.
··

CONCEPT OF HOPE

Besides recognizing the continuing influence of the past and confronting the realities of the present, the nurse and the client must also look to the future. Frequently because of the nature of the client's health care needs and problems, the future looks bleak. Reluctance to face the future can inhibit the client's progress toward an optimal health state. When the nurse attempts to use the nurse-client relationship to instill a realistic but positive attitude toward the future, the focus is on

the development of hope. Hope may also be understood as attention to the spiritual needs of the patient, because much of hope is grounded in faith that there is a possibility for good to occur in the future.

Definitions of hope

Hope is often mentioned yet is not easy to define. Fromm[10] has said:

> To hope means to be ready at every moment for that which is not yet born, and yet not become desperate if there is no birth in our lifetime. There is no sense in hoping for that which already exists or for that which cannot be.

From a nursing point of view Haase et al.[12] state:

> Hope is an energized mental state involving feelings of uneasiness or uncertainty and characterized by a cognitive, action-oriented expectation that a positive future goal or outcome is possible.

Both of these definitions emphasize the lack of certainty for the hoped-for event but, at the same time, the need to fully expect that it will actually happen. It is also important to remember that hope depends on the perceptions of the person who is hopeful. Others may view their hope as futile, but the individual continues to expect the best. This phenomenon has found its way into literature. Fiction frequently revolves around a seemingly hopeless situation that works out well because of the faith of the hero or heroine.

Faith and hope

Faith is closely related to hope. Faith is the reliance on a power greater than the self to intercede in one's behalf. Faith can assist the person to maintain a hopeful attitude even in the face of enormous difficulties. Nurses have often felt uncomfortable dealing with the client's spiritual needs. This is frequently because they have not resolved their feelings about this part of their life experience. Self-examination to identify one's own feelings and attitudes about spirituality and faith will assist the nurse to interact with patients about these needs. Additional discussion of nursing and spirituality is included in Chapter 9.

Components of hope

Morse and Doberneck[26] analyzed the concept of hope. Based on client interviews, they identified seven components of hope:

- A realistic initial assessment of the predicament or threat
- The envisioning of alternatives and the setting of goals
- A bracing for negative outcomes
- A realistic assessment of personal resources and of external conditions and resources
- The solicitation of mutually supportive relationships
- The continuous evaluation for signs that reinforce the selected goals
- A determination to endure

Each of these components was present during interviews of four different groups of clients: clients waiting for heart transplants, spinal cord–injured clients, breast cancer survivors, and breastfeeding working mothers.

Dimensions of hope

Dufault and Martocchio[6] describe six dimensions of hope. The *affective* dimension focuses on sensations and emotions. This encompasses all of the possible feelings that might accompany hope, including the relative certainty of the outcome, the desirability of the outcome, and the anticipated feelings related to the event. The *cognitive* dimension includes the process by which the person thinks through and analyzes the object of hope. It may involve defining what is hoped for, exploring whether the hope is realistic, differentiating hope-promoting and hope-inhibiting factors, and using facts imaginatively to make the outcome seem more possible than not. The *behavioral dimension* relates to the actions that the person takes to make the hoped-for event happen. Hope can also increase energy for performing activities unrelated to it.

The *affiliative* dimension addresses relatedness and hope. This includes relatedness to other people as well as to spirituality and to other living things. It may focus on the behavior of others, such as seeking or receiving help from another. Others may serve as sources of hope by providing cues and information, taking action to assist the person to achieve a goal, or providing affirmation, listening,

supporting, and encouraging. The *temporal* dimension refers to the experience of time related to hope. Some hopes depend on a specific time frame, such as "I hope I pass the exam next week and get an A in this course." Others are more indefinite. For instance, one may recall a particularly happy vacation and hope to return to the same place and repeat the good times in the future. Past, present, and future interact in hoping. One may hope to or hope not to repeat past experiences in the future, using the present as a frame of reference. Finally, the *contextual* dimension relates to the person's own life situation as it affects hope. Some situations can lead to hope, hopelessness, or both depending on the person's response. Hope and hopelessness are not mutually exclusive. For instance, if the student who hopes to pass an examination and receive an A in the course fails instead, there may still be hope for a B. The hope is modified based on the context.

Nursing interventions

Table 6-2 identifies nursing interventions related to each of the dimensions of hope.

CRITICAL THINKING *Question* ....

How might hope be relevant to the nursing care of a terminally ill client? Can you think of a health care situation in which hope becomes irrelevant? How would these situations be influenced by the client's cultural background?
....

Nursing strategies related to hope

When an individual experiences stress, including the stress of illness, hope tends to support coping and recovery while despair interferes with the person's return to a state of wellness. Miller[24] has suggested nursing strategies to foster hope. The first is to assist the person to maintain close relationships with "significant other" people. This may be done by spending time interacting with the client's family and friends. In institutional settings it is also important to provide privacy for the client and visitors.

Many times clients are placed in situations over which they have little or no control. An extreme example of this is the use of life support systems in an intensive care unit. The person feels more secure,

TABLE 6-2   Nursing interventions related to the dimensions of hope

DIMENSION	NURSING INTERVENTION
Affective	Provide an opportunity for expression of feelings
	Respond empathically
	Assist in coping with feelings
Cognitive	Clarification
	Provide information
Behavioral	Encourage appropriate dependent, independent, and interdependent actions
	Enhance self-esteem to decrease feelings of helplessness
Affiliative	Support helpful relationships
Temporal	Help to see the relationship between past experiences and hope
Contextual	Help to create a supportive, hopeful environment

Modified from Dufault K, Martocchio BC: Hope: its spheres and dimensions, *Nurs Clin North Am* 20:379, 1985.

and therefore more hopeful, if the nurse acts in a competent and professional manner. Miller states that the nurse should be "a protector and comforter" to accomplish this. In addition, illness may be viewed as a challenge and an opportunity to grow by learning new coping skills. The nurse can help the patient develop these new ways of managing stress. At the same time adaptive coping mechanisms that have helped the client in the past should be reinforced. Sometimes the nurse needs to assist the client to apply a familiar behavior to a new situation.

A problem-solving approach can be helpful. The client is taught to assess the situation, including personal strengths and weaknesses. This must include both factors that are internal and those that are external to the client. Once the assessment is completed, alternative approaches to problem areas can be identified and compared. Goals should then be established with outcomes that are achievable and easily identifiable. As the client begins to experience goal achievement, hope is created or reinforced. Whenever possible, family members should be involved in this process so they can share the client's hopeful experience.[24]

In the Clinical Example at right the nurse applied the concept of hope to assist the client.

CONCEPTS OF AUTONOMY AND MUTUALITY
Sick role behaviors

When the individual initiates contact with the health care system, whether for preventive or curative reasons, this person is immediately given the label of *patient* or *client*. The behaviors that are associated with these labels are socioculturally determined. In contemporary Western society the client is expected to assume a passive, dependent role relative to caregivers. In part this probably reflects the regression that is associated with illness and the persistent association of health caregivers with the experience of illness. The association is then that one sees a health professional when one is sick and regressed and, therefore, dependent.

The response to this expectation is reciprocal. The health care professional expects the client to be "cooperative," that is, to follow directions without questions and accept recommendations gratefully. The client in turn expects the caregiver to solve the health problem as quickly and inexpensively as possible and also to be made comfortable if discomfort is present. Both of these expectations include a rather magical component; the fantasy is that if the client is cooperative enough and the professional provides the right treatment, wellness will ensue quickly.

More recently this relationship has been changing subtly. The client is beginning to develop an awareness of reasonable expectations of the health care system. The client as consumer has also become more critical of the care that is provided. This is necessitating complementary changes within the health care system. There is beginning to be more encouragement for the development of the client-caregiver team, in which both participants contribute to the health care process. This is where an understanding of the concepts of autonomy and mutuality becomes essential to the development of the nurse-client relationship.

CLINICAL EXAMPLE

Ms. W. was a 58-year-old woman admitted to the hospital for a biopsy of a breast lump that was found to be malignant. A modified radical mastectomy was done. Following the surgery Ms. W. became very withdrawn, refusing to see visitors, including her husband and daughter. She also ate very little, slept poorly, and refused to participate in her treatment.

Ms. J., the primary nurse assigned to provide nursing care to Ms. W., studied the data that were collected before surgery. She noted that the client was a successful businesswoman who owned her own flower shop. Her first marriage ended in divorce, and she had married her present husband 2 years ago. She was very close to her 30-year-old daughter, who was expecting her first child in 3 months. Based on this information the nurse decided to set aside at least 15 minutes each morning and afternoon to be with Ms. W.

Ms. J. explained her plan to Ms. W., who accepted it passively. At first she spent the 15 minutes with Ms. J. turned away from her and refusing to respond to verbal communication. One day Ms. J. remarked about the beauty of some roses that she had seen on the way to work. Ms. W. appeared to be interested, because she looked directly at the nurse. Ms. W. decided to risk requesting a verbal response and asked Ms. W. where florists find roses in the winter. The client explained this and then abruptly began to cry. Ms. J. sat with her and reflected that thinking of flowers seemed to make her feel sad. Ms. W. then poured out her fears that she would die, that she would not have enough energy to continue to operate her shop, and that her husband would probably reject her because she was physically ugly.

Ms. J.'s analysis was that Ms. W. was experiencing feelings of loss and hopelessness. She asked the physician to explain to the client that her prognosis was very good. The nurse encouraged Ms. W. to talk with the physician about breast reconstruction. She also arranged for a visit from a member of Reach for Recovery, a self-help group of women who have been treated for breast cancer. This volunteer was able to answer many of the client's questions about what to expect in the future. Gradually Ms. W. was able to share her fears with her family. They were also supportive. The nurse knew that hope had been restored when Ms. W. asked her how soon she could knit so she could make baby clothes for her new grandchild.

Definitions of autonomy and mutuality

These concepts are considered together, because they tend to interact in the context of the relationship. *Autonomy* is concerned with the ability to be self-directed. *Mutuality* involves a process of sharing with another person. Both are important in the helping relationship and should be considered by the nurse as an integral part of care planning.

Superficially it might seem that autonomy and mutuality are mutually exclusive; however, this is not usually the case. It is more helpful to look at each of these concepts on a continuum and then consider the interaction of the two. It is also important to keep in mind that individuals change in their degree of openness to autonomy or mutual behavior depending on circumstances.

Autonomy

Autonomy, or the capacity for self-direction, can be helpful to the client. People who seek health care are generally concerned about loss of control over their own destinies. In areas requiring the application of specialized skill, the person does, in reality, lose control. However, it should be possible to find aspects of almost any situation that the client can control; the client would thus maintain a degree of autonomy. For instance, the person who is about to travel to Asia cannot control the fact that he must receive immunizations and that these will be painful. However, if he is given the choice of which arm the injections will be given in, he can maintain control over how bothersome the pain will be to him. This may seem like a trivial consideration, but it can be extremely meaningful to a client who may see the health care system as overwhelming and uncaring.

Paternalism and maternalism Frequently there is an assumption by health care personnel that the client is incapable of participating in his own treatment. With the exception of those who are very young or unconscious, this is seldom the case. Jewell[16] proposes that patients participate in their care formally and informally. Formal participation takes place when there is a process of negotiation between the patient and the nurse about the plan of care. Informal participation involves the nurse's getting to know the patient as a person, thereby gaining understanding of the person's likes and dislikes, hopes and fears.

The belief that care providers are the best judges of client needs is called *paternalism*, when it takes the form of authoritarianism, or *maternalism*, when it is evidenced by infantilizing treatment. Paternalistic or maternalistic approaches limit or eliminate autonomous client behavior. Moore[25] has observed that health care providers who label clients as noncompliant are often paternalistic and have failed to explore the reason for the client's refusal to follow the prescribed treatment. This problem can be avoided if the client is a partner in planning for one's care. Fromer[8] asserts that autonomy may be diminished by:

• Limited available courses of action
• A coercive atmosphere
• Insufficient information concerning alternatives.

Courses of action may be limited by the individual's health problems; however, the last two limitations on autonomy frequently relate to the behavior of health care providers. Coercion may be overt or subtle. Nonverbal cues such as tone of voice or emphasis may have a powerful impact on the client's decision-making process. Consider the Clinical Example above.

Although the nurse presented the same information about both alternatives, she did not present it objectively. She was attempting to influence the client to select the course of action that the nurse had decided was best for her. This is an example of limiting autonomy through a paternalistic approach.

Fromer suggests that paternalism may be justified on some occasions. However, this would only be in situations in which the client is not able to make a voluntary decision, such as when unconscious or irrational, and would only continue until the client could act autonomously. She further states, "If an error of judgment is to be made, it is far better to make it on the side of liberty than paternalism."[8]

 CLINICAL EXAMPLE

Ms. L. was a 20-year-old unmarried woman who had just delivered her second baby. Ms. J. was her primary nurse. As part of a postdischarge home visit, Ms. J. initiated a discussion of birth control with Ms. L. She discussed the use of a contraceptive implant at great length, stressing its reliability and the absence of a need to remember to use it. She briefly mentioned possible complications. When Ms. L. asked about oral contraceptive medication, Ms. J. responded, "Well, you could take the pill, but—" and proceeded to describe in detail the possible problems associated with oral contraceptive medication. She then briefly described the advantages of oral contraceptives over other birth control methods.

People who choose nursing as a profession are often nurturing people who enjoy caring for others. This is a valued characteristic of nurses. However, when this need to care *for* becomes too emphasized in the nurse's behavior, the patient is deprived of autonomy. The Clinical Example at right illustrates this situation.

CRITICAL THINKING *Question*

Based on your understanding of managed health care, discuss the following statement: autonomy implies freedom of choice, therefore it is impossible to be autonomous and a consumer of health services in a managed care system.

Advocacy The role that the nurse assumes to promote the client's autonomy and to foster mutual responsibility in the relationship is that of *advocate*. Advocacy implies concern for the rights of the other and active protection of these rights. The nurse as advocate assists the client to become informed about health care alternatives and provides support in carrying out decisions that have been made. This role may lead to conflict for the nurse when the client selects an alternative that is not the preferred option of other members of the health care team. This example illustrates such a situation:

Mr. S. was an 85-year-old man who was admitted to the hospital for evaluation of appetite loss, weight loss, and abdominal cramping. An abdominal mass was discovered

CLINICAL EXAMPLE

Mr. Y. was a 79-year-old man who was referred to a home health care agency following hospitalization for a cerebrovascular accident. Although his speech was hesitant and his gait was halting, he had responded well to physical and speech therapy and was expected to recover most of his functional ability.

Ms. D. was the nurse who was assigned to care for Mr. Y. She had recently joined the home health agency after many years of experience as a maternity nurse. She had decided that she would like a more varied experience and looked forward to practicing her nursing skills in a new role. Ms. D. believed that a nurse should focus on making clients comfortable and assisting them to meet their physical needs.

The passive exercises that had been prescribed for Mr. Y. were uncomfortable. As soon as he complained, Ms. D. would move on to the next step in the exercise regimen. When he tried to communicate his needs, she compensated for his slow speech by finishing sentences for him. Sometimes she even anticipated what he was about to say, eliminating the need for him to try to talk at all. Two weeks

after Ms. D. began visiting Mr. Y., her supervisor accompanied her on a visit to evaluate her performance. It was obvious that there was a positive interpersonal relationship between Mr. Y. and the nurse. However, the supervisor was disturbed to find that Mr. Y. had lost some range of motion since his discharge from the hospital. She also noted that Ms. D. frequently spoke for him.

When they returned to the office, the supervisor shared her observations with Ms. D. She also suggested alternative approaches that would foster the client's autonomy, such as explaining to him that his exercises would cause some discomfort if they were to be effective and to suggest comfort measures that would help with any residual achiness. The hardest behavior for Ms. D. to change was her tendency to interrupt and to speak for the client. She decided to enlist his assistance and asked him to stop her if she tried to talk for him. Mr. Y. liked the idea that he could help the nurse with a problem that she had and became very assertive in letting her know when she was not letting him express himself.

---

and exploratory surgery recommended. Mr. S. had a history of serious cardiac disease and was considered to have only a fair chance of surviving an operation. The physician strongly recommended that Mr. S. agree to surgery. He suspected that Mr. S. had a malignant tumor and predicted a life expectancy of less than a year. Mr. S. consulted with his children and decided that he preferred to go home and live as comfortably as he could with palliative treatment. He asked Ms. B., his primary nurse, what she thought of his decision.

As an advocate Ms. B. recognized that Mr. S. had made a very difficult decision and was requesting her support. She also knew that the physician did not approve of the decision. She told Mr. B. that she agreed with his right to choose the alternative that seemed best to him. She then approached the physician and suggested that referral of Mr. S. to a home care service would be helpful. His response was to request that Ms. B. try to persuade Mr. S. to agree to the operation. She assertively responded that she did not regard that as her role with the client, but she would be glad to help arrange for postdischarge nursing services. She then talked with her nursing

supervisor about her interactions with Mr. S. and his physician. The supervisor indicated that she supported Ms. B.'s nursing actions.

In this situation Ms. B. was able to fulfill her role of advocacy, supporting the client's right to make an autonomous decision. It is important to remember, however, that the health care system is basically paternalistic. The nurse who advocates for a client's rights may risk creating conflict in the work situation. For this reason it is strongly recommended that a nurse who contemplates challenging health care team recommendations discuss this plan with a trusted mentor. It is important that the nurse fully understand and accept the consequences of her own actions for herself and the client before she acts. However, it is certainly hoped that nurses will be able to support each other in protecting the client's basic right to autonomy.

Advocates work to *empower* clients. Smith[31] speaks of "patient power." This is "a person's ability to influence or control his care during sickness." When a person has lost power as a result of a health problem, the nurse may work toward empowering him by initiating interventions that:

• Improve body image
• Enhance self-control
• Increase knowledge
• Reinforce identity
• Foster an appropriate level of dependency
• Focus on realistic goals

Empowerment of clients allows them to take control of the health care process to the extent that they are able to do so.

The promotion of client autonomy should not be construed to mean complete client self-direction. This would involve abdication of all professional responsibility. If an individual were capable of independently meeting all of his own health care needs, there would be no need for caregivers. However, this is not the case. Everyone, including caregivers, needs help maintaining an optimal level of wellness. One demand on the helping relationship then is to establish a therapeutic level of autonomy.

Assertiveness Development of a therapeutic level of autonomy may be compared to the development of assertiveness. Assertiveness refers to the right of the individual to behave in a way that meets his needs as long as he does not intrude on the needs and rights of others. It is distinguished from passive behavior, in which the individual disregards his own needs and rights, and aggressive behavior, in which he disregards the needs and rights of others. The autonomous client will be assertive in communicating his needs and in helping to plan nursing care. The nurse needs to support the growth of assertive behavior in the client, thereby facilitating mutuality in the relationship. Nursing interventions to foster assertiveness are explored further in Chapter 7.

Mutuality

The process through which the client assumes an appropriate level of autonomy without blocking the provision of necessary health care services is mutuality. Wills[43] has described the components of the nurse-client alliance:

• Mutual negotiation of activities necessary to reach the client's goals
• Active work toward mutually contracted goal behaviors

• A supportive egalitarian relationship that facilitates achieving the contracted goals

A helping relationship is most helpful when each participant is contributing positively to meeting the client's health needs. The client and the helping person each have strengths that can facilitate the growth of the relationship. The nurse has a body of theoretic knowledge that helps identify the problem and alternative approaches to it. The client has knowledge of himself and of his own unique biopsychosocial needs that could significantly influence his response to a nursing intervention. For optimal results both of these contributions must be considered in planning care.

In mutual health care planning the emphasis is on the consideration of the client as a unique individual. In this sense mutuality is possible with any client of any age or level of consciousness. For instance, the nurse who is caring for a newborn baby whose mother has a fever would take steps to prevent the passing of an infection from mother to baby. This baby would be treated differently from other babies in the nursery. The modification would be based on the nurse's knowledge of the unique needs of this client and would therefore be mutually determined. The client need not verbally participate in the care planning as long as the plan recognizes his individuality.

The following examples may provide further differentiation between the presence and absence of mutuality in a helping relationship:

During a routine physical examination Ms. C. had a positive blood test for syphilis. She was asked to return to the medical clinic for treatment. The physician left an order for an injection of penicillin. The nurse administered the penicillin to Ms. C. when the client arrived at the clinic. Ms. C. went into shock and died.

Mr. E. saw his doctor because he had a sore throat. The doctor took a culture of Mr. E.'s throat and found that the client had a streptococcal infection. The doctor then asked the nurse to give Mr. E. an injection of penicillin. The nurse asked Mr. E. if he had ever taken penicillin before. Because he could not remember, she performed a skin sensitivity test. The test showed that Mr. E. was allergic to penicillin. Another antibiotic was ordered.

The lack of mutuality in the first example was literally fatal. In the second example, when the client was unable to verbally provide the necessary information, the nurse used an alternative method of gathering information that possibly saved the client's life.

Mutuality in a helping relationship facilitates goal achievement. Goals that are based on the client's individual needs will most likely be accepted by the client. There is the greatest likelihood of success when the client actively participates in setting the goals. There is the least likelihood of success when the goals are based on a "textbook" approach to the client's problem with no consideration for individuality. Failure to foster mutuality can sabotage successful goal accomplishment and undermine the helping relationship.

SUMMARY

The nurse-client relationship is a basic element of a successful health care experience for the client. It is based on the principles of the helping relationship. The nurse is responsible for using knowledge of the relationship process and its related concepts to help the client meet health goals. This requires self-awareness and an understanding of one's own value system, which can be achieved by the values clarification process. Concepts relevant to the relationship process include trust, empathy, caring, hope, autonomy, and mutuality.

Trust is an essential element of a successful mother-child relationship and is the first task in personality development. In some ways the nurse-client relationship resembles the mother-child relationship. It, too, must be based on trust to be successful and growth promoting. Trust implies the ability to rely on others and to depend on them to be genuine. Consistency, reliability, and honesty enable the nurse to be perceived as trustworthy.

Empathy provides the relationship with depth and meaning. It is the ability of the nurse to recognize and understand the feelings of others and to communicate this. It is differentiated from sympathy, in which the nurse loses objectivity because of an inability to sort out the client's feelings from her own. The four steps of the empathy process are identification, incorporation, reverberation, and detachment. Levels of empathic responses can be categorized on a scale.

Caring or love is inherent in the purpose of the helping relationship. However, nurses may experience conflict because of the sexual connotations of love. In the context of the nurse-client relationship love or caring refers to unconditional acceptance of the client. Caring focuses on interpersonal connection and identification of what matters. It also involves respect and concern for the other. It fosters growth and promotes health. Touch is a powerful way of communicating caring, and touch can be used judiciously by the nurse to transcend barriers to verbal communication.

Hope inspires the person to work toward future goals and provides energy to meet those goals. It is closely related to faith, which refers to the belief that a spiritual force will assist the person. The nurse supports hope by encouraging the client to set realistic goals and to recognize progress. The six dimensions of hope are affective, cognitive, behavioral, affiliative, temporal, and contextual, and they are closely related to nursing interventions.

The concepts of autonomy and mutuality are closely related. Autonomy refers to the ability to be self-directed; mutuality involves a process of sharing with another person. Autonomy may be limited by the paternalistic or maternalistic behaviors of the nurse. Advocacy is a nursing role that enhances autonomy. Assisting the client to become assertive is a nursing intervention that leads to autonomy. Mutuality occurs when each participant in the relationship contributes to meeting the client's health care needs. Nursing care is based on knowledge of the client's characteristics and preferences.

DISCUSSION QUESTIONS

1. Recall an experience during a nurse-client relationship that was particularly meaningful to you. Identify the personal and professional growth that occurred for you as a result of that experience. How is this likely to affect your future behavior?

2. Ask yourself the questions that Carl Rogers posed to people who wish to help others. Identify the ones that cause you discomfort. Select one of these, and develop a plan for personal change. Set specific goals so you can evaluate your progress.

3. Using Uustal's description of values as "general guides to behavior, standards of conduct that one endorses and tries to live up to or maintain,"[40] list five of your own values. Analyze these in terms of their importance to you and whether you would feel comfortable stating them to (1) a group of casual acquaintances, (2) colleagues in school or at work, (3) close friends, or (4) your family. What are the factors that influence your willingness to affirm your values?

4. Reflect on a situation in which your value system is in strong disagreement with that of a client. Consider alternative ways to deal with the situation.

5. Describe mothering behaviors that would help the infant develop trust.

6. Identify a public figure whom you consider to be trustworthy or untrustworthy. Describe the specific characteristics of this person that led to your conclusion. Consider both verbal and nonverbal behaviors.

7. You are assigned to care for a hospitalized 4-year-old child who has been subjected to a number of painful procedures. He bursts into tears every time a nurse approaches his bedside. Describe the steps you would take to develop a trusting relationship with this child.

8. Compare the experience of empathizing (or sympathizing) with an elderly male client in a chronic care facility and empathizing (or sympathizing) with an unwed and pregnant adolescent girl.

9. What are the implications for nursing of the research findings that highly empathic people tend to withdraw from situations in which others are experiencing pain and where they do not feel confident in their ability to help?

10. Discuss the influence of contemporary attitudes regarding sexuality on the expression of caring by the nurse.

11. How would you respond if a client said to you, "This is your job. You're just here because you're paid to do this"?

12. Compare and contrast two clinical situations: one that demonstrates effective use of touch, and the other in which touch is not helpful.

13. A client says to you, "Nothing you do can help me. I'm a sinner, and God is punishing me." Describe the nursing interventions you would take.

14. Identify a situation about which you are hopeful. Discuss each of the six dimensions of hope related to this situation.

15. Do you agree or disagree with the assertion that the health care system is basically paternalistic? Give the rationale for your answer, including descriptions of specific incidents that support your argument.

16. Discuss the risks involved for the nurse when she assumes the role of client advocate in a paternalistic system.

17. Describe nurse-client behaviors that would indicate mutuality during each phase of the nursing process.

EXPERIENTIAL & SIMULATED LEARNING EXERCISES

1. Values clarification number 1

PURPOSE: To develop self-awareness concerning values related to nursing and to develop interviewing skills.

PROCEDURE: Students should pair off with another student whom they do not know very well. Each student is to interview the other for approximately 10 minutes, asking questions related to nursing and values. Students should be instructed to use communication techniques that allow the interviewee to respond to each question completely. Both participants should also be aware of their feelings toward each other and the questions asked.

SAMPLE QUESTIONS:

1. Why did you decide to attend a school of nursing?
2. How do you feel about that decision now?
3. What do you like most about nursing?
4. What do you like least about nursing?
5. How can you change the thing that you like least?
6. What are your career goals?
7. What is a good nurse?
8. How much education is needed for entry into nursing practice?
9. Should nurses engage in collective bargaining?
10. Is nursing a profession?

DISCUSSION: Ask pairs to share with each other what they learned about themselves and about the other person. They should also give feedback about the interview styles used and compare the style of each individual. Then bring the whole group together to discuss the relationship of values to the questions and answers.

2. Values clarification number 2

PURPOSE: To sensitize students to moral/ethical issues in nursing that frequently cause values conflict for the individual nurse.

PROCEDURE: Students work individually on this exercise. Each student should indicate in writing agreement or disagreement with a statement that relates to a common moral/ethical dilemma. The students should record their immediate responses to the statement as it is read aloud by the group leader. Written copies of the statement may then be distributed. Students should make two columns on their papers labeled "Pros" and "Cons." They should then write all the reasons they can think of in favor of or against the statement in the appropriate columns. They should then rephrase their response to the statement by writing, "I believe . . . because . . ."

DISCUSSION: In the discussion the leader should ask whether anyone changed their opinions after considering the pros and cons. Did anyone waver in the response, even though it finally remained the same? Were the participants able to come up with as many reasons disagreeing with their opinions as those that agreed? Finally, request that students volunteer to share their responses with the group, pointing out that part of valuing is publicly stating your belief. The sharing should be structured so that beliefs and reasons are simply stated, not debated.

SAMPLE STATEMENTS:

1. Suicide is a valid option for some people.
2. A 16-year-old should be able to have an abortion without her parents' knowledge.
3. It is all right to give medicine to an irrational person without his consent.
4. Elderly people should be cared for by their families.
5. People should be allowed to have as many children as they want.
6. Nurses should give highest priority to activities ordered by doctors.

3. Trust walk

PURPOSE: To experience a trusting relationship.
PROCEDURE: Assign students in pairs. Blindfold one member of the pair. The other is to lead the blindfolded person on a short walk, preferably including some time outside. After 5 minutes the students should exchange roles.

DISCUSSION: Focus on the feeling of having to depend on another person, and relate this to the role of the client. Ask what behaviors on the part of the leaders did or did not encourage trust on the part of the follower.

4. Empathic listening

PURPOSE: To enable the student to identify the level of empathy revealed in various responses and thereby become more sensitive to his or her own empathic behavior.

PROCEDURE: Read the speaker's statement. Then read each of the following statements and ask each student to critique them as category 1, 2, 3, or 4 (on the line provided), according to Kalisch's model.[17]

Speaker I: "My big brother is mean. He's always accusing me of something I didn't do."

Listener responses:

_____ a. "You're upset because you think your brother accuses you unfairly."

_____ b. "Do you do things that provoke your brother?"

_____ c. "That's too bad, a big guy picking on a little kid."

_____ d. "You wonder if your brother really loves you when he accuses you like that."

_____ e. "Why do you think he accuses you?"

_____ f. "I know just how you feel; my big brother used to do that to me."

_____ g. "Want to go to the ball game this afternoon?"

_____ h. "Why don't you tell your mother?"

_____ i. "You feel helpless when your big brother accuses you of something you know you did not do."

Speaker II: "That class sure is boring."

Listener responses:

_____ a. "You resent having to be in a class you don't like."

_____ b. "What is that book you are reading?"

_____ c. "You're feeling bored in your class."

_____ d. "You feel trapped into being in a class you don't like."

_____ e. "That's too bad—boring classes are a waste of time."

_____ f. "You're angry because the class is not more interesting."

_____ g. "Why don't you drop the course?"

_____ h. "Maybe if you talked to the teacher and told her how you feel, she'd change some things."

_____ i. "When are you going to sign up for spring term?"

_____ j. "Your complaining really upsets me."

DISCUSSION: Ask the students to share the level that they assigned to each response. The discussion should focus on the rationale for the decision. The group should strive to reach a consensus on the level for each statement.

5. Autonomy/mutuality

PURPOSE: To assist the student to understand the effect of a paternalistic attitude on autonomous behavior.

PROCEDURE: Students should be divided into groups of three. Each group is given a brief description of a situation. Sample situations follow. One student is to play the role of the client, one the nurse advocate, and one a paternalistic health care provider. Each of the providers separately should discuss the situation with the client. They should then discuss together their respective perceptions of the situation and preferred outcomes. Agreement may or may not result from this discussion. If available, videotape would facilitate analysis of this experience:

1. The client is a 90-year-old woman who is refusing to go to a nursing home.
2. The client is a 35-year-old quadriplegic man who refuses to eat.
3. The client is a 58-year-old man who refuses to take his antihypertensive medication because it has caused him to be impotent.
4. The client is a 12-year-old girl whose parents have refused to allow chemotherapy for her malignant sarcoma.
5. The client is a 21-year-old woman who is experiencing diffuse, dull, lower abdominal pain and refuses a pelvic examination.

DISCUSSION: The discussion should focus on the client's responses to the approaches and the feelings of the two providers as they debated with each other. The participants' behavior may be categorized according to whether it was passive, aggressive, or assertive. Students should consider how they might have changed their approaches to the situation. Reasons should be identified for agreement or disagreement at the end of the experience. Did the client experience any sense of mutuality? What health care provider role did the paternalistic person assume, and how did this influence the nurse-advocate's behavior? Finally, the participants should address the issue of whether the focus of the interaction was on the client's needs and feelings or on achievement of the client's compliance with the recommended therapeutic approach.

REFERENCES

1. Aiken L, Aiken J: A systematic approach to evaluation of interpersonal relationships, *Am J Nurse* 73:863, 1973.
2. Anderson N: Human interaction for nurses, *Supervisor Nurse* 10:44, 1979.
3. Anderson N: Exclusion: a study of depersonalization in health care, *J Humanistic Psychol* 21:67, 1981.
4. Benner P, Wrubel J: *The primacy of caring: stress and coping in health and illness,* Menlo Park, Calif, 1989, Addison-Wesley.
5. Cronin SN, Harrison B: Importance of nursing caring behaviors as perceived by patients after myocardial infarction, *Heart Lung* 17:374, 1988.
6. Dufault K, Martocchio BC: Hope: its spheres and dimensions, *Nurs Clin North Am* 20:379, 1985.
7. Ehmann V: Empathy: its origin, characteristics, and process, *Perspect Psychiatr Care* 9:77, 1971.
8. Fromer MJ: Paternalism in health care, *Nurs Outlook* 29:284, 1981.
9. Fromm E: *The art of loving,* New York, 1956, Harper & Row.
10. Fromm E: *The revolution of hope: toward a humanized technology,* New York, 1968, Harper & Row.
11. Gladstein GA: Counselor empathy and client outcomes. In Gladstein GA, editor: *Empathy and counseling: explorations in theory and research,* New York, 1987, Springer-Verlag.
12. Haase JE et al.: Simultaneous concept analysis of spiritual perspective, hope, acceptance and self-transcendance, *Image J Nurs Sch* 24:141, 1992.
13. Hagerman Z: The patient who is unable to love, *Nurs Clin North Am* 4:691, 1969.
14. Hawks JH: Should nurses give moral advice? *Image* 16:14, Winter 1984.
15. Hoffman G: The concept of love, *Nurs Clin North Am* 4:664, 1969.
16. Jewell SE: Patient participation: what does it mean to nurses? *J Adv Nurs* 19:433, 1994.
17. Kalisch B: What is empathy? *Am J Nurs* 73:1548, 1973.
18. King I: *Toward a theory for nursing,* New York, 1971, Wiley.
19. LaMonica EL: Construct validity of an empathic instrument, *Res Nurs Health* 4:389, 1981.

20. Larson PJ: Comparison of cancer patients' and professional nurse's perceptions of important nurse caring behaviors, *Heart Lung* 16:187, 1987.
21. Locsin RC: Machine technologies and caring in nursing, *Image J Nurs Sch* 27:201, 1995.
22. MacKay RC: What is empathy? In MacKay RC et al., editors: *Empathy in the helping relationship*, New York, 1990, Springer.
23. MacKay RC, Hughes JR, Carver EJ: A model of empathy in the helping relationship. In MacKay RC et al., editors: *Empathy in the helping relationship*, New York, 1990, Springer.
24. Miller JF: Inspiring hope, *Am J Nurs* 85:23, 1985.
25. Moore KN: Compliance or collaboration? The meaning for the patient, *Nurs Ethics* 2:71, 1995.
26. Morse JM, Doberneck B: Delineating the concept of hope, *Image J Nurs Sch* 27:277, 1995.
27. Raths L, Harmin M, Simon S: *Values and teaching*, Columbus, Ohio, 1966, Charles E. Merrill.
28. Rogers C: Empathic: an unappreciated way of being, *Counseling Psychologist* 5:22, 1975.
29. Routasalo P, Isola A: The right to touch and be touched, *Nurs Ethics* 3:165, 1996.
30. Simon SB, Howe LW, Kirschenbaum H: *Values clarification: a handbook of practical strategies for teachers and students*, rev ed, New York, 1978, Hart.
31. Smith FB: Patient power, *Am J Nurs* 85:1260, 1985.
32. Stotland E et al.: *Empathy, fantasy and helping*, Beverly Hills, Calif, 1978, Sage.
33. Stotland E, Sherman SE, Shaver KG: *Empathy and birth order*, Lincoln, Neb, 1971, University of Nebraska Press.
34. Tanner CA, Benner P, Chesla C, Gordon D: The phenomenology of knowing the patient, *Image J Nurs Sch* 25:273, 1993.
35. Thomas M: Trust in the nurse-patient relationship. In Carlson C, editor: *Behavioral concepts and nursing intervention*, Philadelphia, 1970, JB Lippincott.
36. Tommasini NR: The use of touch with the hospitalized psychiatric patient, *Arch Psychiatr Nurs* 4:213, 1990.
37. Travelbee J: *Interpersonal aspects of nursing*, Philadelphia, 1971, FA Davis.
38. Truax CB, Carkhuff RB: *Toward effective counseling and psychotherapy: training and practice*, Chicago, 1967, Aldine.
39. Tyner R: Elements of empathic care for dying patients and their families, *Nurs Clin North Am* 20:393, 1985.
40. Uustal DB: Values clarification in nursing: application to practice, *Am J Nurs* 78:2058, 1978.
41. Watson J: *Nursing: the philosophy and science of caring*, Boston, 1979, Little, Brown.
42. Weiss SJ: The language of touch, *Nurs Res* 28:76, 1979.
43. Wills EM: Nurse-client alliance: a pattern of home health caring, *Home Healthc Nurse* 14:455, 1996.
44. Wolf ZR, Giardino ER, Osborne PA, Ambrose MS: Dimensions of nurse caring, *Image J Nurse Sch* 26:107, 1994.

Suggested Readings

Alligood MR: Empathy: the importance of recognizing two types, *J Psychosoc Nurs Ment Health Serv* 30:14, Mar 1992.

The author suggests that researchers need to differentiate between empathy as a personality trait and empathy in the clinical sense.

Bandman EL: Our toughest questions—ethical quandaries in high tech nursing, *Nurs Health Care* 6:483, 1985.

Questions are raised regarding the role of the nurse in assisting clients and families to make decisions related to technology and health care. The author raises provocative issues that need to be considered carefully by nurses as they analyze their own value systems.

Benner P, Wrubel J: *The primacy of caring: stress and coping in health and illness*, Menlo Park, Calif, 1989, Addison-Wesley.

This book is a rich source of information about the role of caring in nursing practice. It should be a part of the professional library of every practicing nurse and nurse educator.

Bennett JA, DeMayo M, Saint Germain M: Caring in the time of AIDS: the importance of empathy, *Nurs Adm Q* 17(2):46, 1993.

The authors describe a study of the role of empathy in nurses' willingness to provide care to clients who have AIDS. They found that more empathic nurses were more willing to work with these clients.

Dufault K, Martocchio BC: Hope: its spheres and dimensions, *Nurs Clin North Am* 20:379, 1985.

These authors present a scholarly analysis of the concept of hope and present it as a dynamic process. Nursing interventions are described related to the dimensions of hope. This article is highly recommended for both students and faculty.

From MA: Utilizing the home setting to teach Watson's theory of human caring, *Nurs Forum* 30:5, 1995.

The author describes the application of Watson's carative factors by RN-BSN students who were assigned to care for dying patients in their homes.

Fromer MJ: Paternalism in health care, *Nurs Outlook* 29:284, 1981.

This nurse ethicist presents an informative discussion of the concept of paternalism as it relates to client autonomy. The ethical dilemma of paternalism is explored in a way that challenges the reader to examine personal values. Examples of client situations that involve paternalism are presented.

Fromm E: *The art of loving*, New York, 1956, Harper & Row.

This book is a classic in which love is examined from a philosophic perspective by a noted psychologist. The author conveys a deep respect for humanity and the belief that love of others and of self is essential for a meaningful life.

Groer M: Psychoneuroimmunology, *Am J Nurs* 91:33, Aug 1991.

The author discusses possible relationships among psychologic, neurologic, and immunologic body responses. She relates these to the positive effects of nursing interventions such as touch.

Hinds PS: The relationship of nurses' caring behaviors with hopefulness and health care outcomes in adolescents, *Arch Psychiatr Nurs* 2:21, Feb 1988.

This study validated that caring behaviors by nurses had a positive effect on hopefulness in adolescents who were hospitalized for treatment of substance abuse. The author identified positive and negative influences on hopefulness at three points in the course of the treatment episode.

Jenny J, Logan J: Knowing the patient: one aspect of clinical knowledge, *Image J Nurs Sch* 24:254, 1992.

The authors explore the concept of knowing the client as it relates to caring. This study focused on the importance of knowing the client during the process of weaning from a ventilator. They concluded that knowing the client is an antecedent of caring.

Kalisch B: What is empathy? *Am J Nurs* 73:1548, 1973.

This author describes the concept of empathy and discusses the application of empathy to the nurse-client interaction. She identifies and thoroughly describes five levels of empathic functioning and includes a scale that can be used to rate the level of empathy achieved by a nurse during an interaction.

MacKay RC, Hughes JR, Carver EJ, editors: *Empathy in the helping relationship*, New York, 1990, Springer.

This book is an excellent reference for nurses who are engaged in research on empathy. It offers complete reviews of the literature, as well as suggestions for areas needing further research.

Morse JM et al: Exploring empathy: a conceptual fit for nursing practice? *Image J Nurs Sch* 24:273, 1992.

In a thought-provoking article, the authors challenge the relevance of the concept of empathy to nursing practice. They suggest that other strategies such as sympathy, pity, consolation, compassion, and commiseration may be more appropriate and offer suggestions for future research.

Pepin JI: Family caring and caring in nursing, *Image* 24:127, 1992.

The author compares the caring provided by family caregivers to that given by nurses. She discusses two dimensions of caring: love and labor. She states that recent formulations of caring have focused on love and excluded labor.

Rogers C: *On becoming a person*, Boston, 1966, Houghton Mifflin.

This book includes a series of essays and lectures that present many of the beliefs underlying the theory of client-centered therapy. It is recommended to the nursing student because of the deeply humanistic approach of the author and the focus on the feelings and experiences of both the client and the therapist as they participate together in a helping relationship.

Rogers C: Empathic: an unappreciated way of being, *Counseling Psychologist* 5:22, 1975.

In this article Rogers updates his work on empathy. He describes the empathic process, relating it to the other characteristics of the therapist-client relationship. This article is highly recommended for novices and experienced therapists. It is written sensitively with great regard for the humanity of client and therapist.

Simon SB, Howe LW, Kirschenbaum H: *Values clarification: a handbook of practical strategies for teachers and students*, rev ed, New York, 1978, Hart.

The authors present the basic concept of values clarification. Although the format is developed for use by primary- and secondary-level teachers, it is easily adaptable for use by those who work with adults. The bulk of the book is devoted to presentation of various values clarification exercises. These would be appropriate for use by an individual or with a small group of students or practicing nurses.

Thorne SE, Robinson CA: Guarded alliance: health care relationships in chronic illness, *Image* 21:153, 1989.

This is a description of a study of the nature of the third stage of the relationship between the client with a chronic illness and the health care provider. The core dimensions identified are trust and competence. Four relationship types are identified.

Truax CB, Carkhuff RB: *Toward effective counseling and psychotherapy: training and practice*, Chicago, 1967, Aldine.

This classic book presents a research methodology for validating the characteristics most closely associated with successful counseling: accurate empathy, nonpossessive warmth, and genuineness. Although directed toward psychotherapists and trainers of therapists, the book is readable and applicable to the experience of students in a helping profession. It is rich with clinical examples and quotes from many noted theorists in the fields of counseling and psychotherapy.

Uustal DB: Values clarification in nursing: application to practice, *Am J Nurs* 78:2058, 1978.

This article is written by a recognized authority on the use of the values clarification process by nurses. It is a good introductory overview of the theory, explaining the process and its relevance for nurses. Also included are 10 values clarification strategies that assist the reader in applying the process with the dual benefit of integrating the concepts and beginning to identify one's own values.

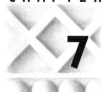

7 The Course of the Helping Relationship

Talk to me
speak to me
of memories
you care for
and moments
that you've shared
and days when love
was more important
than tomorrow.

touch me with
your words
that I might feel
  what you feel
that I might love you
as you need to be loved

Laurence Craig-Green
Perhaps*

LEARNING OBJECTIVES

After studying this chapter, the student should be able to:

- Identify and describe each phase of the helping relationship.
- Identify the current phase of a helping relationship in which the student is participating.
- Collect data and prepare a plan for the first meeting with each assigned client.
- Describe the components of an interpersonal contract.
- Establish a mutually agreed on verbal contract with an assigned client.
- Identify feelings experienced by the client and the student during the course of the helping relationship.

---

* From Craig-Green L: *Perhaps,* Hollywood, Calif, 1973, i.d.t.t.c.

- Discuss the therapeutic use of confrontation, immediacy, self-disclosure, and humor.
- Characterize her own behavior in a specific situation as passive, aggressive, or assertive.
- Describe the elements of assertive behavior.
- Differentiate between angry and hostile behavior.
- Distinguish between dislike of a person and dislike of an aspect of a person's behavior.
- Discuss appropriate demonstrations of affection in the context of the helping relationship.
- Compare and contrast the helping relationship with the social relationship.
- Describe therapeutic nursing interventions with the client who is fearful, angry, hostile, crying, or seductive.
- Discuss the process of terminating a helping relationship.
- Terminate a helping relationship by applying knowledge of the termination process.
- Analyze the manifestations of the relationship concepts of trust, empathy, caring, hope, autonomy, and mutuality during each phase of the helping relationship.

The relationship process is usually divided into four sequential parts or phases, and each phase is characterized by identifiable tasks. Although there may be some overlap between phases, each one builds onto the next. As a group of phase-appropriate tasks is accomplished, there is readiness for movement to the next phase. The nurse can use knowledge of this sequence of phases and tasks to examine the progress of the helping relationship.

PREINTERACTION PHASE

For the nurse the relationship begins before the first face-to-face interaction with the client. In most clinical situations the nurse has access to some information about the client before they meet. This may be as limited as name, address, and age or as complex as a medical record compiled over a period of years. However, by reviewing whatever information is available it is possible to formulate some preliminary ideas about the anticipated relationship.

In this as in each phase of the relationship, the focus is on each of the participants. In terms of the client the nurse must review pertinent theoretic information and past clinical experiences. If the client is an 85-year-old woman who immigrated to the United States from China and is living in a retirement home, it would be wise to review the normal biopsychosocial process of aging. In this case, one would note that her separation from her family is unusual for an elder from China. The Chinese culture places great value on age and expects that younger family members will provide care for the elders. The nursing assessment would explore whether she had family members in the United States and how the decision was made for her to live in a retirement home.

When preparing to provide nursing care to an elderly person, it could also be helpful for the nurse to consider the available information in light of past clinical experiences with aging people, particularly in terms of nursing interventions that did or did not prove effective. Obviously, it is not possible to make specific plans at this point, because the important aspect of the uniqueness of this client has not been experienced. However, the nurse can and should begin to think about potential areas of concern, which then need to be assessed as the relationship progresses.

During this period of time the nurse also has an opportunity to be introspective. It is essential to identify initial reactions to the client even before the individual is seen. For instance, if the nurse who is to interact with the 85-year-old woman is tied down because of financial responsibility for aging parents, resentment toward the parents may influence the nurse-client relationship. This would then block the nurse's ability to be helpful.

Stereotyping or stigmatizing of the client may take place at this time. Stereotyping is the attribution of a set of characteristics to a group of people, such as the idea that Latin Americans are romantic. A stigma attributes a negative characteristic or set of characteristics to a group of people. The belief that people with mental illness are not able to behave responsibly and therefore are dangerous is a stigma. Stereotypes and stigmas are conveyed during the developmental process through association with family and friends and participation in the cultural system. They may operate very subtly, so it is important for the nurse to be aware of her own belief system and to validate it with real experiences with real people. To limit irrational responses during the rest of the relationship it is important to be aware of one's own feeling responses to prospective clients.

Some anxiety is generally present in the nurse during this phase. At mild levels this sharpens thinking and enhances planning for the first interaction. More intense anxiety, however, may interfere with planning by leading to the use of coping or defense mechanisms that inhibit clear thinking. Assistance from an instructor or supervisor may be needed to identify the source of high anxiety and to deal with it. Asking for help in this situation is not a sign of weakness or incompetence. Rather, it indicates self-awareness and openness to others—both of which are positive characteristics that are desirable in the nurse.

The final task of the preinteraction phase is to plan for the first interaction with the client. The nurse should think about the location of the meeting. If one has control of the setting, it should be as comfortable, attractive, and private as possible. A definite period of time (with some flexibility allowed) should be set aside for the meeting. It is also wise to identify the specific information that is to be covered during the first interaction and to outline this mentally.

This is the only phase of the relationship during which the nurse is the sole participant. In the next phase the client becomes actively involved for as long as the relationship lasts.

INTRODUCTORY OR ORIENTATION PHASE

The first meeting between nurse and client sets the tone for the rest of the relationship; therefore it deserves special attention. The plans made during the preinteraction phase should provide a foundation for a successful first meeting.

Introductions

In any interpersonal relationship it is important for each person to identify the other by name. This is perhaps even more crucial in a helping relationship. Yet it is not unusual to observe staff members, including nurses, approaching clients whom they have never met before and not introducing themselves. This can be particularly confusing in settings where staff members wear street clothes. However, even when in complete uniform the nurse should not assume that a client will identify her by reading her name tag. The client may be unable to read or see well or be embarrassed to use a name when unsure how to pronounce it. At the same time the nurse can learn how to pronounce the client's name, an action that is very meaningful, particularly to people with unusual names. Most important, when two people share their names with each other, they are reciprocally offering a part of themselves, indicating an openness to relate to each other and to share further. Within this culture name sharing is also seen as an expression of friendliness. Adults trying to make friends with small children will almost invariably say, "Hello. What's your name?" Thus exchanging names with a new client may also be seen as a friendly gesture.

Stating one's name should be followed by an explanation of one's role, particularly in relation to the client. One example would be: "I am Sarah J., a nursing student. I will be talking with you while you wait to see the doctor." This gives the client an idea of what to expect from the nurse. The client's understanding will need to be validated as the relationship progresses. Beginning students commonly have difficulty with introduction and try to avoid it. It is anxiety provoking to take on a new role, especially when one is just beginning to learn and has doubts about whether the expectations of the role can be met. It is therefore necessary to make an effort to initiate introductions. As the role becomes more familiar, this process becomes easier.

CRITICAL THINKING *Question* ....

Bowie[4] has studied the relationship between status and terms of address. The terms that the nurse selects when addressing the client communicate whether there is

Continued

CRITICAL THINKING *Question —cont'd*

recognition of the client's status. This applies to use of title and last name, as well as the use of pronouns. Consider the possible responses of a client who is a 75-year-old physician to being called "Dr. Smith," "Ms. Smith," or "Mary." Might the response differ according to sociocultural background? Would the client's age make a difference? Are there any other factors that would influence the terms of address selected by the nurse?

The choice of pronouns is another important aspect of addressing clients. Compare and contrast possible responses to a nurse saying, "Are we ready for our bath?" or "Are you ready to take your bath?" Identify other examples of the use of pronouns that enhance or block therapeutic communication.

....

The contract

Another important task during the first meeting is establishing the contract. A contract is simply an agreement between the nurse and the client that describes the nature and content of their relationship. Any contract includes the obligations that are to be met by each of the participants. Mutual establishment of a contract sets a tone for a collaborative helping relationship in which the client participates fully in setting goals and evaluating the effectiveness of nursing interventions.

Zangari and Duffy[18] describe the relationship between the contract and the nursing process. They list the following steps:
1. Nurse initiates database collection.
2. Nurse and client describe their expectations to each other.
3. Mutual agreement is reached on both long- and short-term goals.
4. Contract is established, including distribution of responsibility for each goal.
5. Nurse informs other staff and, if the client agrees, the client's family of the contract and enlists their collaboration.
6. Nurse and client evaluate progress toward goal achievement.
7. Nurse and client revise the contract if goal modification is needed or terminate it if goals have been achieved or the client is discharged.

They also point out that contracts can include options, allowing for more flexibility in the approach to care delivery.

Components of a Nurse-Client Contract

The roles and responsibilities of the nurse and client
The location, frequency, and length of meetings
The overall purpose of the relationship
The duration of the relationship
Indications for termination
Confidentiality

In the helping relationship the contract is usually a verbal one. The mutual expectations that are generally included in the contract are summarized in the box above. Initiating the discussion of a contract may feel awkward the first few times the nurse tries it. It is not necessary and may even be obstructive to use the term *contract* directly with the client. What is important is to gain the client's agreement to the terms of the relationship.

Roles of the nurse and client

Discussion of the nurse's role and responsibilities usually leads to development of the contract. For instance, the nurse may say, "I have explained that I shall be assigned to the Pediatric Clinic for 3 months to learn about the health care of children. I have enjoyed talking with you this morning and would like to meet with you and your children each time you come to the clinic between now and April 30." At this point the client should be allowed to respond. The nurse may then elaborate and clarify other aspects of her role, such as a course requirement that she do a health-teaching project. In return the client should be given time to state personal health goals as they may apply to the relationship, with the nurse validating whether these are areas in which she can help. She can also gradually introduce the other elements of the contract, giving the client an opportunity to respond to each point as it is raised.

Timing is important in introducing the discussion of the contract. There needs to be enough time allowed at the beginning of the conversation so that participants will have developed a beginning awareness of each other as people and will have begun to feel comfortable in talking together. Sometimes anxiety will cause the inexperienced nurse to initiate the discussion of the contract too early in the interaction, possibly resulting in the client's rejection of a continuing relationship. However, another response to anxiety may be to wait until almost the end of the time, thus leaving the discussion of the contract incomplete or superficial. A guideline for the novice nurse would be to introduce this topic at about the midway point of the first interaction, leaving ample time for clarification.

Location, frequency, and length of meetings

Although the nurse should have some idea about the location, frequency, and length of meetings, there should be a mutual decision reached between the nurse and the client. Agreement on these factors gives a sense of reliability and legitimacy to the relationship; each participant is then able to plan for the meeting with a sense of security in expecting the other to be present. Knowledge of the length of the meetings may be reassuring to clients who have difficulty handling vague situations. Time limits should be maintained. Attempts to maneuver this factor are discussed under the working phase of the relationship. Means should also be established for notifying the other if one participant is unable to keep an appointment. It is generally a good idea to reconfirm the time of the next meeting at the end of each session even if there has been no change in the original agreement.

Overall purpose of the relationship

The nurse should give the client an idea of why she is involved in the relationship and what the client should or should not expect from her. For example, a client seeing a nurse practitioner should expect her to interview him and perform a physical examination. He should not expect her to perform surgery, which in most states is an activity restricted to physicians. The nurse must also find out what the client expects from the relationship. Most people who relate to nurses do so by choice, generally because they are seeking help for some health need. At times nursing students approach individuals and invite them to participate in helping relationships. These clients also choose whether to participate. It is important to determine the client's rationale for choosing to relate to the nurse. When the nurse and the client have each presented their own reasons for initiating the relationship, they can work toward mutually determining the purpose of the relationship. This becomes the foundation for the work of future meetings. It is not unusual for it to take the participants more than one session to reach agreement about the purpose of the relationship. Also, by mutual agreement, the purpose may be modified as the relationship progresses.

Duration of the relationship and indications for termination

Sometimes there are conditions external to the relationship itself that determine how long it should last. For instance, the duration of a relationship between a nursing student and a client may be limited by the length of the semester or clinical rotation. A relationship with a hospitalized person may be terminated when the client is discharged. Some relationships are terminated by death. In instances such as these the nurse and the client have little control over the duration of the relationship. It is important to include validation of known external conditions during the first session, so that the client as well as the nurse will be aware of the limits and prepared for termination.

There are also times when the duration of the relationship is not subject to external controls. In this case the nurse and the client should agree on the indications for termination. These indications are derived from the established purpose for the relationship, so that when the goals for the relationship have been accomplished, termination will take place. For example, a community health nurse and a client who is newly diagnosed as diabetic may agree to terminate their relationship when the client has learned to care for himself physically, accepted his illness psychologically, and resumed his normal lifestyle socially.

Way in which confidential material will be handled

The nature of the nurse-client relationship is (and should be) conducive to the client's confiding in the nurse. Curtin[7] asserts that the promise of confidentiality is implicit in the nature of the therapeutic relationship. Possession of personal information about clients is a serious responsibility. Information is a source of power. As Curtin has pointed out, the amount of power given is directly related to the intimate or vital nature of the information possessed.

This gives the health care provider great control over the client. Therefore clients have a right to expect nurses to handle this information with respect and discretion. Confidentiality in a professional relationship implies that client information will be shared only with appropriate others and in appropriate places in a professional manner. Inappropriate others include friends, parents, and spouses—anyone who is not directly involved in the care of the client. It also implies that when information is shared, it will be done with the purpose of facilitating the care that the client receives. Students should specify that aspects of the relationship will be shared with the instructor and classmates as a part of the learning experience.

It is important to discuss confidentiality with the client. Sometimes the client assumes that the relationship with the nurse is secret. When he discovers that the nurse has written notes in the chart or has talked with a physician, the client may feel betrayed and lose trust in the nurse unless he has been warned that this will happen. Sometimes the client approaches the nurse and offers to confide a matter of extreme importance "If you promise not to tell anybody, not even my doctor." The nurse should be aware of this trap and *never* agree to these terms. If the client's message is that he just took a bottle of sleeping pills, the nurse is in a dilemma. She has agreed not to tell. The client may not have really taken the pills and may be testing her reliability, yet he may have taken them and be in need of immediate medical attention. Of course in this situation the physician would be informed, but more subtle variations of this situation may be much more difficult to resolve. A better way to handle such a situation would be not to agree to maintain unconditional secrecy but to reserve judgment on who to tell until the client has shared the information. He should be warned in advance that it may be necessary for his welfare to share his confidence with another health-team member.

Summarizing the contract

It is usually helpful for both participants to summarize the elements of the agreement at the end of their first interaction. This may include writing down the important facts, such as the nurse's name; meeting dates, times, and locations; and termination date if known, and then giving them to the client for future reference. The purpose of the relationship and the expectations of each participant should be reviewed and any misunderstandings clarified.

Beginning client assessment

Once the contract has been established, the nurse and the client can concentrate on expanding their knowledge of each other. This is a major task of the initiation phase of the relationship and continues beyond the first session. The nurse is organizing the information gathered about the client through the process of nursing assessment. As the assessment proceeds the nurse becomes aware of the uniqueness of the client as an individual and begins to see him as a real person rather than as a "client." The client will be performing his own assessment of the nurse and will be comparing her with his preconceived ideas of what a nurse should be. He may also engage in some "testing" behavior at this point; this type of behavior is one way of measuring the nurse's sincerity and interest. For instance, if he doubts the nurse's concern about him, he may wait somewhere other than their agreed-on meeting place to see if she will look for him. Another time he may refuse to talk much to see if she will stay for the whole time anyway. As the client develops trust in the nurse and learns by her consistent demonstration of interest in him that she is trustworthy, the need for testing behavior will decline. At this point the client is beginning to perceive the nurse as an individual rather than as a "nurse." When both participants view each other as unique individuals, they are ready to begin building more specific goals for their relationship based on the interaction between the unique aspects of their personalities. At this point they have begun to move into the working phase of their relationship.

By the end of the orientation phase the participants are no longer strangers to each other. Through evidence of mutual commitment to the relationship, trust is beginning to develop. Two originally autonomous individuals have developed a degree of mutuality by agreeing on the terms and purpose of the relationship. As they begin to appreciate each other's uniqueness, they begin to care about each other—in a very tentative way at first. As caring develops, the potential for empathy

grows. The initial anxiety has been alleviated, and they are now beginning to be able to assess each other's anxiety levels accurately. Their roles within the relationship have been clarified, and both hope that the relationship will be a rewarding one. All of this signifies that the relationship is entering the maintenance or working phase.

MAINTENANCE OR WORKING PHASE

The nurse-client relationship now enters the period of time when interaction is maintained for the purpose of accomplishing the mutually agreed-on tasks (work). Therefore this phase is generally designated the *maintenance* or *working phase* of the relationship.

Patterns of growth and resistance

The relationship may feel more comfortable to the participants during this phase because they know each other and some degree of predictability has developed. However, it is also a time of intensive work. If the relationship is proceeding productively, there should be periods of growth demonstrated by positive behavioral changes. These periods of growth alternate with times of resistance during which the client continues with or goes back to his earlier behaviors. The Clinical Example illustrates such growth and resistance behavior.

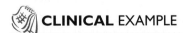 **CLINICAL** EXAMPLE

Ms. J. was an 80-year-old woman who had been hospitalized with a fractured hip. Because of a permanent restriction of her mobility and because no family members were able to care for her, the decision was made that she should be discharged to a nursing home. Ms. B., the staff nurse who had cared for Ms. J. consistently throughout her hospitalization, was aware that the client would need understanding help in accepting the loss of her home and many of her possessions. Ms. J. trusted the nurse and with encouragement was able to share her feelings of anger, sadness, and helplessness and to cry. The client stated that she felt better after expressing these feelings. However, the next time Ms. B. approached her she was withdrawn and distant, responding briefly and only when addressed directly.

This type of response is not unusual following the exposure of painful feelings to another person. Such self-disclosure may lead to feelings of vulnerability, shame, and self-consciousness, and at times it may be necessary to limit the amount of personal information the client shares. Superficially, a response such as Ms. J.'s could be interpreted as anger, resulting in confusion and reciprocal anger on the part of the nurse. Whenever a behavioral change is observed, it is important to validate the meaning of the change with the client and to assess the change in the context of the mutually agreed-on goals for the relationship. In this situation Ms. B. was able to communicate her continued concern for and acceptance of Ms. J. This alleviated the client's anxiety, and the nurse and client began again to work together.

Facilitating expression of feelings

An important aspect of the nurse's role during the maintaining phase of the relationship is to encourage open expression of feelings on the part of the client. This frequently involves a change in behavior. Sociocultural factors generally determine the extent to which feelings may be verbalized, in what situations, and by whom. It is therefore essential that the nurse take into account the assessment of the client's sociocultural background when helping the client verbalize feelings. If this is a new experience for the client, a great deal of patience and understanding will be required. The nurse may also be unaccustomed to confrontation with intense feelings of another and become so involved with her own reciprocal feelings that she fails to respond to the client objectively. The nurse must examine her own responses and increase her self-awareness so that her feelings are less apt to cloud her perception of the client's situation. Frequently help is needed in acquiring this self-awareness. Supervision from faculty or more experienced staff members should be requested if feelings seem to be blocking nurse-client communications.

During the working phase the nurse may facilitate the client's exploration and expression of feelings by the use of the therapeutic communication techniques described in Chapter 5. In addition, Carkhuff[6] has identified three other activities that the helping person can use with discretion to assist the client in dealing with feelings: confrontation, immediacy, and self-disclosure.

Confrontation The nurse may choose to use confrontation when she is aware of inconsistencies in the client's behavior and believes that it would be beneficial for the client to be aware of this. Carkhuff identified three types of inconsistency that might occur:

1. Inconsistency between the client's view of himself as he is and his description of what he would like to be
2. Inconsistency between the client's verbal and nonverbal communication
3. Inconsistency between the client's perception of himself and the nurse's perception of him

Confrontation of inconsistent behavior can be useful to the client if it is presented in the context of a trusting relationship and in a caring way. Hostile confrontation has no place in a helping relationship. If the client is unable or unwilling to recognize the inconsistency, it is generally best not to push the issue but return to it at a later time if the behavior occurs again.

Frequently as people change and grow their self-concept changes more slowly than does their behavior. Confrontation can assist the client to recognize the growth that is taking place. The following example demonstrates this:

CLIENT: I feel fat and dumpy.
NURSE: The last time we met, you told me you had lost 15 pounds and gone down a dress size. I really see the difference.
CLIENT: I guess you're right, but I still *feel* fat sometimes.

Confrontation may also be used to initiate discussion of an issue relevant to the relationship, as demonstrated in this example:

NURSE: You say these meetings are important to you, yet you come late each time.
CLIENT: I figure you have better things to do with your time.
NURSE: The meetings are important to you, but you don't believe they're important to me?
CLIENT: Yeah—except you're here and I'm not. Seems backward, doesn't it?
NURSE: It sure does! (Both laugh.)

Sensitive use of confrontation can open up the relationship and allow the participants to explore new areas. It involves some risk taking for the nurse, but it also has the potential for great rewards.

CRITICAL THINKING *Question* ···············

Confrontation can be helpful when used within a trusting nurse-client relationship. Identify situations in which confrontation would probably not be helpful. What are the factors that must be considered when using confrontation as a communication skill? Are there groups of individuals who would not be likely to respond well to confrontation from a nurse? How might you tell that someone does not appreciate being confronted?

··

Immediacy Immediacy refers to focusing the interaction on the present situation between the nurse and the client in the relationship. The nurse-client relationship may represent the client's interactions with other significant people. By discussing behavior within the relationship the client can be assisted to understand his interactions with other people as well. Successful use of immediacy by the nurse is closely related to the level of empathy that has been achieved. The nurse must be able to perceive the client's feeling tone while also analyzing the status of the relationship and then reflect the connection between these elements back to the client. An example of this process follows:

NURSE: You've been very quiet today.
CLIENT: Um-hm.
NURSE: I wonder if you are upset with me for missing our last session because my car broke down?

Acknowledgment by the client in this example that he was upset about the nurse's absence could then lead to a discussion of how he acts when he is upset with people. As the nurse gains skill in interpersonal relationships, she will find many opportunities to use here-and-now situations as learning experiences for both herself and the client.

Self-disclosure Self-disclosure refers to the nurse's revealing personal experiences, thoughts, ideas, values, attitudes, or feelings in the context of the relationship. The purpose is not to provide a therapeutic opportunity for the nurse but to provide the client with a model or with evidence that his experiences can be understood by others. Careful use of self-disclosure can add to the mutuality of the relationship as the client comes to view the nurse as a real person who can therefore understand his real problems and concerns. Young[17] has noted that similarities between the nurse and the client contribute to genuineness and empathy, decreasing social distance and increasing self-disclosure.

Limited self-disclosure may be helpful in the beginning stages of the relationship when the client may request information about the nurse, such as hometown, marital status, years until graduation, and other related facts. The nurse should respond to these requests with discretion, giving only information that she is comfortable in releasing and that would facilitate the progress of the relationship. This is illustrated in the following examples:

Example 1: Ms. J., a nursing student, is visiting Ms. R., an elderly client who lives by herself in a senior citizen apartment complex.
MS. R.: This is my cat, Fluffy. I don't know what I'd do without her. She means so much to me.
MS. J.: I know just what you mean, Ms. R. My cat, Midnight, meets me at the door every night when I come home. I look forward to seeing her.

Example 2: Ms. J. next visits Tom W., an 18-year-old who is in a back brace following a football injury.
TOM: It's nice having you come to visit. I get really bored being around the house all day. Do you have a boyfriend?
MS. J.: You feel like you're drifting away from your friends now that you can't go to school?

In the first example Ms. J. offered information about herself that enhanced the closeness between her and Ms. R. In the second example she chose not to answer Tom's question, because she perceived that his real need was to discuss his loneliness and ways to reestablish himself with his peers.

Auvil and Silver[3] have analyzed self-disclosure in a relationship to the phases of the nurse-client relationship. During the orientation phase self-disclosure should be limited to that needed to communicate warmth and a wish to become involved. As the relationship progresses into the working phase, self-disclosure can assist the client to perceive the nurse's values and select attributes on which he may pattern his own behavior. Finally, sharing one's own feelings during termination helps both the client and the nurse to fully appreciate the value of the relationship.

At times it may be necessary to deflect a client's insistent requests that the nurse disclose personal information that is not related to the relationship. Auvil and Silver suggest several approaches to this dilemma. These include:

1. Benign curiosity. The nurse inquires about why the information might be important to the client: "I wonder why you want to know that."
2. Redirection or refocusing. The nurse ignores the request for personal information and refocuses on the topic that was being discussed before the request was made: "I don't think we had finished talking about your visit with your aunt."
3. Interpretation. The nurse requests the client to look at the reason for taking the focus of the discussion away from himself: "I've noticed that when we start to talk about your problems at school, you change the subject to talk about me."
4. Ask for clarification. The nurse asks the client the reason for requesting a particular piece of information at a particular point in time: "You're asking about my relationship with my husband. I wonder if something has happened recently that has led you to bring that up."
5. Feedback and limit setting. The nurse informs the client about her reaction to his trying to persuade her to share personal information: "I'm uncomfortable when you try to find out about my social life, because this is a professional rather than a social relationship."

Although these approaches may seem awkward at first, practice will enable the nurse to use them more naturally. It helps to keep in mind that the purpose of the relationship is to assist the client with health care problems. Therefore it is important to maintain the focus of the interaction on the client.

Use of humor in the relationship The inclusion of humor in the nurse-client relationship might seem inappropriate. People often seek health care because of serious, frightening, and often life-threatening problems. They expect to be taken seriously. However, using humor judiciously can help the client gain perspective on his problems. By reducing stress it also has a positive physiologic effect on the person; the physiologic effect of stress reduction is described in Chapter 9. Acceptance of the therapeutic value of humor has resulted in the creation of humor rooms in some hospitals.[5] These rooms are stocked with comedy videotapes and films, joke books, cartoon collections, clown equipment, and any other aids or props that will cause the clients and staff to laugh.

Opportunities for humor often arise spontaneously in a nurse-client relationship. Sharing laughter can cause the nurse and client to feel closer to each other, promoting the development of empathy and caring. Enjoying a humorous situation can also help the client cope with fears and anxieties related to his condition. See the Clinical Example below.

Several therapeutic uses of humor have been identified by Davidhizar and Schearer.[8] The first is stress management. This is characterized by relaxation and decreased interpersonal tension. It may be used as a coping mechanism, assisting the person to adapt to change, and in this case humor is most helpful to people who have used it for coping in the past. As a communication technique humor can decrease interpersonal distance. As a relationship-building strategy it can help increase the participants' self-esteem. Humor is a tool to promote physical healing. It also promotes psychologic healing.

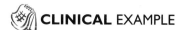 **CLINICAL EXAMPLE**

Mr. J. was recovering from the above-the-knee amputation of his right leg. He was feeling discouraged about his progress in physical therapy. Ms. T., his primary nurse, tried to persuade him to talk about his feelings, but he refused to do so. As she was leaving the room, Ms. T. slipped on a wet spot on the floor. She regained her balance after nearly falling, and Mr. J. said, "When I get the hang of using my new leg, I want the next dance." They laughed together and were then able to discuss Mr. J.'s problems in physical therapy.

Although humor has many positive applications in the nurse-client relationship, it must be used with care. Sometimes humor is experienced as hostile. If the client does not understand the reason for the humor, it can be frustrating, and some people just do not have a well-developed sense of humor. Humor that focuses on a person's ethnic or cultural background or on an unusual physical characteristic is usually inappropriate in a health care situation. Raines[15] has suggested questions that can be used to assess a client's use and appreciation of humor. These include:

1. How often do you find yourself looking at the humorous side of a situation when dealing with everyday problems?
2. Since you have been ill, do you find yourself using humor more, less, or about the same?
3. Which of the following activities do you find amusing or enjoyable?
   a. Watching comedy movies
   b. Watching cartoons
   c. Watching comedies on television
   d. Hearing jokes
   e. Telling jokes
   f. Reading joke books
   g. Being around funny people
4. Does it make you feel better or worse if the people around you have a sense of humor?
5. Can you think of a time when humor has made you feel better?
6. Do you like telling jokes or funny stories?
7. Can you think of a time when humor made you feel worse?

She suggests additional questions that the nurse can consider to complete the assessment, and these include:

1. What cues have been given that the client would be receptive to humor?
2. What cues have been given that the client would not be receptive to certain kinds of humor, or are there certain areas about which the client is sensitive?
3. Is the client's physical or emotional state such that humor might be annoying or indicate a lack of caring?
4. What are the specific problems for which a humorous approach could be used?

5. Are there cultural aspects to consider in using humor?

Based on a complete assessment of the client's use of humor, the nurse can use her own sense of humor to make the relationship more pleasurable for the client and herself.

Responding to the client's feelings

Self-disclosure, immediacy, and confrontation, as well as humor and self-awareness, can all be valuable tools for the nurse while assisting clients to deal with their feelings. Feelings that commonly arise and must be dealt with during a helping relationship include fear, anger, hostility, dislike, sadness, affection, and sexuality. These are discussed now.

Responding to the fearful client Fear may be defined as a response to a threat. It is differentiated from anxiety by the individual's ability to identify the threat underlying fear, whereas the source of anxiety is usually hidden. Most people who are clients of the health care system experience some level of fear. Health care clients face threats to lifestyle, self-concept, physical integrity, and any other aspect of biopsychosocial functioning. Even a routine physical examination causes the fear that some area of dysfunction may be revealed, and this fear is enhanced by the constant reminders from the media of the many health problems to which people are vulnerable. Hospital admission brings another set of fears related to unfamiliar surroundings, intrusions on personal space, strangers, and complicated procedures. Even discharge from the hospital creates fears about perceived changes in ability to function, mastery of self-care activities, and responses of significant others to the recovering person.

Behavioral manifestations of fear are similar to those of anxiety as described in Chapter 9. It may be helpful to the client to have fear recognized and accepted by the nurse. Some clients will want to talk about their fears to identify the threats to which they are responding. Other clients may prefer to remain silent but to have someone close by offering nonverbal support. Some people want detailed information about what is happening to them; others desire only a general explanation. As the nurse assesses the individual's response to a stressful situation, the individual's preferred way of dealing with the immediate threat should be respected and supported. When the feeling of fear is under control, it is usually helpful to the client to talk about the experience and memory of it. The nurse can help the client in assessing his ability to cope with threatening situations and in identifying coping behaviors that may be helpful in future similar circumstances.

Responding to the angry client Anger is an emotion that may be frightening to the individual, because it involves the potential of being destructive to the self and others. As part of the normal development process each person evolves ways of handling anger to minimize this destructive potential. One such method is to direct anger at objects less threatening or less capable of retaliation than the real object. For instance, a client who is angry at her husband for not visiting may snap at the nurse rather than phone her husband to tell him how she feels. She thereby releases some of her anger and avoids a confrontation with her husband, a more significant person to her than the nurse.

Others may turn anger inward, blaming themselves for their problems and experiencing guilt. With these individuals any external expression of anger is too threatening, and the self becomes the best alternative object. In the example of the client whose husband fails to visit, the client may express her anger by saying that she was not cheerful enough the last time he visited and thereby drove him away.

Silence is another way of handling angry feelings. The silent angry client fears that if he speaks at all, his angry feelings will pour out. Anger may be inferred by his facial expression, but this inference would need to be validated with the client.

Some people who are unable to express anger directly choose indirect means to express it; this may be labeled as *passive-aggressive behavior.* For instance, some people behave in a way that superficially looks like intense kindness. Phrases such as "She's too nice to be believed" and "killing with kindness" refer to this type of behavior. Although the person's overt intent is to be nice to the other, there is an underlying current of anger. This may be recognized by a sense of discomfort or an angry response to the person's actions that may at first seem unprovoked. Other passive-aggressive expressions may include forgetting important things such

as a person's name or an appointment. Of course it should be remembered that some people have poor memories. The behavior becomes significant within the context of the relationship. The nurse's own feelings in response to a client provide an important clue about the issues that need to be addressed in the interaction. If the nurse feels angry and cannot identify a reason to be angry that is unrelated to the client, she should consider the possibility that the client is behaving in a passive-aggressive manner.

Anger often arises in the course of the nurse-client relationship and may be bewildering to the nurse until she identifies its source. An individual who is submitting to any level of medical care has to some extent placed himself in a dependent position. People who highly value their independence may become angry in response to this feeling of dependence. On the other hand, a person who likes being dependent may become angry if he is encouraged to assume a more independent role in his care. In either case the nurse will probably notice this anger expressed within the context of her relationship with the client.

Clients may also become angry if they think the nurse has become too close to them. This may occur if the nurse asks for too much self-disclosure before the client is ready or if she fails to prevent the client from revealing too much. Anger in this case is a way of telling the nurse to keep her distance, because the client is uncomfortable.

At times nursing care inevitably involves discomfort for the client. Changing a surgical dressing or giving an injection causes physical pain. Asking the questions necessary to complete a thorough assessment may cause psychologic pain. A normal response when a person is subjected to physical or psychologic discomfort is anger. Therefore the nurse should be prepared to cope with anger created by these circumstances. In addition, the nurse may unwittingly cause discomfort for the patient at times. For instance, a previously resistant client may indicate readiness for health teaching. The nurse may decide to spend extra time to capitalize on the readiness, making her late for the appointment with her next client. The client who had to wait may then be angry, because waiting was uncomfortable.

Anger generally occurs in response to the frustration and anxiety that result when an individual is unable to fulfill a need or reach a goal. The more important the need or goal is to the person, the more intense will be his frustration and the angrier he will appear. Even if the source of the frustration seems trivial to the nurse, it must be remembered that the client's perception of the situation determines the extent of the angry response.

Lancee et al.[11] studied the amount of anger experienced by psychiatric clients related to the way in which nurses placed limits on unacceptable behavior. They found that the least amount of anger was felt when the nurse was empathic. Somewhat more anger was felt when the nursing action was explained to the client, and the most anger occurred when the nurse used an unempathic approach such as belittling the client. This study demonstrates the effect that the nurse's way of communicating with the client can have on the client's behavior.

Assertiveness Both the nurse and the client who are having difficulty expressing anger constructively may benefit from learning and applying the principles of assertiveness training. Anger is frequently expressed passively or aggressively rather than assertively. Translated into transactional analysis terms, anger is frequently expressed at the child or parent level rather than at the adult level. Passive or aggressive expression of angry feelings tends to generate an angry response. This often leads to escalation of feelings, resulting in an argument and no resolution of the original problem. Anger presented in an assertive manner is stated rationally; it is expressed with feeling but not in a manner that will degrade the other person. As in the following example, the individual states the feeling that is being experienced as well as the reason for the feeling, the expectation of the other person, and the consequences of failure to change:

Ms. L., the head nurse, was aware that she was becoming increasingly angry at Ms. D., a staff nurse. Ms. D. was 15 to 20 minutes late every time she was scheduled to work. Ms. L. arranged a counseling session with Ms. D. and stated, "I am angry at you because you are consistently late for work. This adds to my work and the work of the other nurses, because we have to repeat the report for you when you arrive, putting us all behind schedule. I expect that you will arrive at work on time. If you have a problem that is causing your lateness, I need to know so I can help you

find a way to resolve it. As you know, chronic lateness is a reason for dismissal, but you are a good nurse and I would prefer not to have to dismiss you."

Although the message was probably upsetting to Ms. D., it was delivered firmly and directly, with no attempt to attack her as a person. The head nurse made it clear that it was Ms. D.'s behavior that made her angry and that she was willing to assist her to find help in changing her behavior. She also informed her of the consequences of failure to change.

Alberti and Emmons[1] have identified seven components of assertive behavior: direct eye contact; erect body posture with appropriate distance and leaning toward the other person; appropriate gestures; congruent facial expression; moderate tone, inflection, and volume of voice; timing; and content. Content includes the directness and spontaneity of what is said plus accepting responsibility for the feelings that are expressed.

In describing an assertiveness course that was taught to senior nursing students, Palmer and Deck[12] identified five assertive behaviors that group members often needed to remind each other about:

1. Using *I*'s in statements
2. Using words that are congruent with the state of mind, such as using "I think" to express a thought or "I feel" to express a feeling
3. Using stronger words that imply greater control rather than weaker ones
4. Developing awareness of self-devaluing statements
5. Communicating assertively, including slow, deliberate speech and attending to nonverbal communication.

Anger must be dealt with individually in each situation in which it occurs. The nurse needs first to validate that the client is indeed angry. It may be reassuring to the client that the nurse is prepared to accept the expression of this feeling. Open expression of feelings of anger in an assertive way that does not result in later feelings of guilt is healthy behavior and should be encouraged. Next, it is helpful to look at the circumstances that have led to the anger. If the nurse is involved in the situation, it can be clarified by discussion with the client. Both can share the feelings and responses to the other that they experienced during the interaction. It may then be helpful for the nurse to demonstrate for the client an assertive approach to the problem. After discussing feelings and responses once again, the client should be encouraged to try out the alternative behavior in a role-play situation with the nurse, followed by more feedback. If the client begins to try to be assertive in other situations, the nurse should be sure to give encouragement and recognition for the change in behavior.[1]

Other approaches that enhance assertiveness have been suggested by Palmer and Deck.[13] *Thought substitution* refers to the replacement of negative or self-defeating thoughts by positive or self-enhancing ones. This needs to be done consciously, so the nurse should assist the client to identify both negative and positive thought patterns. Learning to be skilled at *negotiation* involves application of assertive behavior. In this case the person has a particular objective in mind and must acquire the assistance of another to achieve it. The person must be able to describe the objective, its benefits, and the help that is required. *Equalizing internal messages* may be helpful when the client subordinates his own needs to those of others. It requires him to consciously remind himself of his rights and those of the other so they may be balanced in a rational way.

If the client's anger is not directed at the nurse, she can still assist him to manage it appropriately. Listening and helping the client identify the reason for the anger are of paramount importance. Providing a description of the situation can also help the client express any residual feelings to an understanding and receptive person. The assertiveness training process can then be implemented. It is important for the nurse to return to the client after he has practiced a new behavior to see if he is satisfied with it and to help identify alternatives if he is not.

Learning to express feelings of anger constructively can be a painful process and requires understanding and patience on the part of the nurse. It may be particularly stressful for the beginning nurse who is developing an awareness of her own methods of handling anger.

Responding to the hostile client Many individuals behave in a hostile manner when confronted with a new situation. This may be particularly true if past experiences in similar situations have been negative. Hostility may provide the person with a degree of protection by keeping others at a safe distance.

Unfortunately, there is generally also the result of making others less willing to offer help or to approach the client. A cyclic self-defeating pattern then develops, whereby the client seeks help in a hostile manner, is rejected by the potential helpers, and feels justified and reinforced in a negative view of the health care system.

Green[9] has identified several behaviors that may indicate hostility. The person may have a need to retaliate verbally or nonverbally. This may include "rudeness, criticism, insults, sarcasm, repetitive complaining," and various physically assaultive behaviors. Withdrawal that is characterized by a threatening or resentful attitude is often experienced as hostile, and it is also suggested that some physiologic disorders may be at least partially related to hostility. These illnesses, which include hypertension and headaches among others, represent the stress imposed by relating to others in a hostile manner. The physiologic effects of stress are explored further in Chapter 9.

Hostility generates a hostile response. Green[9] has referred to it as "anger with a hook." There is frequently also a feeling of dislike toward the hostile person. Nurses may experience difficulty in dealing with attitudes of hostility on the part of their clients or themselves. Hostility is rarely a component of a trusting or caring relationship. If it does occur in one of these situations, it becomes necessary to search for occurrences within the relationship that might have destroyed trust. An example of this might be an instance in which the client becomes aware of a breach of confidentiality and loses trust in the nurse. Approaches to the hostile client are consistent with those that tend to facilitate the development of trust. Time and patience will probably be necessary to establish even the beginning of trust with a hostile client. The nurse may well respond with hostile feelings; self-awareness and security in her professional role are essential for the nurse who is working with a hostile client. The nurse's own feelings must be identified and correlated to the client's behavior. Because hostile clients often seek out vulnerable areas and verbally attack them, the nurse needs to have professional role security. A beginning nurse can feel devastated by an attack directed at professional competency unless the communication is placed in the context of the client's situation.

Responding to feelings of dislike Dislike may be linked to hostility, because these reactions often occur together. It is difficult to like a hostile person. Likes and dislikes are intimately related to a person's life experiences. It may be difficult to identify why another person is liked or disliked. Nurses have a responsibility to try to understand their responses to clients and to learn how this affects their ability to care for people. It may not be realistic to expect to like every client who is ever contacted, but it is imperative to try to identify reasons for positive and negative responses to people. Over time it may be possible to modify some reactions of dislike through increased self-understanding. Clients may also demonstrate dislike for particular nurses. This should be accepted as the client's right, but it should also be assessed as to possible causes.

Individuals can usually sense that another person dislikes them. Frequently dislike of a particular aspect of behavior is confused with dislike of the whole person and it is important to clarify this point with clients. Caring for a person or being cared for is in no way a commitment to like everything the other individual does or says. One must be explicit in conveying this message to a client. The Clinical Example at right may clarify this concept.

Clients often need the reassurance that Ricky needed regardless of age. Behaviors associated with illness are often behaviors that people dislike in themselves and expect others to dislike as well. If the client is experiencing a negative self-concept, it is difficult for him to feel liked. The nurse must then put forth extra effort to help the client accept himself as worthwhile and likeable. If the nurse does like the client as a person, this can usually be communicated through a consistently caring approach and may be verbalized directly. For instance, the nurse may say, "I really like you as a person, and I would like to help you change the things about yourself that you dislike." If the nurse is experiencing dislike toward a client, however, it may be better for the nurse to arrange for another person to work with the client. This is definitely a situation wherein discussion with a supervisor is recommended to better identify the nurse-client problem and to initiate growth-producing changes.

Responding to sadness As a client grows to trust the nurse he may decide to share with her

 CLINICAL EXAMPLE

*T*hree-year-old Ricky T. accompanied his mother when she brought his new baby sister to the well-baby clinic for her first checkup. While she was interviewing Ms. T., the nursing student noted that Ricky was "patting" the baby quite hard and that his mother told him to stop. Ricky then looked quite dejected and sat alone in a corner. The student also discovered that Ricky had been toilet trained but was now less consistently successful in getting to the bathroom in time. Ms. T. said that she disciplined him for wetting himself by verbally scolding him and withholding snacks. She said that he seemed to understand, because he often said, "Ricky bad boy" when he had misbehaved. The student explained that Ricky may have been responding to the stress of the new baby and to the fear that his mother would no longer love him. She encouraged Ms. T. to demonstrate her love for Ricky in addition to setting consistent limits on his misbehavior. She also discussed Ricky's tendency to see himself as "good" or "bad" based on his behavior and his mother's response to him. He needed to be helped to see that his mother could dislike his behavior while continuing to love him.

experiences that are painful for him to remember. For instance, an elderly widow may reminisce about her relationship with her husband. She will also be sharing her feelings of sadness over having lost this relationship. Any loss, past or present, creates feelings of sadness.

There is also an element of sadness in change, even long-anticipated change. High school or college graduation, for example, contains elements of relief, joy, and sadness. A young woman who is pregnant for the first time may feel awed and happy about her condition but also sad about giving up a degree of independence to become a mother. The nurse needs to recognize this and to communicate to the client that these feelings are normal and acceptable.

Sadness generally leads to the urge to cry. Socioculturally, crying is not always acceptable. In our culture this is particularly true for men. It is considered to be feminine and not quite respectable for a man to cry. However, it is also very uncomfortable to try not to cry when one is feeling sad. If a client appears to be about to cry, the nurse can sometimes facilitate the crying by verbally recognizing the client's discomfort and suggesting that crying may help.

Nurses also have to deal with their own socioculturally derived feelings about crying. Frequently the initial impulse in response to a person who is crying is to encourage him to stop with platitudes such as "It will be all right" or "It's not that bad." To make the nurse more comfortable the client may then stop crying, thereby feeling still more uncomfortable himself. A more helpful response is a simple assertion that crying is all right, perhaps accompanied by a touch. It is important to remain with the client until he regains control and to offer to talk with him about whatever has distressed him. These indications of acceptance are reassuring to the client and help to build his trust in the nurse as a compassionate person.

The nurse who is a warm and caring person will probably feel very sad about the life situations of some clients. If the nurse is moved to tears, it is best for her to be honest with the client about the feelings that are being experienced. A statement such as "What you just told me makes me very sad" may be appropriate. If the nurse is able to accept feelings of sadness and share them openly with the client, this could facilitate the client's expression of feelings. To leave the room abruptly after the client has related a moving experience would convey rejection and create a communication block between the nurse and the client. If the nurse has spontaneously shared intense feelings with a client, it would be advisable for her to review the situation carefully following the interaction. The focus of the interaction should remain on the client's feelings and needs. If in confronting self-behavior the nurse feels that this has not been the case, consultation with an instructor or supervisor could be helpful.

Responding to feelings of affection As the relationship develops and the bonds of trust between client and nurse grow, feelings of mutual affection also develop. This can make the relationship pleasant and facilitate growth. It can also create problems for the nurse when the client's expressions of affection infringe on the limits of a professional helping relationship. It is the responsibility of the nurse to set limits in this area.

The setting of limits in the professional relationship is also referred to as maintaining *professional boundaries*. It refers to avoiding social relationships with clients, as well as other types of involvement such as business partnerships. Pilette et al.[14] point out that it may be difficult to identify boundary violations because they are often related to the nurse's own needs. They recommend careful self-assessment so the nurse can seek supervisory assistance in dealing with boundary problems.

A professional relationship is necessarily different from one that develops in a social setting. Social relationships develop on a basis of relative equality. Responsibility for the progress of the relationship is shared by both participants. Each person expects the other to respond with help in time of need. There is reciprocal sharing of problems. The duration of the relationship is not usually determined, and meetings may or may not be predetermined. Sometimes there is a formal termination, but it is not uncommon for a social relationship to fade away as the interest or proximity of the participants changes.

Compare this type of relationship with the helping relationship that has an explicit contract and planned meetings. Perhaps the most important difference is in the balance of responsibility for the progress of the relationship. The nurse always retains responsibility for maintaining the goal-directed nature of the relationship and for continually assessing progress toward the mutually determined goals. Because these goals are established around the health needs of the client, it is inappropriate for the nurse to share her own needs and problems with the client.

As affectionate feelings grow a conflict can arise because of the difference between the two kinds of relationships. Both participants are more familiar with, and feel more comfortable in, a social relationship. The client may begin to feel vaguely guilty about asking for so much help from the nurse and giving none in return. The nurse may feel uncomfortable encouraging the client to disclose his experiences, thoughts, and feelings openly while sharing less of herself. It may seem to both that their feelings of mutual affection are suspect when a more equal or social relationship does not evolve.

A further danger for the nurse in this situation is the loss of objectivity. An objective approach is essential in a professional relationship. The nurse may find herself becoming angry at others who set limits on her client or who question the progress of the relationship. Crying in response to feelings of sadness may be an attempt to meet her own needs and not those of the client. The nurse may avoid looking at goal achievement within the relationship, protesting that such an approach is unfeeling. It is important to be aware that such reactions are indications that the relationship is veering off course.

CRITICAL THINKING *Question* ················

Most professional codes of ethics prohibit personal relationships between care providers and clients. What are the reasons for this? Is it ever all right for a nurse to have a social relationship with a former client? Should a nurse ever date or marry a former client? What is the rationale for your opinion?

···

Heinrich[10] has described three stages of emotional overinvolvement by a nurse. The first is the stage of initial attraction. The nurse feels drawn to the client, and she gradually begins to treat the client more like a friend. Co-workers may notice increased emotion related to the client or unusual fascination with the details of his problem. The second stage, conflict, is characterized by anger and guilt when the nurse realizes that she is too attached to the client. This guilt may stand in the way of seeking peer support. The third stage is withdrawal—the nurse withdraws from the client suddenly with no explanation. This is very destructive to the client's ability to trust, and the nurse should be assisted to explain the situation to the client.

Consistent supervision is one way of avoiding this pitfall. This is optimal for any nurse involved in ongoing helping relationships, but it is particularly crucial for the novice who has not yet learned enough about herself to be sensitive to incipient problems.

Responding to sexual feelings The experience and expression of affection are closely linked to sexuality. As the nurse and client come to care about each other, one or both may feel sexually attracted to the other. To maintain the professional helping focus of the relationship, these feelings must be recognized but not acted on. The nurse who is attracted to a client will probably find it helpful to share her feelings with a trusted, more experienced nurse who can guide her in her approach to the client. Seductive behavior by the nurse can be very uncomfortable for a client who does not wish to reciprocate and can create an obstacle to progress in the relationship.

If the nurse and client are sexually attracted to each other, the nurse will again need supervision in deciding how to approach the situation. Modifying the relationship to a social one is not ethical for the reasons discussed earlier. It is difficult to ignore sexual feelings, especially when the nurse may be providing very intimate physical care to the client. If the attraction prevents the nurse and client from being able to interact at a professional level, it may be best for the nurse to arrange for a colleague to care for that client.

Probably more common than either of these situations is the one in which the client is sexually attracted to the nurse who does not feel a reciprocal attraction. This situation may be aggravated by the image that is projected by the media of the nurse as a sex object. Combined with the intimacy of the nurse-client situation, this can lead the client to believe that the nurse will be receptive to a sexual approach. Client behavior may range from off-color stories to remarks about the nurse's physical attributes to inappropriate touching and lewd suggestions. Several possible explanations for seductive client behavior have been suggested by Assey and Herbert.[2] These include a need for friendliness and warmth, attention seeking, a demonstration of anger, and a plea for reassurance about sexual attractiveness. Understanding the behavior in the appropriate context can help the nurse to react without becoming defensive. The best approach for the nurse to take is one that is immediate, honest, and sincere. For instance, one might say, "That kind of remark makes me uncomfortable. Let's discuss something else" or "I would prefer that you not touch me (talk to me) that way." It is important to remain composed and to respond assertively. If a client persists with inappropriate sexual behavior, the nurse can confront the problem directly and suggest that the client may want to discuss the need to relate to people through sexual rather than other means.

Assey and Herbert also describe several steps for the nurse to take when she is providing care for a seductive client. They are:

1. *Introspection.* This includes self-awareness of feelings and obtaining objective feedback from others.
2. *Self-monitoring.* This focuses on awareness of one's behavior, as well as asking peers about their behavioral observations.
3. *Confrontation.* This involves pointing out seductive behavior to the client and sharing one's thoughts and feelings about it.
4. *Limit setting.* This means informing the client of the consequences of continuing the seductive behavior.

The nurse should strive for self-awareness in terms of both responses to sexual overtures from others and the possibility of behavior that is unconsciously seductive, thus inviting a sexual response. A problem that may arise for male nurses in particular is that of an accusation by a client that the nurse made overt sexual advances. If the nurse perceives that a client is unusually seductive or is inviting sexual activity, the nurse should arrange to have a colleague of the opposite gender present while interacting with that client. It would also be wise for that nurse to avoid providing intimate physical care for that client.

The expression of sexuality may also be related to the development stage of the client, and it should be assessed by the nurse in that context. For instance, an adolescent or young adult may be experimenting with gender-role behaviors and may try approaching a nurse who is viewed as a trusted, caring person. In this case the nurse should approach the client in an honest, caring way and offer to talk about some of the dilemmas presented by this stage in life, as demonstrated in the Clinical Example at right.

It was important for Ms. N. to preserve Phil's self-esteem while clearly stating her response to him. Based on his age and behavior she assessed that he needed counseling about heterosexual relationships and offered that to him, thereby reassuring him that she still cared about him and wanted to continue their relationship. Situations involving sexual behavior, like many other situations between nurses and clients, can provide opportunities for growth and increased self-awareness. It is the responsibility of the nurse to guide the relationship in a positive direction and to use the feelings expressed by both participants in a productive manner.

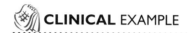 **CLINICAL** EXAMPLE

Ms. *N. was a nursing student who was assigned to a general surgical unit. Her client was Phil, a 16-year-old boy who was recovering from an appendectomy.*

PHIL: *You know, Ms. N., I really like you. You're always nice to me.*

MS. N.: *Why, thank you, Phil. I like you, too.*

PHIL: *You do? Hey, cool! (pause) Ms. N.? Will you rub my back?*

MS. N.: *I just rubbed your back.*

PHIL: *I know. Do it again.*

MS. N.: *Let's talk for a while instead.*

PHIL: *Okay, I do like you.*

MS. N.: *So you said. What shall we talk about?*

PHIL: *Will you go out with me after I leave here?*

MS. N.: *That's very flattering, Phil, and I know it took a lot to ask me, but no. I'll be your nurse while you're in the hospital, but when you leave, we'll say goodbye.*

PHIL: *You don't like me.*

MS. N.: *I do like you in a special way as a special person. Because I like you, it wouldn't be fair for me to tell you I'd go out with you when I don't plan to do that. What I could do is talk with you about how to approach girls so you'll feel more comfortable doing that in the future.*

PHIL: *Okay. I sure was nervous.*

The maintenance phase progresses under the consistent guidance of the nurse, who takes the initiative in ensuring that the goals for the relationship are not forgotten. Over time goals may be modified, original goals dropped, and new ones added. This is optimally done as a mutual process between the nurse and client. The time will come when the originally determined criteria for termination will be met. Goals may be accomplished, or the nurse or client may no longer be able to maintain contact. The relationship then moves into the final phase.

TERMINATION PHASE

The end of a successful helping relationship is always met with ambivalence. The satisfaction felt by both participants over having accomplished their mutual goals is balanced by the realization of the impending loss of a person with whom meaningful experiences have been shared. Termination of a relationship is emotionally painful, partially because of these conflicting feelings. If in addition there is doubt about the effectiveness of the relationship, termination may be even more difficult. This emphasizes the importance of setting and adhering to realistic goals.

Termination and interpersonal growth

The process of terminating can also be a growth experience for the nurse and the client. There is an opportunity for crystallizing the real meaning of the relationship to both individuals. A review of goal accomplishment can stimulate a feeling of achievement. This may be facilitated by sharing reminiscences of how it was at the beginning compared with how it is at the time of termination.

If the nurse and client have been close and trusting enough to be able to share feelings and to relate to each other openly, they will be able to benefit by sharing feelings related to termination. People respond to termination of a helping relationship as they respond to any loss. Frequently past losses are relived during termination. Intense feelings of anger, fear, and sadness often occur. This is particularly true if the individual has not resolved losses that were experienced in the past, as in the Clinical Example.

This client exhibited a response to the proposed termination of his relationship with the nurse that appeared to be out of proportion to the situation. When the nurse reviewed with her supervisor the data she had gathered during her nursing assessment of Mr. T., she questioned how adequately he had been able to resolve the losses he had experienced in the past. Mr. T. was able to direct his loss-related feelings at the nurse whom he trusted. When termination was accomplished, both the nurse and client had grown in understanding of themselves and each other and were able to recall their relationship as a meaningful experience.

Behavioral responses to termination

Sene[16] has identified three frequently encountered behavioral responses by clients to termination. The first is regression, manifested by increased anxiety, recurrence of previous maladaptive behavior, lateness or absence from sessions with the nurse, and verbalized doubt about the worth of the relationship. A

second group of behaviors may be recognized as related to withdrawal from the relationship; this includes a demand to stop meeting immediately, absence from sessions, superficial interaction, or denial that the nurse's help is needed. The last type of behavior is characterized by attempts to intensify or extend the relationship. The client may act helpless, bring up new problems, and attempt to persuade the nurse to make his decisions. The nurse should be alert to the likelihood that some of these behaviors will occur when termination is introduced and should recognize them as characteristic of the client's usual pattern of behavior when reacting to a loss. She can then help the client to explore this behavior and to grow by learning new and more productive ways to respond.

Feelings related to termination need to be expressed. This cannot be delayed until the last meeting because of the risk that time will run out with this important task left incomplete. When termination is finally recognized as inevitable, the nurse and client are apt to respond with anger. The

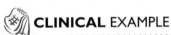

CLINICAL EXAMPLE

Mr. T. was a 69-year-old diabetic man whom the community-health nurse was visiting for health teaching and dressing changes on a small ulcer on his foot. Mr. T. and the nurse had established rapport quickly, and both looked forward to their meetings. The nurse had learned that Mr. T. was the last surviving member of his family, having lost his parents, wife, and son, all through sudden, accidental death. He was, however, socially active with numerous friends whom he saw at the local senior citizens center where he was very involved. The nurse had not observed any signs of depression or undue preoccupation with his past losses.

The foot ulcer eventually healed, and Mr. T. was well versed on how to manage his diabetes. He had been reliable in seeking medical attention when it was needed. The goals of the relationship appeared to have been met, therefore the nurse initiated the process of termination. Mr. T. responded with fear ("Please don't leave me alone.") followed by rage ("You never did really care about me."). The nurse was surprised and puzzled. She assured Mr. T. that she would see him again, and after he had calmed down, she returned to her agency.

nurse's anger will likely be directed at the circumstances that make the end of the relationship necessary; the client's anger will be directed at the nurse, whom he sees as the instigator of termination. This anger needs to be expressed. The client should be encouraged to tell the nurse how he feels. It is acceptable for the nurse to tell the client that termination makes her angry too but that she also realizes it is a necessary result of the relationship. Intense anger on the part of the nurse, which may arise from a loss of objectivity, should be directed at the appropriate object: in most cases the instructor or supervisor.

As angry feelings are shared and accepted, feelings of sadness emerge. These are closely linked to the caring that has developed between the nurse and client as they have grown to appreciate each other as individuals. It is healthy to be able to share these feelings as well. This is the time to talk about memories. It is also the time to look ahead to the future. Continuation of the accomplishments reached in the relationship should be discussed to reinforce the fact that the experience has had meaning. It is often helpful to the client to have some idea of what the nurse will be doing after the relationship has ended. This provides a sense of the nurse's continuity as a person. It is also helpful to discuss what the client plans to do in the future. Summarizing the high points of the relationship and its meaning to the nurse and client also tends to bring about a feeling of satisfaction. The nurse will need to initiate these exchanges. If she does so, the client will generally follow her lead. This is not the time to be nondirective or impersonal. The experience of termination is real to both participants, and it is an opportunity for each to learn about how he or she and others deal with loss.

Both the nurse and the client may experience anxiety as they anticipate termination. This may lead to some of the avoidance behaviors described earlier. Nursing students who are unaccustomed to initiating the formal termination of a relationship may feel particularly anxious. This may lead to postponing discussion of impending termination until there is insufficient time to allow the client to work out the feelings associated with the experience. It is the responsibility of the nurse to be sure that this phase of the relationship is addressed as completely as the others. Nurses should be aware of their usual behaviors in response to anxiety and be alert to the occurrence of these near the end of a relationship. Whenever a nurse experiences anxiety related to nursing interventions, supervision should be sought. This will help the nurse to identify and experience the opportunities for personal growth that can be realized through the successful termination of a meaningful relationship.

The end of a helping relationship (particularly a close one) often results in a wish to exchange gifts as a tangible remembrance of the experience. Most people feel pleasure when a gift is given because of the caring involved. In social relationships this is a usual occurrence and is only significant because of the mutual pleasure involved. In a helping relationship, however, there is a need to examine the exchange of gifts more closely. Consider the Clinical Example.

CLINICAL EXAMPLE

1. **M**s. D., a nursing student, had been assigned to visit an elderly lady for a semester. She was angry that she had to terminate and therefore never quite got around to talking about it until the last day. As soon as she told the client that it was her final visit, she reached into her handbag and presented the client with a needlepoint coin purse that she had made. The client had no opportunity to respond to the statement about termination. She thanked the student politely for the gift and said she had enjoyed seeing her. For the rest of the visit they chatted about superficial topics.

2. **A**nother nursing student had been working with Ms. Q., an elderly lady who was accustomed to having her way. The student had regularly reminded Ms. Q. that she would only visit until the end of the semester. Ms. Q. had plied the student with small gifts throughout their relationship. At the final meeting she greeted the student with a beautifully wrapped package; it contained a sterling silver vase that the student had admired once. The student thanked Ms. Q. sincerely and proceeded to remind her that this was their last visit. Ms. Q. responded furiously that the student was ungrateful and heartless. The student returned the vase, but Ms. Q. sulked until the end of the visit.

In each of these situations the giving or receiving of a gift was not based on a sound rationale. In the first the student effectively blocked the client's expression of feelings about termination. She may well have been unaware of this motive. However, the situation could have been avoided had the student expressed her own anger to her instructor, thereby handling her own feelings so that she would be able to handle those of the client as well. When the nurse feels the impulse to give a gift to the client, she should examine her motives carefully and, if in doubt, ask the advice of a person external to the relationship.

In the second situation the client cherished the hope that she could in effect bribe the student to continue visiting. She saw the student's acceptance of gifts, particularly the vase, as indicative of an obligation beyond that contracted at the beginning of the relationship. The student had never validated this with the client and had perceived her as a nice lady who liked the student. Therefore when a client offers a gift, it is important to validate the motivation for doing so. It is never a good idea to accept a valuable gift from a client.

Sensitivity is crucial when the issue of gifts arises. The exchange of small remembrances at the very end of the last meeting can be a good experience for the nurse and the client. Such an exchange must be based on the nurse's assessment of the relationship, and it is also recommended that it be discussed with the instructor or supervisor. It is important to remember that a person who receives a gift and is unable to reciprocate usually feels badly. Also, there is no obligation whatsoever in a professional relationship to exchange gifts.

Termination implies finality. This is usually the case at the end of a nurse-client relationship. It is important that this fact be reflected in the termination process. Cultural differences must be taken into account when one is choosing the words of termination. In some sections of the United States "see you later" is taken quite literally; in others it is interpreted as a final "goodbye." Language used in terminating should be consistent with current and local communication patterns. The difficulty, and also the gratification, of terminating may be avoided by making empty promises to get together in the future. Some clients cling to these superficial promises, however, and they generally fade quickly from the nurse's mind as she becomes involved

with new clients. This is not fair and may even be cruel to a person with limited social contacts. Giving a client an address or phone number or promising to write periodically fits into the same category. To be most helpful to the client termination should be complete and final, as the word itself indicates.

The cycle of the nurse-client relationship is completed countless times by each nurse during her professional life. Each relationship is unique. Each offers the nurse a new opportunity to grow in her interpersonal skills and to gain in self-awareness. If the nurse resists slipping into a routine and approaches each new human relationship as a challenge to her interpersonal ability, she will be rewarded by knowing that she has made significant contributions to the optimal wellness of most of those whom she has tried to help.

SUMMARY

This chapter and Chapter 6 have not been intended to serve as a recipe for how to put together a successful relationship. The specific "how's" and "why's" are much too unique to each interpersonal relationship to make such an effort advisable. The framework for relationship development and the concepts that have been presented are intended to provide basic information that may be applied to most helping relationships. Use of these concepts by a beginning nurse learning about interpersonal relationships should help the nurse develop the ability to provide effective nursing care. Awareness of the characteristics of the various stages of the relationship will enable the nurse to plan care within a rational, theoretic framework and to anticipate some potential problems before they arise.

The first phase of the nurse-client relationship is the preinteraction phase. At this time, the nurse prepares for the first meeting with the client by reviewing available information, reviewing related nursing concepts, and planning for the setting of the meeting. The client becomes involved in the relationship during the introductory or orientation phase. An important task during this phase is establishing the nurse-client contract. This provides basic guidelines for the rest of the relationship, including goals and expectations of the participants. Confidentiality of client information is clarified.

During the maintenance or working phase of the relationship, the nurse and client work toward accomplishment of the goals that were identified by them. One important role for the nurse is to help the client express feelings. Nurse characteristics that facilitate client openness include confrontation, immediacy, and self-disclosure. Humor may also be helpful. The nurse may need to help the client manage difficult feelings. Many health care clients are fearful. Some clients become angry and may benefit from learning to be assertive. Hostile clients need a patient approach to help them develop trust. Clients may become sad in response to memories or to their current situation. Clients who express affection, including the expression of sexual feelings, for the nurse need a sensitive but clear response.

The last phase of the relationship is termination. The client should be reminded of the basis for ter-

mination throughout the relationship. Termination may be related to discharge from a health care setting, to achievement of the client's goals, or to the departure of the nurse. It provides an opportunity for summarizing the accomplishments that have taken place and for the participants to share their plans for the future. It is helpful for the nurse to share feelings and learning related to the relationship. Termination implies the end of the relationship. Plans for future contact between the nurse and the client are not part of termination.

The theoretic concepts introduced in Chapter 6 can be expected to be manifested somewhat differently, depending on the developmental stage of the relationship. Table 7-1 summarizes the progress of trust, empathy, caring, hope, autonomy, and mutuality relative to relationship phases.

TABLE 7-1   Correlation of relationship concepts with relationship phases

	ORIENTATION	WORKING	TERMINATION
Trust	Limited. Based on past experiences. Begins to grow as contract is established.	Grows as commitment to the relationship is tested and validated. Demonstrations of concern are facilitating.	Falters as termination becomes a reality but reasserted if well established during working phase. Tendency to be trusting in future similar situations.
Empathy	Difficult because of lack of awareness of the person as an individual.	Occurs more frequently as participants communicate more openly and learn to interpret nonverbal cues. Facilitates growth of self-understanding.	Helps toward successful termination, because feelings can be shared and understood more easily. Allows more accurate expression of feelings.
Caring	Expressed as an initial positive feeling toward another person—not specific to the individual. Relatively superficial.	Grows steadily as participants gain in appreciation of each other and share meaningful experiences together.	If termination is successful, feeling of caring will be shared by participants as part of termination process.
Hope	Expressed as a generally positive attitude toward beginning a new relationship together.	Experienced as progress toward goal accomplishment is recognized and positive responses are shared.	Sharing plans for the future extends hope that has been fostered in the relationship.
Autonomy	Both individuals essentially autonomous. Little data about contributions that each could make to the relationship.	Some autonomy given up by each participant in favor of area of expertise of other person. Sharing becomes important.	Both resume earlier autonomy as relationship is given up. Ideally, autonomous behavior of each is enhanced by behaviors learned during the relationship.
Mutuality	Limited. Tentative beginnings of sharing at an information level. Need for careful validation.	High level. Sharing of information and feelings. Deep appreciation of the uniqueness of the person. Teamwork. Interdependence.	Given up as each participant returns to more independent functioning.

DISCUSSION QUESTIONS

1. Describe how the client's self-concept influences his communication patterns within the context of the relationship.

2. Think about the last experience you had as a consumer in the health care system. What feelings did you experience? Critique the relationship behaviors of the health care providers with whom you had contact.

3. Write your own description of the ideal nurse. Share your description with one other classmate. Compare your ideas about the characteristics of your ideal. Are they realistic? Are they open to modification? Are they achievable for you? What would you need to do to become your ideal?

4. Some dislike the idea of contracting with clients because they find it dehumanizing. Do you agree or disagree with this point of view? Discuss your rationale.

5. Discuss which phase of the relationship seems most difficult to you.

6. Compare your last interaction with a client to your last talk with a friend.

7. Discuss your own methods of coping with losses in the past.

8. How do you usually respond when you are in a situation that makes you feel uncomfortable?

9. Think about the most recent time that you were angry. Was your response passive, assertive, or aggressive? Were you satisfied with your response? If not, how would you have liked to change it?

10. How would you respond differently to a seductive person who is (1) a colleague at work, (2) a client, (3) a stranger on the street, or (4) someone you just met in a singles' bar.

11. Identify the aspects of your own behavior that could be termed seductive and the situations in which you behave seductively.

12. Critique the following nurse-client interaction, including your rationale for your position:

> The client is Maureen, a 16-year-old who has been admitted to the hospital for an initial workup of juvenile onset diabetes. Ms. R. is a nursing student assigned to Maureen.

MAUREEN: (excitedly) Ms. R., I have the best news! I've been waiting for you to get here. My boyfriend's the only one who knows, and you have to promise not to tell anyone else. Promise?
MS. R.: OK.
MAUREEN: I'm pregnant, and my boyfriend says we can get married as soon as I leave the hospital. Isn't that great!

13. You are a nurse working in a sexually transmitted disease clinic. Your teenage son's friend comes in for treatment. He looks shocked when he sees you and says, "Oh, wow, I didn't expect to see you here! Please don't tell my parents." How should you respond?

14. Select a particular type of hospital unit and design a "humor room." Include the way you would decorate the room, the furniture you would select, and the materials you would supply. Relate your choices to the type of client for whom the room is designed.

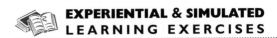 ## EXPERIENTIAL & SIMULATED LEARNING EXERCISES

1. Assertiveness number 1

PURPOSE: To experience and identify passive, aggressive, and assertive behaviors.

PROCEDURE: Divide the class into groups of five. For each exercise, one student is to act as observer/recorder; one should play the role of the antagonist; and one each should act passively, aggressively, and assertively. The recorder should be reminded to be aware of both verbal and nonverbal communication. Students should be given a written description of the situation and instructed to role play each type of behavior in turn using the antagonist as the object of the behavior. If time allows, each student should be given an opportunity to experience each type of behavior.

SAMPLE SITUATIONS:

1. You are assisting a physician with a sterile procedure and note that she has contaminated her glove. She continues with the procedure.

2. You are taking a break in the coffee shop with a peer. She begins to discuss very personal information that a client has just shared with her.

3. You have requested your vacation to coincide with that of your spouse. The head nurse tells you that you may not have the week off.
4. A client's husband angrily confronts you with numerous complaints about the nursing care that his wife has received in the hospital.
5. A client who knows you are a new graduate requests a more experienced nurse to change her dressing.

DISCUSSION: During the discussion following each situation, each student should share the feelings aroused by the various behaviors. The antagonist should focus on the responses evoked by each of the actors. The observer/recorder may elaborate and provide feedback on whether the behavior identified by the participants was communicated and whether the verbal and nonverbal behaviors were congruent.

2. Assertiveness number 2

PURPOSE: To provide the student with experience in positive behavioral change and to enhance self-awareness.

PROCEDURE: Request that each student select a situation in which he or she finds it particularly difficult to be assertive. The student should then fantasize an assertive response to that situation. When the response seems adequate in fantasy, the student should explain the situation to a friend and rehearse the new response with the friend. It is important to be aware of feelings while rehearsing and to elicit feedback from the friend about the effectiveness of the new behavior. When the student feels reasonably comfortable behaving assertively with a friend, the new behavior should be tested in the real situation.

DISCUSSION: Students who are pursuing this guided fantasy/rehearsal approach to assertiveness should be encouraged to discuss their experience in a small group. This engenders group support and reinforces the growth of the new behavior.

3. Contracting

PURPOSE: To practice the development of a mutual, verbal, nurse-client contract.

PROCEDURE: Divide students into groups of three. One person should be assigned the role of the nurse, one of the client, and the third should be the observer. The client is a parent who is bringing a toddler to an outpatient clinic for a routine immunization. The nurse's assignment is to role play the establishment of a contract with the client. (Assume that they will meet at least four more times.) The observer should take notes on the verbal and nonverbal behavior of the participants.

DISCUSSION: The observer should provide feedback on (1) the nurse's communication techniques, (2) the degree of mutuality in the contract, and (3) the specific elements of the contract in terms of adequacy and clarity.

4. Termination

PURPOSE: To rehearse the termination process.

PROCEDURE: This exercise may be performed by the student alone or in a small group. The student should be seated facing an empty chair. The chair should represent the individual with whom the student will soon be terminating a relationship. The student should tell the imagined person whatever he or she would like to say when termination actually takes place. This exercise may also be done following termination if the student is left with many unresolved feelings.

DISCUSSION: If the exercise is done in a group, the other group members may provide feedback about their reaction to the termination process. They should be encouraged to share their own feelings and experiences. If the exercise is done alone, the student should share the experience with the supervisor or the clinical group to receive support and feedback.

REFERENCES

1. Alberti RE, Emmons ML: *Your perfect right: a guide to assertive behavior*, San Luis Obispo, Calif, 1974, Impact.
2. Assey JL, Herbert JM: Who is the seductive patient? *Am J Nurs* 83:530, 1983.
3. Auvil CA, Silver BW: Therapist self-disclosure: when is it appropriate? *Perspect Psychiatr Care* 22:57, 1984.
4. Bowie I: Terms of address: implications for nursing, *J Adv Nurs* 23:113, 1996.
5. Buxman K: Make room for laughter, *Am J Nurs* 91:46, 1991.
6. Carkhuff R: *Helping and human relations*, vols I and II, New York, 1969, Holt, Rinehart & Winston.
7. Curtin LL: Privacy: belonging to oneself, *Perspect Psychiatr Care* 19:112, 1981.
8. Davidhizar R, Schearer R: Humor: no geriatric nurse should be without it, *Geriatr Nurs* 13:276, 1992.

9. Green CP: How to recognize hostility and what to do about it, *Am J Nurs* 86:1230, 1986.

10. Heinrich KT: What to do when a patient becomes too special, *Nursing* 22:63, Nov. 1992.

11. Lancee WJ, Gallop R, McCay E, Toner B: The relationship between nurses' limit-setting styles and anger in psychiatric inpatients, *Psychiatr Serv* 46:609, 1995.

12. Palmer ME, Deck ES: Teaching assertiveness to seniors, *Nurs Outlook* 29:305, 1981.

13. Palmer ME, Deck ES: Teaching your patients to assert their rights, *Am J Nurs* 87:650, 1987.

14. Pilette PC, Berck CB, Achber LC: Therapeutic management of helping boundaries, *J Psychosoc Nurs Ment Health Serv* 33:40, 1995.

15. Raines CF: Humor. In Creasia JL, Parker B, editors: *Conceptual foundations of professional nursing practice*, St Louis, 1991, Mosby.

16. Sene BS: "Termination" in the student-patient relationship, *Perspect Psychiatr Care* 7:39, 1969.

17. Young JC: Rationale for clinician self-disclosure and research agenda, *Image* 20:196, 1988.

18. Zangari ME, Duffy P: Contracting with patients in day-to-day practice, *Am J Nurs* 80:451, 1980.

Suggested Readings

Assey JL, Herbert JM: Who is the seductive patient? *Am J Nurs* 83:531, 1983.

> These authors deal with this troubling topic using sensitivity and respect for the feelings and needs of both the client and the nurse. Information is given regarding recognition and validation of seductive behavior. Practical suggestions for intervention are provided. This article should be very helpful for students who are perplexed about how to deal with their clients' sexuality.

Billings CV: Come here, nurse! *Am J Nurs* 86:915, 1986.

> This nurse-consultant describes several interventions that might be effective in the care of a demanding client. She emphasizes the need for flexibility and creativity. Her practical suggestions will be helpful to students and practicing nurses.

Brockopp DY, Kreis K: Not by any other name, *Am J Nurs* 85:510, 1985.

> The authors doubt that nurses can establish effective interpersonal relationships if they use inappropriate forms of address. Examples are provided. Using individual titles for the nurse and the client indicates a willingness to become involved and take on responsibility for the relationship.

Colorado Society of Clinical Specialists in Psychiatric Nursing: Ethical guidelines for confidentiality, *J Psychiatr Nurs Ment Health Serv* 28:43, Mar 1990.

> This section of a larger description of ethical guidelines presents considerations related to nurses and adult clients, minor clients, peers, research subjects, and students. It is a concise overview of the many situations in which confidentiality is a concern.

Gay S: Over the wall, *Am J Nurs* 91(8):82, 1991.

> The author describes a clinical experience that led her to understand the importance of taking time to communicate with clients. The article will enable students to see the relevance of classroom learning to the clinical setting.

Grau L, Chandler B, Saunders C: Nursing residents' perceptions of the quality of their care, *J Psychosoc Nurs Ment Health Serv* 33:34, 1995.

> This report of a pilot nursing study assessed the satisfaction of nursing home residents with the care that they received. They were more positive about care provided by professional staff and least satisfied by care from nurses' aides. Satisfaction was related to the quality of interpersonal relationships.

Hall BA, Allan JD: Self in relation: a prolegomenon for holistic nursing, *Nurs Outlook* 42:110, 1994.

> This is a thought-provoking article that challenges nurses to provide holistic, caring nursing care even in health care environments that may not be supportive. It is highly recommended as a stimulus for discussion about what is possible in the "real world."

Holm K et al: Effect of personal pain experience on pain assessment, *Image J Nurs Sch* 21:72, 1989.

> This study revealed that nurses who had experienced a higher intensity of personal pain perceived greater levels of suffering in others than those who had had less intense pain experiences. This demonstrates the impact that one's past experiences can have on interpersonal relationships.

Menzel TE: We couldn't come to terms with Hank—until he signed a contract, *Nursing* 22:50, 1992.

> This article describes an experience with a manipulative, noncompliant client with quadriplegia and his family. It demonstrates the advantage of developing a mutually agreed-on contract for nursing care.

Moritz DA: Understanding anger, *Am J Nurs* 78:81, 1978.

> The author concisely relates the concepts of anger to clinical nursing practice. Included are examples from the author's own experience, analyses of the examples, and suggested nursing approaches to the angry client.

Schwartz-Barcott D, Fortin JD, Kim HS: Client-nurse interaction: testing for its impact in preoperative instruction, *Int J Nurs Stud* 31:23, 1994.

> The results of this study demonstrated that nurse-client interaction before surgery can alleviate postoperative anxiety.

Sene BS: "Termination" in the student-patient relationship, *Perspect Psychiatr Care* 7:39, 1969.

> This article is highly recommended for its thorough exploration of the termination process. Although it focuses primarily on the psychotherapeutic relationship, the principles discussed apply equally to all helping relationships.

Smoot SL, Gonzales JL: Cost-effective communication skills training for state hospital employees, *Psychiatr Serv* 46:819, 1995.

> This study applied the interpersonal concepts developed by Carkhuff with particular emphasis on empathy in a communications training program for psychiatric unit staff. The findings indicated that empathic communication was a cost-effective approach.

Steckel SB: Contracting with patient-selected reinforcers, *Am J Nurs* 80:1596, 1980.

> This article describes a method for implementing the nursing process through use of an outcome-oriented contract. It is unique in that the contract incorporates a behavior modification approach in which the client selects the rein-

forcers. This is a collaborative method of providing nursing care and merits further attention from nursing faculty and nurses who are in clinical practice.

Taylor C: Rethinking nursing's basic competencies, *J Nurs Care Qual* 9:1, 1995.

This thought-provoking article focuses on the increasing emphasis on intellectual and technical competence by nurses to the detriment of interpersonal skills. Nurses are challenged to reverse this trend.

Treistman JM: Teaching nursing care through poetry, *Nurs Outlook* 34:83, 1986.

The many examples of women's poetry in this article richly illustrate the author's premise that nurses need to maintain a connection with humanity. This unique approach to nursing education helps to focus students on the meaning of relationships in their own and their clients' lives.

Warner SL: Humor: a coping response for student nurses, *Arch Psychiatr Nurs* 5:10, Feb 1991.

The author describes the ways in which nursing students who were involved in a psychiatric nursing clinical experience used humor as a coping mechanism. Faculty members will find this useful in understanding their students' reactions and assisting them to cope.

Small Groups and Group Process Dynamics: An Overview

Now, who shall arbitrate?
   Ten men love what I hate,
Shun what I follow, slight what I receive;
   Ten, who in ears and eyes
   Match me; we all surmise,
They this thing, and I that; who shall my soul believe?

Robert Browning
Rabbi Ben Ezra

LEARNING OBJECTIVES

After studying this chapter, the student should be able to:

- Define the term *group*.
- Compare and contrast different types of groups.
- Identify the stages of group development.
- Describe the characteristics of each phase of group development.
- Describe the process dynamics of groups in terms of roles and functions
- Discuss the role of the nurse in different group situations.

A s described in the preceding chapters, individuals grow and develop through their interpersonal interactions. These interactions often occur within a group situation. A *group* can be defined as two or more people involved in face-to-face interactions with a common purpose or goal. In a group effort there is a pooling of individual energies and resources aimed at goal accomplishment. *What* the group purpose is and the effectiveness of *how* the group works together are examined and enhanced through the analysis of group dynamics.

Nurses frequently work in groups and deal with groups of clients; nursing is an interdependent profession. The nurse works alongside other nurses, professionals from other disciplines, and paraprofessional personnel to provide care. Involvement on multiple committees, group presentations, and task forces is part and parcel of the role of the nurse. Interactions within groups occur at all levels of nursing. In addition, efficient utilization of time can be fostered through the use of client/patient groups to provide educational information, instruction in certain procedures, or therapy. Knowledge of the many aspects of groups and group work can facilitate the role of the nurse.

This chapter provides an overview of task groups and therapeutic groups. The phases of group development and the characteristics of each phase are discussed. The behavioral dynamics of the group process include the roles and functions of the members of groups. Some implications for nursing and groups conclude the chapter.

TYPES OF GROUPS

When any person speaks about groups, a vast number of ideas come to mind. Most often the image of a group depends on the person's life experiences with groups. People interact in many groups: they may belong to a family, a community, a club, a job crew, a self-help group. Generally groups are divided into two major categories: *task groups* and *therapeutic groups*. All groups meet to fulfill some common objective, which may be implicit or explicit. The nature of the goal-problem influences the type of group and its life span. Task groups and therapeutic groups differ in terms of focus, specific purpose, techniques used to facilitate group goals, roles and functions of group members, and the people involved.

Task groups

When a specific job needs to be done, when a particular problem is to be solved, or when specific decisions are to be made, a *task group* is often used. This is a type of group that has as its primary purpose the completion of some directive, often but not always one that will meet the goals of a larger group or organization. A task group is a work group. Its focus is on getting the job done. Examples of task groups include a nursing team, a political campaign committee, a computer users' group, and a bowling team. These groups focus mainly on the content of the task at hand (the *what* that needs to be done). This content work involves proposing, discussing, evaluating, and making decisions related to ideas and facts that contribute to getting the job done. Basic functions of the members of a task group include initiating ideas, giving suggestions and opinions, clarifying issues, record keeping, summarizing content, and planning for the next meeting.

Leadership can be defined as using multiple processes to influence the activities (of individuals and the group as a whole) toward attainment of the goal in a given situation.[2] The leader may come from within the group via formal or informal mechanisms; this type of leadership is called an *emergent leadership*. More often someone will be designated or appointed from outside the group to provide leadership; this has been termed *imposed* or *organizational leadership*. In situations when an appointed leader does not have the support of the group, a leader may still emerge from among the group membership.

There are a number of variables that can enhance the way in which a person may lead the group. Characteristics of the leader include self-awareness, maturity, assertiveness, advocacy, and accountability. In addition, acknowledgment of some level of expertise is evident.

The leader role and its functions vary with the structure, organization, and composition of the group. Nursing process is the strategy most often employed by nurse leaders. Additional strategies employ aspects of organization, teaching/learning, decision making, change, conflict management, and evaluation.[2] The ability to appropriately choose and utilize any of these strategies in a given situation facilitates fulfilling the role of the leader.

Some of the functions of the leader include assisting the group to:

1. Become aware of or decide on its purpose and goals

2. Become aware of its resources, strengths, and limitations
3. Focus on the process of working together
4. Explore alternatives
5. Evaluate its progress and goal accomplishment

Leadership involves the effective utilization of the group's total resources. This applies in both task groups and therapeutic groups.

The goals of the task group are accomplished in the context of its potential power, and this power is often seen in terms of the strength of its leader. Five different kinds of power can be distinguished. The first is called *legitimate power*. This is the power of an authority relationship resulting from the person's position, such as director of a department. *Referent power* is that power derived from association with someone else or some idea. It is more of a sense of influence, because the person identifies with and respects the other; for example, if the nurse works with the person who has received a national award, she may be viewed as having more power by virtue of reflected power of the other person. A third type of power is *expert power*, which is power that exists because of one's expertise and knowledge in an area.

The fourth type of power is called *reward power*. Individuals within an organization who provide rewards (such as salary enhancement, promotions, and so on) may be viewed as having specific power. Reward power can only be exerted if the recipient of the proposed reward values what is being offered. Often the recipient of a reward feels controlled and is compliant with the rules of "the company game." The last type of power is *coercive power*, and this is the power of punishment or negative sanctions. Coercive power invokes coercion and allows no means of escape from what the powerful person wants short of leaving the situation totally.[7]

The amount of power any individual has depends on:

1. The position of the person within the larger organization, which brings authority and legitimate power
2. The status or prestige of the group to which the person belongs
3. The special expertise or competency that others attribute to the person
4. The personal feelings of others toward the person that provide referent power

5. The person's ability to provide or administer rewards and punishment[2,7]

Any combination of these five power bases is possible to enhance goal accomplishment. In many cases the leader's influence depends on a combination of sources of power.

To illustrate the relationship of leader power to group task accomplishment, consider the following situation:

Ms. T., a staff nurse who has just received her nursing license, attended a workshop on nursing care planning. She decided that the nursing care plan format used in her hospital unit was inadequate to sufficiently communicate the client's nursing care needs. In particular there was no provision for including a nursing diagnosis.

On returning to work Ms. T. requested a meeting with Ms. J., the head nurse. She told Ms. J. about the workshop and volunteered to help revise the nursing care plan format. Without realizing that Ms. J. did not accept the use of nursing diagnosis, Ms. T. described the deficiency caused by failure to use a nursing diagnosis at great length.

Ms. J. said that she would form a committee to assist Ms. T. with a revision. Ms. T. put forth great effort to assemble her task groups and accomplish her objectives, but the group members usually forgot about meetings. If they did attend, they sat silently while Ms. T. presented her ideas.

Ms. T. finally returned to Ms. J. to report on the lack of progress. Ms. J. suggested that she probably needed more experience before trying to make changes.

Ms. T. was unable to lead effectively because (1) she had little status in the organization, (2) she had not yet demonstrated her competency to her colleagues, (3) the head nurse had negative feelings toward her proposal, and (4) she had no power to reward or punish her group members. In fact, the members had probably perceived the head nurse's lack of support for the project and were more concerned about pleasing her.

The behavior of the leader influences the behavior of other members of the group. The major types of group leadership are (1) autocratic leaders, who are directive and make unilateral decisions; (2) democratic leaders, who involve the group; and (3)

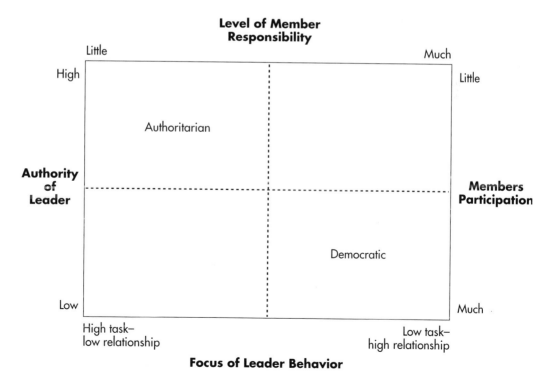

Fig. 8-1 Factors related to type of leadership in a group. (Courtesy Elizabeth Anne DeSalvo Rankin, Professor, University of Maryland School of Nursing, University of Maryland at Baltimore.)

laissez-faire leaders, who have loose control over the membership of the group. Each of these types of leadership may be most effective depending on the task, the structure of the group in terms of size and composition, the personal attributes of the members, and motivational factors.

Basic leadership behavior includes the components of task behavior (i.e., things done to get the job done) and relationship behavior (i.e., things done to assist people to work together to do the task).[8,11] The type of leadership is related to these components in that as one demonstrates more autocratic leadership, the emphasis falls more on the task behaviors. If the leader demonstrates a more democratic style, the emphasis shifts to the relationship behavior (Fig. 8-1). As such, the behaviors of the members are also modified. Although varying degrees of each are possible, a balance between these features promotes completion of the tasks at hand.

Within a group there are different primary *roles* that people assume, generally those of leader, member, or both. The roles that the individuals perform may be defined in terms of a set of expectations held by others about the appropriate behaviors for a specific position. These expectations help the person know what to do. One of the problems of Ms. T. in the preceding example was that she was unaware of the expectations of others concerning her role. People learn about roles through interactions with others where expectations for a role are communicated. These influential people become the person's *role set*, and the actual process of

Expectation → Communication → Perception → Action/actual role behavior

is termed the *role episode*. When different types of roles are performed by people within the group, there is said to be *role differentiation*. For example, the leader functions differently than the follower in certain respects.

Problems may also occur with roles, because individuals often hold many roles simultaneously. Three role-related problems are role conflict, role ambiguity, and role overload.[2] When expectations for one role are incompatible with expectations for another, *role conflict* occurs. An example is the demands made on an individual who is both the charge nurse of the intensive care unit and the mother of a toddler who is ill.

A second kind of role problem occurs when there is a lack of clarity about expectations for a role or a discrepancy between expectation and knowledge available to carry out the role. This is termed *role ambiguity*. An example is the nurse who makes most client care decisions independently when working the evening shift but must clear all decisions with the team leader on the day shift.

The third type of problem related to roles is that of *role overload*. When expectations and demands of a role exceed the abilities of the person to adequately perform, or when a multiplicity of roles with many demands is too great for one individual, role overload occurs. This problem is experienced by the nurse who is assigned to be the team leader and has a client assignment equal to that of other team members.

The completion of the task and decision-making process can also be facilitated in terms of the organization of the group meetings. If the group is focusing on a large topic, smaller pieces can be dealt with at separate meetings. Preplanning is necessary, and a system for designating when the smaller pieces are to be discussed can be helpful. This can be managed by using an agenda, which is a list of topics for consideration at a meeting with a specified time frame and specific sequencing. With an agenda the focus of the meeting is established, and the direction of the discussion is, to a certain extent, modulated.

The first feature of an agenda is agenda integrity.[3,11] This means that it is the responsibility of the entire group (leader and members) to see that all items on the agenda are discussed in the meeting for which they are scheduled and items *not* on the agenda are *not* discussed. Commitment to agenda integrity is necessary to ensure that time and efforts are properly invested and that important, timely decisions get made. In establishing an agenda time factors must be considered. Temporal integrity refers to beginning on time, keeping to the agenda schedule, ending on time, and maintaining a long-range schedule. Thus the group learns that time constraints are important. The idea of temporal integrity suggests that some items should be scheduled before others and some be allocated more time than others.

Closely related to this idea are three additional rules: the *rule of halves*, the *rule of three quarters*, and the *rule of thirds*.[3] To establish the agenda the rule of halves can be applied. This rule states that in general, no items shall be entered onto the agenda unless they are forwarded to the person setting the agenda before one half of the time between meetings. Thus important items are sure to be on the agenda, given priority, and allocated adequate time.

The person scheduling the agenda can arrange the items according to the rule of thirds so that the most important items are scheduled for the middle third of the meeting. By that time everyone likely to attend the meeting has arrived, and a break can then be scheduled at the two-thirds point of the meeting after major business has been completed.

Last, the rule of three quarters is implemented to ensure that by the three-quarter point between meetings, all members have been sent all relevant materials. As a result members can be prepared for discussion, make informed decisions, and know when specific items will be discussed. Such an organization can clearly promote task accomplishment.

Thus far this chapter has focused on the accomplishment of the goal of the group. This focus on *what* is to be accomplished is but part of the picture; *how* the group functions or the dynamics of the process of the group are significant features in goal accomplishment. All groups do some process work to create and maintain a climate conducive to achieving goals. The process dynamics are related to the group norms, the expectations and patterns of behavior in the group, and the phase of the group development. Group process dynamics will be discussed later in the chapter with the phases of development of the group.

Therapeutic groups

Like task groups, therapeutic groups meet for a specific purpose. However, their purpose is usually related to the processes of personal-emotional growth, developing human relationship skills, and coping with certain problems. Examples of such therapeutic groups include encounter groups, laboratory training groups (T-groups), counseling groups, and therapy groups. These groups differ in terms of their goals, the techniques used, the people involved, and the role of the leader.[12]

Encounter groups or personal growth groups meet for the purpose of gaining insight into the self and making closer contact with the self and others. The intense group experience is intended to assist relatively healthy individuals to learn about personal-emotional growth and development. Many structured and unstructured encounter exercises and nonverbal techniques such as sensory-awakening exercises are used. These groups emphasize experiential learning with spontaneity of feelings versus cognitive-rational techniques. The groups are time limited, with many occurring in the form of retreats or marathon meetings.

Laboratory training groups, also called T-groups, emphasize a cognitive-rational approach to teaching human-relationship skills and education through task accomplishment related to specific organizational problems. The focus is on the analysis of the group process related to how the problem solving occurred. Trainers (leaders) set up the experiences and foster the analysis and discussion.[10]

Group counseling also focuses on a type of problem solving, such as educational problems, social disruptions, or vocational planning. Such groups deal with conscious problems and the resolution of specific, short-term issues. A variety of educationally based techniques are used. The role of the counselor is to structure activities and foster a climate where both productive work and group interaction will occur.

 CULTURAL CONSIDERATIONS

The cultural backgrounds of group members should be considered when the nurse designs a counseling group. If members are of cultures that have very different belief systems or norms about appropriate responses to life events, it will be extremely difficult to address their concerns in a group. Because there are also differences within major cultures, it is wise to conduct an interview with prospective group members to assess potential cultural barriers to communication.

There may be situations in which the members are deliberately selected because of their cultural differences. For instance, a group that was intended to sensitize the members to the positive aspects of contact with diverse cultures would be most effective with a membership that represents a variety of cultural backgrounds.

Nurses are frequently called on to lead group counseling sessions. The following situation provides an example:

Ms. S. was a community health nurse who worked in a lower-income urban area. A local church sponsored a day-care program for preschool children. Ms. S. visited the day-care program once a week. She noticed that although the children ranged in age from 2 to 5 years, they were always involved in the same activities. Four teaching aides were employed in the program. Ms. S. approached the program director and shared her observation. The director described her own role overload and stated that she agreed the various age groups should have separate programs, but she did not have time to work with the staff to develop this approach. Ms. S. volunteered to meet with the staff to discuss levels of psychomotor, cognitive, and social development and assist them in planning age-specific programs; her offer was accepted. Based on the group discussions she led, the program was modified. The staff later asked her to conduct other staff development programs for them on topics related to child health care.

Counseling groups, laboratory training groups, and encounter groups are all specific in focus. Such groups deal primarily with healthy individuals within a short-term time frame.

Group therapy is somewhat different than the aforementioned therapeutic groups. Group therapy is established when several individuals with specified psychologic disruptions come together for treatment under the direction of a psychotherapist. The goal of group therapy is often more "person specific" and is generally related to changing certain behaviors, self-awareness, and establishing more functional coping patterns. Individuals participate to resolve their specific problems within a setting (the group) where there are possibilities for support, caring, direction, confrontation, and testing-out or practice of new behaviors. Attention is often given to past behavior, fears, barriers to interpersonal relationships, and unconscious factors depending on the theoretic framework of the therapist (and group).[12]

The frame of reference for the therapy group may be psychoanalytic, a transactional analysis focus, interpersonal relationship-based, communication-oriented, client-centered, gestalt therapy-oriented, existentially focused, systems-related, or eclectic (combination of several frameworks synthesized into a working approach by the therapist).[1]

Many therapeutic groups incorporate several approaches to foster cognitive, behavioral, experiential, and emotional growth among the members. Individuals are encouraged to examine the alternatives available to them, examine the choices they can make, and learn how to use or develop their own sense of control.

To facilitate these behaviors, an effective therapeutic group leader demonstrates several leader characteristics. These leaders are willing to model and teach desired behavior, be genuine in dealing with clients, and demonstrate sincere caring and interest in the welfare of others. Courage to confront, follow one's beliefs, and express concerns goes hand in hand with openness and a willingness to explore. A sense of humor, inventiveness, and flexibility to deal with the varied experiences are important to the total group atmosphere. In general the leader of a therapeutic group must be self-aware and self-assured, with a clear sense of self-understanding.[6]

These characteristics alone are not sufficient. Specific skills, many related to therapeutic communication processes, are necessary. Although these skills can be taught to a degree, they must be developed and sharpened over time through experience with groups. Examples of these skills include active listening, empathizing, facilitating, clarifying, questioning, linking ideas, blocking counterproductive behaviors, supporting, and summarizing. In addition, the leader must be skilled in analyzing the situation, synthesizing information and experience, and evaluating the group and individual processes and productivity. If a coleader model is used, working closely with a colleague in all aspects of the therapeutic model is important. Some advantages and disadvantages of coleading appear in Table 8-1.

Other groups

In addition to task groups and therapeutic groups, the nurse may be involved with groups of individuals who gather for some other purpose. Often, individuals gather for mutual support and learning derived from the interaction and exchanges that occur within the group. These groups, referred to either as self-help groups or mutual support groups, are somewhat of a hybrid between task groups and therapeutic groups.

TABLE 8-1   Some advantages and disadvantages to coleadership of therapeutic groups

ADVANTAGES	DISADVANTAGES
Reducing leader "burnout" with shared responsibility	Different philosophic approaches may not mesh well
Sharing the focus where intense feelings are expressed (one coleader and person, one coleader and rest of group)	Distrust or lack of respect leading to lack of support of each other's approaches
Coverage so group can proceed if one coleader must be absent	Competing behaviors between coleaders
Sharing in the analysis–evaluation of each session-experience	Resistance to implementing each other's ideas
Serving as sounding board for each other	Inadequate joint planning in advance of each session
Assisting in the maintenance of objectivity	Inadequate postsession review regarding analysis–evaluation
Providing support to each other	Being at odds with each other
Coleader skills complementing each other and strengthening the approaches	Coleader deficits becoming compounded if both have the same areas of weakness

Such groups may convene to share concerns or to effect personal change, such as Al-Anon or Narcotics Anonymous. In other groups, a major function is direct activism or change on a larger scale, such as the environmental group Greenpeace or the National Alliance for the Mentally Ill. For all of these groups, the major functions include advocacy and education. A comprehensive overview of self-help groups, including definitions, functions, and the nurse's role in advocacy, appears in Chapter 10.

THE DYNAMIC PROCESSES AND DEVELOPMENT PHASES OF A GROUP
Group set

A variety of factors predispose a group to function in a particular way. These are termed the *group set*, and they include goals, values, norms, climate, and historical factors.

For a gathering to be a group it must have a goal, a manifest statement that describes the specifics the group aims to attain within or by a specific time.[9] Regardless of the type of group, goals influence its function. Goals function to facilitate the stability of a group and the evaluation of its processes and task completion. Each goal is tied to the value system of the group that prescribes certain preferred ways to achieve desired ends.

The value system of the group, related to individual member values, then functions in the establishment of the group norms. Group norms involve the standards of behavior, including those that are acceptable and those that will not be tolerated, that rule the functioning of all members of the group. Norms may be explicit or implicit, and members may or may not be consciously aware of what the norms are in actuality.[11]

The overall group climate, the atmosphere within the group, created by the group and each individual within it, will influence how the group works together. The historical factors of the group related to its existence over time also influence its functioning. Ongoing groups have established norms, traditions, and procedures that require incoming participants to adapt to the existing models of behavior. Sometimes past history serves to decrease time spent exploring norms; sometimes it fosters continuance of behavioral patterns or norms that may not be the most efficient or functional. With newly developed groups the norms are tested by being continually developed, explored, and challenged.

The intangible group set variables previously discussed exist concomitantly with structural group set variables. Each group, as it is established and as it exists over time, has a particular organization, size, composition, and set of characteristics. These structural factors are influenced by the particular theoretic framework within which the group is organized.

If, for example, the orientation is interpersonal and the aim is to learn more about relationships with spouses, couples will make up the group, a coleader model might prevail, and a small group of from four to six couples will be included. Thus the organization involves pairs, the size is 10 to 14 (including coleaders), the group is heterogeneous (male and female), and the special characteristics of members are that they are partners. In contrast, if the group is a therapeutic group for rape victims, the theoretic framework is more likely a crisis format, and the group will be organized around the therapist (usually a female), homogeneous, small in number (usually no more than eight), and each member sharing the characteristic of past experience as a victim.

The structural group-set variables have a large influence on the less tangible group-set norms, values, climate, and history that in turn influence the group structure. Thus all of these variables are dynamic in their influence on each other and the functioning of the group, called the *group process*.

CRITICAL THINKING *Question* ················

Select any group of which you are a member. Identify and describe the elements of the group set in that group.
··

Group process

The term *group process* describes the internal functioning of any type of group with all of the dynamic interactions among its members. Group process is examined in terms of the task performance, activity patterns within the group, interpersonal relationships, and communications. In addition, the behaviors, roles, and issues that surface during the group meetings are important process factors.[7,11] It is important to note that many of the specifics that occur in groups (in terms of interpersonal relationships and communications) are essentially the same as those discussed in previous chapters pertaining to the individual. The concepts related to those areas apply to groups as well.

When examining the group process, one of the primary tasks is separating the content and the process of the group. Content focus is related to the actual topics of discussion and facts; process focus is related to the inferred meanings attached to the topic or the basics for the topic.[1] For example, discussion about problems of authority (content) reflect that there is a struggle for leadership going on in the group (process). Four out of eight students arrived late for a clinical conference that was being presented by one of their peers, and when confronted about their lateness by the student who was designated as group leader, the spokesperson for the late group said, "It's really the instructor's fault. She gives us such heavy assignments we can't get to lunch. The same thing happened to me when I presented. I guess you were off sick that day." What is said in the group (content) has meaning for what is going on in the group or how the group is functioning (process).

Based on the pattern of content-process, the theme of the meeting will arise. The theme is the major concept-idea that serves as a thread to link the parts of the meeting into a more or less unified whole. There may be more than one theme occurring at a time, yet themes are usually closely related. The activity patterns observed in the group and the level of task performance will be related to the process work at any point in time.[4,5]

The communications, interpersonal relationships, and roles within the group are also related to the process and greatly influence the process in a reciprocal way. Among the easier aspects of group process to observe are the patterns of communication and relationships. Through observing who speaks to whom, what the topic is, when each person speaks, how the communication is delivered in terms of the type of communication, and the tone and nonverbal aspects, an individual can begin to identify specific patterns within the group. Also, who does not speak, who is not spoken to, who interrupts whom, and who rescues or supports whom are important aspects of the process. All of these shed light on who influences whom within the group, as well as the leadership and follower patterns of interaction. These aspects of the group process can be noted by using a sociogram, a diagrammatic representation of interactions in the group (Fig. 8-2) that notes to whom comments are directed, where reciprocal conversation occurs, and when comments are directed to the group as a whole. Diagramming the seating arrangement and flow of the conversations assists in exam-

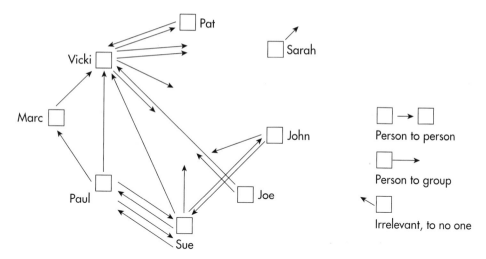

Fig. 8-2 Sociogram.

ining patterns of interaction that emerge over time. In Fig. 8-2 Paul and Sue interact as a dyad, and Vicki is spoken to by six of the seven other members and directs many of her responses to the group as a whole. Sarah, on the other hand, does not participate in the group and offers only one irrelevant comment.

Group roles The interactions in the group may be viewed in terms of the purposes that the behaviors serve. Some behaviors primarily serve the individual's needs without regard to the group. These behaviors are related to *self-oriented roles*. Examples of such roles and the related behaviors include:

• **Self-protector:** defensiveness
• **Intellectualizer:** facts without feelings
• **Town crier:** self-acclamation and adulation
• **Snob:** better than you, above-all-that attitude
• **Invisible man/woman:** silent, nonparticipant
• **Confused:** never understands, so never has to carry the load
• **Yes man:** going along with everything, uncommitted to anything or anyone

Such behaviors serve to hinder the group in attaining goals. As long as the behaviors are accepted by others in the group, they will exist and interfere. Only if the group confronts and discusses the behaviors can any change occur. Because these behaviors are often related to trust and anxiety issues, it takes time to effect the change.

The behaviors relevant to fulfillment of the group task or purpose are called *task role behaviors*.[11] As mentioned in the section on task groups, such behaviors are essential to the group. Whether they fall to a member or the leader depends on the type of leadership in the group. Task roles generally include the role of:

1. **Initiator:** defines the problem and suggests procedures to solve problems
2. **Information seeker:** requests relevant information or expression of ideas
3. **Information giver:** offers ideas, facts, information
4. **Clarifier:** clears up ideas, indicating definition of terms
5. **Explorer:** explores alternatives and deeper meanings or ramifications related to alternatives
6. **Summarizer:** puts ideas together and restates suggestions after discussion
7. **Consensus taker:** asks if group is near a decision on possible conclusion
8. **Record keeper:** maintains record of ideas, discussion, and decisions to most efficiently move group along

These roles may be taken on independently or concurrently, or they may be assigned. The roles related to what is to be done and *content work*.

The last category of role behaviors for group members relates to how the job gets done or to the *process work*. These roles are called *maintenance roles*[11] because they facilitate the group climate, interactions, and positive communications. Examples of maintenance roles include:

1. **Standard setter:** checks with group members to see if they are satisfied with how things are going, pointing out implicit and explicit norms
2. **Encourager:** shows responsiveness to others and acceptance of others' ideas, especially nonverbally
3. **Supporter:** actively supports positions presented by others and acknowledges group task performance
4. **Harmonizer:** reduces tensions, assists others to explore differences, and reconciles disagreements
5. **Compromiser:** offers to compromise his or her own ideas and modifies ideas in the interest of group cohesiveness, growth, or productivity
6. **Gatekeeper:** facilitates total group participation and helps maintain flow of communication

Without maintenance roles the process work of the group stagnates, and the task performance is compromised. Although it takes skill and practice to effectively integrate the task and maintenance roles, the group experience can be an enriching one.

Group issues Even when there is a functioning balance between task and process, there are often conflicting issues that arise in each group. These issues tend to be accompanied by an increase in self-oriented behaviors and an undercurrent of tension in the group. The issues cannot be ignored, or the group will become ineffective. Conscious recognition and open discussion of the issues are necessary. Issues generally arise around the areas of trust and identity as the members struggle with the notions of who they are in the group and what behaviors are acceptable. Problems related to needs and goals surface as a differentiation between a member's own goals (what do I want from the group) and the group goals. The person must examine whether the group goals are consistent with personal goals.

Another major issue relates to influence, power, and control. The degree of member comfort with the locus of power and control either produces or reduces tension. Each person must come to terms with how much influence he or she has and who will control what the group does.

The fourth major issue for the group is that of intimacy. Intimacy is related to the degree of trust among members. As a member senses more trust among the others there is more self-disclosure and interaction at a personal level.

Until these issues are dealt with, counterproductive behaviors will be evident in the group. Such counterproductive behaviors include dependency, resistance, fighting, domination, forming coalitions or subgroups, and withdrawal. The occasional evidence of such behaviors may relate to individual issues. The pattern of these behaviors is indicative of problems within the group. Problems do arise during the life of a group, and during these times conflict resolution techniques can be most useful. If the objectivity of the discussion can be maintained, behaviors can be examined in terms of their meaning to the group and alternatives tested to promote the effectiveness of the group.

Group decision making Groups are always making decisions, either consciously or unconsciously. The decisions to be made and how they are made will vary with the dynamics of the group and the phase of group development during which the decisions are made. Group decision-making procedures fall into five categories:

1. **Dumping:** (lack of response): members suggest decisions without discussion of the ideas among the group.
2. **Authoritarian decision:** delegated authority makes the decisions for the group, whose members may or may not advise the leader.
3. **Majority voting or polling:** vote for an approach that is then carried out as the group's decision.
4. **Consensus:** discussion of the issue takes place so members agree to support it and are more or less committed to it.
5. **Unanimous vote:** all members vote in accord to support the decision. This form of decision making is rare.

Any variety of these forms of decision making or combinations of them may be found to be operating in any group.[2]

Group phases

The process of the group evolves over time. The dynamics that occur and the issues and tasks that are addressed all relate to the phase of group development. There are generally five phases in the development of a group, ranging from preaffiliation to termination.[11] These phases are similar to those of the helping relationship described in Chapter 7. Information about each phase is summarized in Table 8-2.

The first phase in the development of the group is the *preaffiliation phase*. During this period members enter the group and behave in accordance with norms from previous group experiences. There are many stereotypic, formalistic activities and an impersonal atmosphere. There are approach-avoidance behaviors related to ambivalence about roles. Self-oriented behavior predominates and issues of trust and commitment are evident. Decisions such as items for the agenda or when to schedule the next meeting are made as the group searches for structure and preliminary commitments. As acceptance of distance is allowed, anxiety reduced, and trust eventually built, evidence of the exploration of ideas within a structure appears to support the clearly stated goals. The group norms begin to emerge. Standard norms such as regular attendance, punctuality, degree of sharing, and focus on exploring and problem solving emerge. Behaviors that encourage group development include active listening, empathy, genuineness, respect, encouraging shared responsibility, and some degree of personal investment.

The next phase is that of *power and control*. Characteristically at this point the group focuses on struggles of power and control. There is concentrated attention to authority relationships such as who influences whom, who makes decisions, and who abides by decisions. Individuals struggle with relationships between their own needs, autonomy, and group needs. Status-related jockeying for power positions occurs as members confront the reality of the group. At this phase there may be aggressive competition for leadership and testing of the strength of authority. Rebellion occurs, and some dropout danger is evident. With active focus on the power issues and clarification of the struggle, conflict resolution is possible. Direct focus on alternatives and their consequences, as well as the active encouragement of the expression of feelings and anxieties, can move the group through this phase. Tempering decisions so that they are not made on the basis of emotions is also a challenge at this point.

The third phase is that of *intimacy*, which is characterized by greater other-orientation and personal involvement. The membership crises experienced during the second phase may continue, but there is more open expression of dependency and emotion-laden struggles. This is a transition stage with inevitable conflicts focused on human relationships, responsibility, and changing positions. Some problem behaviors include nonparticipation, monopolizing, hostility, intellectual belaboring of extremes in questioning, and advice giving.

TABLE 8-2   Phases of group development

PHASE	DYNAMICS
Preaffiliation	Issues of trust vs. mistrust, identity questions, self-oriented behaviors, distance maintained, approach-avoidance behavior, ambivalence, anxiety, impersonal climate
Power and control	Issues of power, influence, and control; struggles regarding autonomy and interdependence; aggressive competition; many self-oriented behaviors exist; emotionality
Intimacy	Increased trust and self-disclosure; dependency vs. independence still an issue; conflicts regarding relationships, responsibility, and identity; high emotional level, yet some task work accomplished
Differentiation	Trust, commitment, and cohesion are evident; freedom of expression regarding acceptance and support; cooperative atmosphere; positive outlook; high productivity
Termination	Separation; summarization and evaluation regarding experiencing of emotionality and self-oriented behaviors noted in preaffiliation stage

The fourth phase is that of *differentiation*. This phase is the working phase of the group. A sense of trust and commitment exists among members. Cohesion is evident, and norms are further developed and solidified. There is a freedom of expression, spontaneity, acceptance of others' ideas, and support. Reciprocity is clearly evident. Change is seen in light of a willingness to take a risk based on mutual support and caring. At this point the group essentially runs itself. Tasks are accomplished in a cooperative manner with shared responsibility. The group has its own identity, and there are few power problems as a positive outlook prevails.

The final phase in the development of the group is that of *termination* or separation. At this point the focus changes to review and evaluation of the task accomplishment and the process of the group. The task of the group is also related to the consolidation of learning, summarization of progress, and discussion of the future goals and plans of the individuals; this parallels the termination work in all relationships. It is a time for letting go. The emotional intensity in the group rises as separation becomes imminent. Behavior evident in the preaffiliation phase may be reenacted, and the leader must be very active in the tasks necessary for positive termination.

IMPLICATION FOR NURSES

Nurses spend much of their professional lives engaged in group interactions. The various models of nursing care delivery rely heavily on group work.[2] Assignments are made to individual nurses who work in conjunction with other health team members (a group) and other nurses on the unit (also a group). Some areas use a functional approach in which everyone relies on others to carry out selected functions so the total task gets done. Others use primary nursing, where the nurse has 24-hour responsibility for the care of assigned clients and all clients' nurses form the group to provide total care and coverage. Still other areas use team nursing models in which a nurse leader directs the activities of members who are assigned to groups of clients. The arrangements vary, but the dynamics still have a point of reference in group work.

A professional nurse is often involved in directing groups of clients, serving as resource person, coordinator, and facilitator.[2] Again knowledge of group dynamics plays an important role in the success of the planning, functioning, and evaluation of such groups.

There is value in group participation for most people. The individual receives validation for thoughts and feelings that might otherwise be regarded as unusual or unique. Support can be received for risking new ideas or different approaches to problems. "Brainstorming" can help the nurse identify alternatives when it seems that all resources have been exhausted. Sharing frustration and pain or joy and satisfaction with empathic colleagues replenishes the nurse's interpersonal resources.

Groups are also a source of strength and power. Individuals separately often accomplish much less than the same people united in a group effort do. Nurses are becoming aware of the need to function effectively in groups to influence the health care system. Political action committees have been organized at state and national levels to channel the political power of nurses. Collective bargaining units are

Group Activities

The following are brief examples of the many group activities in which nurses participate:

Situation I: A *group* of nursing students plans a series of health education classes for a *group* of women who are attending a prenatal clinic. They also present their plans at a clinic *staff meeting*.

Situation II: The *board of directors* of the state nurses' association appoints an *ad hoc committee* to conduct a search for a new executive director.

Situation III: The representatives of a *collective bargaining unit* present nurses' job-related demands to the hospital management's *negotiating team*.

Situation IV: A *nursing care team* in a nursing home organizes a gin rummy tournament for a *group* of wheelchair-bound residents.

Situation V: The staff nurses in a burn treatment center ask a mental health nursing specialist to lead a *peer support group* in which they can share feelings and build solid *team* relationships.

Situation VI: A *small group* of nurses from a variety of hospital units meet regularly to receive peer review of the care they provide to their clients.

organized by state nurses' associations to ensure adequate nursing care for clients and adequate compensation for nurses. Nurses who excel in group leadership skills are needed to maximize the effectiveness of these groups.

CRITICAL THINKING *Question* ....

Select a current issue in nursing or health care, such as managed care or the use of unlicensed assistive personnel as nurse extenders. State your analysis of the implications of the issue for nursing practice. What sorts of group approaches would help nurses address the issue?

....

Knowledge of groups and their functions can also facilitate multidisciplinary sharing of expertise, enhanced examination of alternatives, and dissemination of information to others. Nurses with advanced preparation may also colead or lead therapeutic groups. In these cases in particular experience and knowledge are important. The individuals involved and the depth of the process-focused work require sophistication in handling the delicate emotional issues that often arise during group sessions.

Nurses who are able to apply interpersonal skills in groups, who understand group dynamics and group process, and who work to develop effective group leader and group member skills will be well rewarded. They will be able to facilitate good care of their clients, will be respected by their peers, will be valued as team members, and will be offered opportunities for leadership. The nurse who is able to unravel the complexities of group behavior or who knows when to request help in group analysis will find a whole new set of ways to achieve professional objectives. The development of group participation skills is hard work, but the rewards are great.

SUMMARY

A group can be defined as two or more people involved in face-to-face interactions with a common purpose or goal. There are task groups whose primary purpose is to do a job or make decisions, and there are therapeutic groups where the primary focus is on member interactions, growth, and development. A combined focus on task (content work) and process (relationship work) facilitates goal accomplishment. Therapeutic groups include encounter groups, T-groups, counseling groups, and therapy groups.

Leadership is the use of multiple processes to influence the activities of individuals toward goal attainment. It may come from a designated authority or from within the group. Leadership styles may be autocratic, democratic, or laissez-faire. The style of leadership influences leader authority, member responsibility, leader focus, and member participation. These behaviors are related to roles that are expectations held by others about appropriate behaviors for a specific position. A role set is learned during a role episode. Role differentiation, role conflict, role ambiguity, and role overload are important concepts in relation to behavior and functioning in certain roles. In therapeutic groups leadership behavior includes characteristics such as modeling, openness, caring, courage, inventiveness, a sense of humor, and flexibility. A coleader might also be useful for group therapy groups.

Group process is the internal functions of a group with all of the dynamic interactions among its members. The various factors that predispose the group to functioning in a given way are termed the *group set*. The intangible group set variables include goals, values, norms, climate, and historical factors. Structural group set variables include organization, size, composition, characteristics, and the theoretic framework of the group. These group set variables influence the process in terms of the interpersonal interactions, communications, patterns of activity, and roles apparent in the group. These roles may be self-oriented, task oriented, or group maintenance oriented. Emotional issues as part of the group process usually involve concerns about trust, identity, needs and goals, influence, power and control, and intimacy. The type of decision making is also considered in analyses of group process.

The process dynamics are closely related to the phase of group development. The five phases are preaffiliation, power and control, intimacy, differentiation, and termination. Within each phase the relevant issues, process dynamics, and task behavior vary; these phases parallel the stages of the nurse-

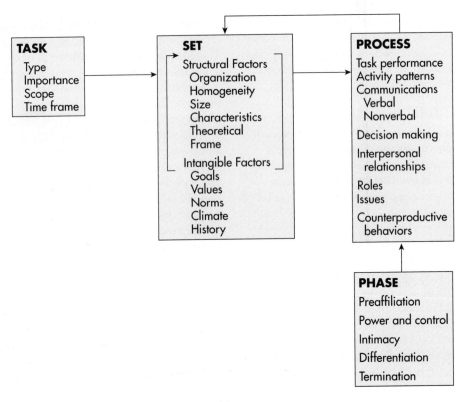

Fig. 8-3 Variables to consider in analysis of the group.

client relationship. Figure 8-3 summarizes the variables to consider in the analysis of the group. Nurses who are able to unravel the complexities of groups will be able to function at a higher level in the multifaceted nursing arena.

DISCUSSION QUESTIONS

1. Identify a situation in which you have experienced (a) role conflict, (b) role ambiguity, (c) role overload. Describe your feelings in the situation, and analyze your task performance. What will you do to avoid similar situations in the future?

2. Explain the *rule of halves*, the *rule of three quarters*, and the *rule of thirds* as they pertain to group behavior.

3. Analyze three major differences between task and therapeutic groups.

4. Define and provide an example of (a) laissez-faire, (b) autocratic, and (c) democratic leadership behavior. Discuss the relationship between leadership style and group task or group relationship behavior.

5. Discuss the rationale for requiring advanced educational and supervised experiential preparation to be qualified for the role of group therapist.

6. Consider your clinical experience group. Identify the group goal, norms, and values.

7. Think about your last clinical conference. Describe one content issue and one process issue that arose during that meeting. Discuss your answer with the other group members.

8. Based on your last experience with a small group identify one task role behavior and one maintenance role behavior that you performed during the meeting. Would you describe yourself as primarily task oriented or primarily maintenance oriented? Validate this perception with a classmate.

9. Compare and contrast the five approaches to group decision making. In your opinion which has

the best potential for member satisfaction? Discuss your selection. What member characteristics might lead you to change your mind?

10. Identify the phase of group development that is typified by each of the following member statements:
   - "I think Mary would be good at that job."
   - "I've never been in a group as great as this one."
   - "Can you get us some information about community resources to fund our project?"
   - "I really don't know why I'm here."
   - "Who made you boss, anyway?"
   - "I've learned so much from all of you."
   - "I think we should kick John out of this group for being late all the time."

Discuss your answers with your clinical group, and reach a group decision about the correct answers. Identify the decision-making process you selected and your rationale for choosing it.

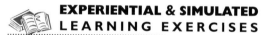

EXPERIENTIAL & SIMULATED LEARNING EXERCISES

1. Planning a group meeting

PURPOSE: To prepare to conduct an initial meeting of a task group.

PROCESS: Divide students into small groups of three to five each. Assign a group task such as (1) planning a baby shower, (2) planning an orientation program for new nursing students, (3) planning a nursing students' speakers bureau, or (4) doing another activity of the instructor's choice. Assign each student to develop an agenda for the first group meeting. Each student should also identify the other arrangements that need to be made.

DISCUSSION: Students should compare their agendas and agree on a consensus agenda. Rationale for agenda items, priorities, sequence of items, and time allotments should be shared. Students should then discuss and agree on the other arrangements that need to be made. A group leader should be selected.

2. Task group experience

PURPOSE: To carry out plans for the initial meeting of a task group.

PROCESS: Based on the plans made in the group meeting planning exercise, students should carry out the arrangements that they agreed on for a first meeting including distribution of the agenda. They should then meet and pursue the assigned task.

DISCUSSION: Students should analyze their group behavior, including:
   1. The adequacy of the planning process
   2. The role assumed by the leader
   3. The roles assumed by the members
   4. Intangible group set variables
   5. Structural group set variables
   6. Degree of task accomplishment

3. Role play of group behaviors

PURPOSE: To experience and identify constructive and destructive group role performance.

PROCEDURE: Prepare small slips of paper, each naming one of the roles listed on pp. 207-208. Divide students into small groups of six to eight. Have each student select a role at random. Assign one student to be leader, and have that student select a leader role that is laissez-faire, autocratic, or democratic. Assign a simple group task such as planning a dinner menu. Instruct each student to act in keeping with the assigned role.

DISCUSSION: Ask students to identify the role played by each group member and to discuss the impact that the behavior had on the group's task accomplishment.

4. How to stop the project

PROCEDURE: Instruct the group to work toward making some decision on an element of a project or task that is relevant to the group. One member is selected by the leader/group to be the recorder. The recorder will be instructed to observe the group and to note when and in what situation a decision blocker is used. A record form that is set up like a grid should be provided. Names of group members are listed on the left side. Five columns appear across the top, labeled as followed:
   1. Ordering/directing
   2. Moralizing/preaching
   3. Criticizing/evaluating
   4. Persuading/arguing
   5. Other (list specific)

Whenever a member uses one of the blocking statements, put a check in the appropriate box and make a note of the situation or statement. Instruct the group to proceed toward the decision for approximately 40 minutes, then discuss the experience for 15 minutes. Before the discussion, the recorder is to share with the group the information on the grid, summarizing the number of times any one blocker was used.

DISCUSSION: In the group, discuss the following:

1. What functions do decision blockers serve?
2. What immediately preceded the use of the blocker and what followed its use?
3. How did the blocker impede the decision-making process?
4. When might a decision blocker be useful?
5. Why are members more comfortable using certain types of blockers more frequently?
6. How can the group move past blockers?

5. Identifying group members' needs

PURPOSE: To examine the needs of individuals in the group to work effectively and productively.

PROCEDURE: The facilitator instructs members to:

1. Make yourselves comfortable and close your eyes.
2. Imagine you are at work with the group and see yourself working. (Pause) What do you need to be more effective?
3. Now travel slowly through the group, seeing/experiencing each member working and answer … What does the group need to work more effectively?
4. Pretend a powerful genie will grant each of you one wish based on a need you identified … What would that be?
5. When you are ready, come back to the present situation and open your eyes.

Each participant writes down their "wish" *in positive optimistic terms*, in as much detail as necessary, using half a sheet of paper, which is then folded and placed in a box. Each participant then draws one wish from the box (not their own) and spends 5 to 10 minutes describing how the written wish can be implemented. Group participants share the ideas.

DISCUSSION: In the group discuss the following:

1. How did it feel to determine how to implement someone else's wish?
2. How did you feel when you heard your wish's implementation shared by someone else?

3. What common themes or issues were raised by the members?
4. What is the value of having to present other people's ideas regardless of whether you think the idea is worthwhile?
5. What did you learn about your group during this activity?
6. How can you use what you have learned to help the group work more effectively to achieve its goals?

REFERENCES

1. Berger J: Expectations, theory and group process, *Soc Psychol Q* 55:3, 1992.
2. Bernard L, Walsh M: *Leadership: the key to the professionalization of nursing*, ed 2, St Louis, 1990, Mosby.
3. Burleson C: *Effective meetings: the complete guide*, New York, 1990, Wiley.
4. Honeycutt A, Richards B: Nominal group process in organizational development work, *Leadership Organization Dev J* 12:24, 1991.
5. Keyton J: Evaluating individual group member satisfaction as a situational variable, *Small Group Res* 22:200, 1991.
6. LaSalle P, LaSalle A: Small groups and their therapeutic force. In Stuart G, Laraia M, editors: *Principles and practice of psychiatric nursing*, ed 6, St Louis, 1998, Mosby.
7. Napier R, Gershenfeld M: *Groups: theory and experience*, ed 4, Boston, 1989, Houghton Mifflin.
8. Reis F: From controlling to flexibility: how to L.E.A.D. In Pfeiffer JW, editor: *The 1992 annual: developing human resources*, San Diego, 1992, Pfeiffer.
9. Stockton R, Rhonde R, Haughey J: The effects of structured group experiences on cohesion, engagement, avoidance and conflict, *Small Group Process* 23:155, 1992.
10. Vinogradov S, Yalom I: *Concise guide to group psychotherapy*, Washington, DC, 1989, American Psychiatric Press.
11. Wilson G, Hanna M: *Groups in context: leadership and participation in small groups*, ed 2, New York, 1990, McGraw-Hill.
12. Yalom I: *The theory and practice of group psychotherapy*, ed 3, New York, 1985, Basic Books.

Suggested Readings

Anderson L: Teams: group process, success and barriers, *J Nurs Adm* 23(9):15, 1993.

This article reviews the importance of teams to total quality management. The theoretical perspectives related to stages, tasks, goals, and interpersonal relationships are reviewed. Major concepts and characteristics, predictors of effectiveness, and the nurse's role in the development of work teams are also presented.

Baker D: The behavioral analysis of interpersonal intimacy in group development, *Small Group Res* 22:76, 1991.

   For the advanced learner to explore the issue of interpersonal relationships and development of group cohesiveness.

Begin J: Building group cohesion through cooperation activities, *Elementary School Guidance and Counseling* 24:90, 1989.

   Pediatric experiences might be developed using an approach similar to that reported by this author.

Brunner N: That was a good meeting! *Orthop Nurs* 12(4):35, 1993.

   Presents information and suggestions for structuring successful meetings, including the participation in group process as an essential aspect of meeting effectiveness and efficiency.

Deffenbacher J et al: A comparison of cognitive behavioral and process oriented group counseling for general anger reduction, *J Counseling Dev* 69:167, 1990.

   Excellent support article for learning more about the topic of anger and handling conflict in groups.

Dinkmyer D: Encouragement: basis for leader training and participative management, *Individual Psychol J Adlerian Theory Res Pract* 47:504, 1991.

   Excellent article for those undertaking leadership positions within groups.

Fargason O, Haddock O: Cross-functional, integrative decision making: essential for effective QI in health care, *Q Rev Bull* 18:157, 1992.

   This article provides an example of decision-making strategies in action in the health care arena.

Kassis J, Boothroyd P, Ben Dor R: The family support group: families and professionals in partnership, *Psychosoc Rehab J* 15:91, 1992.

   This article provides an example of use of a group approach with client groups, in this case families, as well as an example of support groups.

Kroon M, Kreweld D, Rabbie J: Group versus individual decision making: effects of accountability and gender on group therapy, *Small Group Process* 23:427, 1992.

   This article provides information specific to processes that occur within therapy groups.

Lanza M: Total quality management: a golden opportunity for psychiatric clinical nurse specialists, *Clin Nurse Spec* 8:221, 1994.

   This article applies the elements of group process to the total quality management (TQM) role as a key to achieving TQM goals. It also highlights the role of the nurse as the facilitator of the process.

Menneck B, Hoff J, Wayne B: The implications of group development and history for group support systems theory and practice, *Small Group Process* 23:524, 1992.

   Group dynamics is discussed in light of theoretical and practical factors. This article is appropriate for the more advanced student.

Neubauer J: Redesign: managing role changes and building new teams, *Seminars for Nurse Managers* 1:26, 1993.

   This article reviews group process concepts and the importance of process to accomplishing project outcomes. Emphasis is given to the importance of clarification of roles, negotiation, and effective decision making.

Rhorer J, Young M: Surviving your first job, *Healthcare Trends Transitions* 3:24, 1992.

   This article will be especially interesting to the student who will soon be transitioning between the domains of education and occupation.

Rich B et al: Peer consultation: a look at process, *Clin Nurse Spec* 9:181, 1995.

   In this article, the evolution of group process, from an experiential perspective, is described as it is applied to professional growth and development.

Smith G, Hukill E: Quality work improvement groups: from paper to reality, *J Nurs Care Qual* 8(4):1, 1994.

   This article emphasizes the importance of knowledge of group development and group dynamics in maintaining effective, high-performance work teams. In addition, the importance of dealing with both the content and process are discussed.

CHAPTER

9 *Stress and Adaptation*

*Stress is the rain of life, adaptation the umbrella,
and relaxation the sunshine.*

E. A. D. Rankin

LEARNING OBJECTIVES

After studying this chapter, the student should be able to:

- Define *stress, stressor,* and the *stress response*.
- Define the *stress state* in terms of the intensity, scope, and duration of the stress experience.
- Define the concepts of *frustration, threat, conflict,* and *anxiety*.
- Compare and contrast the local adaptation syndrome and the general adaptation syndrome.
- Describe the physiologic, behavioral, and emotional reactions seen in the stress response.
- Define *coping* and *adaptation*.
- Describe each of the major defense mechanisms.
- Analyze the role of the nurse in dealing with clients who are experiencing stress and the processes of adaptation.
- Describe two ways to decrease stress reactivity.
- Analyze one's own responses to stress and strategies used in adaptation.

To determine the nature of the client's needs, to formulate a plan, and to implement nursing care, the nurse must thoroughly assess the client's situation. What is it that the nurse must assess? Part of the answers lies in understanding the stress experience of the person. What does the individual perceive the situation to be? What meaning does it have? What are the related demands, costs, and benefits for the person? How does this person usually react to a situation? This chapter is devoted to the discussion of the phenomenon of stress reactivity, how people strive to cope

with and adapt to stress, and the nursing implications of both. The focus is on stress as a multifaceted experience, involving biologic, psychologic, and sociocultural factors. Several theories are noted to emphasize different approaches to examining the stress state and the ways in which a person responds to life situations.

DEFINITIONS RELATIVE TO STRESS

There are many definitions of stress in the literature. Stress may be defined as a force applied or as a state of tension. When examining the concept from a nursing perspective, *stress* can be defined as a state that occurs when some situation or event places a demand on the person, or causes tension, such that the individual is required (consciously or unconsciously) to respond or take action.[11]

Stress involves both psychologic and physiologic responses to life situations. Whenever an individual perceives a "mismatch" between self and the environment or elements of the environment, stress occurs. The day-to-day challenges and demands motivate the person to grow and develop, to resolve the strains that are experienced, and to overcome the tensions.

However, there are times when the amount of stress becomes more intense or the person's experience is compounded in some way so that it is difficult to resolve the demands. One of the factors that have been studied relating to the stress experience has to do with the notion of change and life experiences.

Any major change that an individual experiences initiates a universal phenomenon: the stress reaction. Regardless of the nature of the change or disruption, a series of demands that challenge the individual to adapt arises. Even though each person may respond differently, certain life events have been identified as stressful for most individuals.

Early researchers identified significant life events that precipitated major personal adjustment to changes. This led to the development of the Social Readjustment Rating Scale by Holmes and Rahe.[8] The events listed on this tool, which are noted in Table 9-1, are assigned a numeric value depending on the amount of adjustment each requires. To obtain a score for the relative stress related to the changes that a person has experienced over the past year, add the life-change units corresponding to the life events that have been checked. A score of 200 or higher is indicative of high-level stress.

Although the work of Holmes and Rahe is noteworthy as one of the initial contributions linking social science research and the stress response, one of the major criticisms of this tool is that it does not take into account the individual perceptions of the impact of the event. The person's appraisal of the negative or positive nature of the event determines the impact. In addition, this tool lists only major life events and does not take into account the daily "hassles" each individual must face. These hassles pile up and compound each other, causing high levels of stress in the individual. Because of the subtle nature of the hassles, their influence is often more profound than that of major life events, causing a decline in the individual's ability to cope and function. The hassles become the straw that breaks the camel's back.

The stimuli or agents that precipitate the demands made on the individual are called *stressors*. The life

TABLE 9-1 Social readjustment rating scale: a schedule of recent life events requiring or reflecting change and initiating a stress response

RECENT EVENTS	LIFE-CHANGE UNITS	RECENT EVENTS	LIFE-CHANGE UNITS
Death of spouse	100	Change in responsibilities at work	29
Divorce	73	Son or daughter leaving home	29
Marital separation	65	Troubles with in-laws	29
Detention in jail/institution	63	Outstanding personal achievement	28
Death of a close family member	63	Spouse began or ceased work	26
Personal injury or illness	53	Began or ceased formal schooling	26
Marriage	50	Change in living conditions	25
Fired from work	47	Revision of personal habits	24
Marital reconciliation	45	Trouble with boss/supervisor	23
Retirement	45	Changes in work hours or conditions	20
Change in health/behavior of family member	44	Change in residence	20
Pregnancy	40	Change in schools	20
Sexual difficulties	39	Change in recreation	19
Gain a new family member	39	Changes in church activities	19
Business readjustment	39	Change in social activities	18
Change in financial state	38	Mortgage or loan less than $10,000	17
Death of close friend	37	Change in sleeping habits	16
Change to different line of work	36	Change in number of family get-togethers	15
Change in number of arguments with spouse	35	Change in eating habits	15
Mortgage or loan over $10,000	31	Vacation	13
Foreclosure of mortgage or loan	30	Minor violations of the law	11

Modified from Holmes TH, Rahe RH: The social readjustment rating scale, *J Psychosom Res* 11:214, 1967.

events previously noted are examples of stressors that are predominantly sociologic, but stressors may also be biologic or psychologic in nature. They may be very specific threats to one's safety or more subtle conflicts, threats to goal achievement, or unmet expectations. Any stimulus in excess or in too small an amount may be stressful if perceived as such. Sensory deficit and sensory overload may be experienced as equally discomforting. When an individual experiences the situation as negative (often the case when under excessive stress), the stress overload is called *distress*.

The nature of the demands placed on the person, the amount of work (energy) necessary to deal with the incoming stimuli, and the resources available are important variables to take into account when investigating a person's responses to the pressures of daily life.[9]

The stress state

Everyone must constantly attempt to handle stress related to both internal and external factors, because stress is very much a component of life. The cumulative reaction occurring as a result of the stress is referred to as the *stress state*.

The stress state is that dynamic process in which the person experiences and reacts to the balancing,

imbalancing, and rebalancing effects of stress. The stress state can be described in terms of the variables of intensity of the stress, the scope of the impact of the stress, and the duration of the experience. *Intensity* refers to the magnitude of the force of the stressor;[11] it may be of low, medium, or severe intensity. The person may easily cope with the situation without too much apparent stress if it is of low intensity. For example, getting a splinter usually does not engender as intense a reaction as does severing a finger. As the intensity of the demand increases, greater energy is needed to maintain functioning.

Scope of the impact of the stress refers to the extent of involvement of the total organism and the spread of the stress state. The scope depends on the force of the stress and may be described as of limited, moderate, or extensive involvement. An example of limited scope would be a carbuncle on the forearm. Compare this with the extensive involvement of a woman during pregnancy when she undergoes physiologic and structural changes of the entire body as well as emotional and sociologic changes. It becomes evident that the energy required to cope increases as the scope of the stress increases.

Duration of the experience refers to the length of time of exposure to the stressor. Continued exposure

 CLINICAL EXAMPLE

A *nurse interviewing Ms. J., a patient in the medical clinic, notes that Ms. J. complains of being tired and of not having as much "get up and go" as before. The nurse continues to talk with Ms. J. to identify things that might possibly cause such a change in energy level. The client is under stress of some kind; there are several demands with which she must cope. Ms. J. works as a teacher's aide in an elementary school. She has two school-age children who are "growing like weeds." The union to which she belongs is about to go on strike, so budgeting money is very important. Also, the family diet usually consists of noodles, cheeses, some meats such as chicken and hamburger, and vegetables such as beans, peas, corn, cauliflower, and squash in season. From this information it seems that nutrition may be a factor as well as all the decisions and functions that Ms. J. must deal with each day. Thus the nature of the demands are prob-*

ably physical and emotional. The client has been able to cope but states that "It's getting worse." Her energy is at a very low level. Attempts have been made to utilize personal abilities to try and deal with the situation, but it is becoming more difficult. The assistance of other family members was sought, and one sister now assists with housecleaning occasionally but doesn't seem to be too helpful. Now Ms. J. is seeking aid from those outside the family. One such measure has included talking with health professionals to try to resolve some of the demands. Attempts to use personal resources were unsuccessful, which has necessitated utilization of energies available through others. Ms. J. cannot do all of the work in dealing with incoming stimuli alone, because her resources and energy stores are nearly depleted.

to a stressor can exhaust one's energy supplies and thus greatly affect one's ability to cope. Duration is described in terms of short, moderate, or long-term exposure. If a child has a 24-hour virus, less strain is placed on his normal functioning than if a severe episode of flu confines him for a week or two. For a short time he is able to draw on body reserves to deal with the situation. After an extended period, however, the child's energy stores become depleted, and his ability to deal with the situation becomes compromised. Thus it can be said that as the span of time (duration) of the stress state increases, the energy required to maintain daily functioning also increases.

The energy requirement for functioning during times of stress will vary from person to person. Although dependent on the intensity, scope, and duration of the stress state, the particular criteria for identifying the levels of each of these characteristics cannot be generalized. A subjective appraisal of the situation is the fulcrum on which the stress experience rests. It must be remembered that an imbalance occurs when the demands of the stressor are perceived and, through the process of cognitive appraisal, are evaluated as demanding, overwhelming, or incongruent with the person's ability to "meet the demand."[14] This perception and appraisal is highly individualized, depending to a great extent on personal factors such as personality traits, values, past experiences, and sociodemographic variables; process factors such as decision-making abilities, mental processes, and coping strategies; and environmental factors such as physical setting, social support networks, and organizational variables.[9,14] These factors mediate the stress experience. As a result, when an event occurs and is observed by two individuals simultaneously, one person may respond by behaving as if very distressed while the other reacts minimally, having experienced only a mild disruption in routine. The event has been perceived and appraised differently by the two individuals.

The *number of stressors* also affects the stress experience. Exposure to several stressors at once presents a greater demand than would a single stressor. More energy and utilization of resources are required to deal with multiple stressors. Similarly, being subjected to a single stressor several times within a short time span depletes energy

TABLE 9-2 Types of stressors

Time dimension

Acute—occurs suddenly, usually of uncommon nature for the person

Chronic—recurring, over a long period of time; long-standing duration

Cognitive process

Hidden—unconscious, unknown stressor linked to a conflict and evidenced by long-standing stress reaction

Unnoticed—somewhat more conscious but generally cognitively avoided to manage stress

Obvious—the connection between the stressor and the stress situation is known

Point of origin

External—originating outside of the person

Internal—originating within the person, often related to conflicts in values, desires, and social interactions

Life experience

Developmental—those events that occur at critical points in one's growth and development

Occupational—those events related to work situations that are stress producing

Social—those stressors that are related to social, interpersonal, and interactional situations and events

stores. Even dealing with the same stressor over a period of time without a reprieve, to allow for a period of time to recuperate from the stress state, will have a similar effect.

In examining the stress state as experienced by the individual it is important to be aware that there are different types of stressors. Stressors may be categorized based on the time factor, cognitive processes involved, point of origin, or life situation. The type of stressor, the nature of the stress state, and stress reactivity of the individual will greatly influence the individual's experience (Table 9-2).

CRITICAL THINKING *Question*

How do you feel when you are stressed? Identify at least three biologic, psychologic, and sociologic behaviors that you recognize in your own responses to stressful situations.

THE STRESS RESPONSE

Appraisal

The stress response involves the entire person within the context of a given situation. When a particular event occurs, the individual mentally processes the information. Any event is actually "neutral" in its occurrence.[9] Then based on past experiences and beliefs a person appraises the situation. *Appraisal* involves the attachment of meaning or a label to what is perceived. Depending on the content of the situation, the event may be labeled as positive, negative, or neutral; this appraisal is made within seconds of the perception of the event. One's perception of the event (mediated by such variables as self-concept and beliefs) then triggers a series of emotions related to the situation.

Basic internal needs, drives, and motives, as well as external, interpersonally motivated pressures, will cause the person to respond in some manner to the perceived situation based on the appraisal. If the event is labeled as having a negative impact, such as a demand or a threat, the stress response ensues.[4] This response is accompanied by the experience of discomfort, either as a feeling of frustration, threat, conflict, or anxiety. These four concepts are important components of biopsychosocial theories of stress and adaptation. They are closely linked, and their effects are frequently observed simultaneously.

CRITICAL THINKING *Question* ················

Ask three different people to define stress and provide an example of something in their lives that they identify as very stressful. Examine the results of this survey for similarities and differences.

··

Frustration

Frustration is a condition that occurs when a course of action cannot be carried out or brought to conclusion. In this event goal attainment and achievement are blocked or delayed. Barriers to goal accomplishment may be internal or external. They may be caused by an environmental factor or an interpersonal situation that seems to deter the person from moving along a chosen course of action. If the barrier is internal, the person may experience a greater frustration just trying to come to a decision as to the course of action. Internal barriers frequently involve cherished values and ideas, and for this reason internal barriers produce situations with which a person has more difficulty coping.

Threat

Threat may be defined as an anticipation of harm. It is the anticipation of an undesirable outcome of a basic biologic need, drive, or motive. The expectation of future harm implies an evaluation, an appraisal of what this present situation portends, based on past experiences. Because of what has been learned in past experiences those situations that have never previously been connected with harm probably will not result in an appraisal of threat; cues previously linked with harm will tend to be threatening. Thus the threat is usually related to actual, realistic, or objective dangers.

When the realities of the situation are more difficult to assess, actual objective danger and threat may not correspond. One example is noted in the tooth-brushing activities of young children. The young child has experienced little connection between tooth decay and dental hygiene. The threat of caries does not seem real. Brushing is merely something the child is told to do. When the child actually develops tooth decay and experiences the discomfort, he begins to relate the lack of brushing one's teeth regularly with a threatening situation.

When threatened, the individual attempts to take some preventive actions. The person anticipates harm and therefore prepares to deal with or avoid it. When the individual is frustrated, on the other hand, the situation requires some form of correction. Stress stimuli may contain elements of both frustration and threat. This point is illustrated in the manner in which people cope with hospitalization for elective surgery. To a certain extent the individual is aware of the threats. The fact that he will be in an unusual environment, separated from family and friends, is known. Daily activities will be changed, and there will be a loss of independence. There may be discomfort associated with the surgery. The person can take some preventive actions. He may find it helpful to bring items from home, such as a radio or a picture of the family, to make the room seem more personal. He can inform friends of the dates of the confinement and of visiting hours. He can bring work to do or books to read to help parallel usual daily activities.

He can even prepare himself mentally for the post-surgical discomfort.

Despite all of this preplanning, however, the person may become frustrated and restless. If a diagnostic procedure is done, hours may be spent away from the now-familiar room. Friends may come to visit and find no one. All the anticipatory plans made by the individual have become ineffective for coping with hospitalization and contribute to a sense of frustration. The threat of the surgery may be handled better than the ensuing frustration because of the gross physical discomfort and incapacitation afterward. These serve as barriers to what little independent functioning the person has while hospitalized. To overcome these barriers different coping strategies, such as taking medication to relieve pain, are necessary. This is just one example of how stress stimuli contain elements of both threat and frustration.

Conflict

Conflict is a third concept relative to stress and adaptation, and it can be defined as the simultaneous presence of incompatible desires or goals. This state arises because the behaviors or attitudes necessary to accomplish one goal are countermanded by those required to complete a second. A conflict makes a threat or frustration inevitable. There can be no completely satisfactory solution to a conflict as long as the person remains committed to both goals. For example, a person who feels ill may be in conflict over seeing a physician. He must either lose a day's work, pay the ensuing expenses, and possibly find relief, or suffer the discomfort of the illness, avoid the expenses of the visit and medications, and go to work but produce less. He can either tolerate the circumstances as they are, give up or modify one (or both) of the conflicting goals, or engage in self-deceptive denial of the entire situation. His choice of a coping strategy should help relieve the conflict, the frustration, and any threat. As long as any of these exist the person will experience a sense of uneasiness called anxiety.

Anxiety

Anxiety is the fourth concept relevant to the stress experiences. It can be a by-product of frustration, threat, or conflict and it is defined as a persistent feeling of dread, apprehension, and impending disaster.[1] Anxiety has two meanings. First, it is a response,

a reaction to certain experiences; anxiety is a state inferred from the manner in which a person acts or from the physiologic changes associated with it. Second, it is an intervening variable, a state brought about by certain conditions; this state in turn produces certain consequences or effects. Everyone experiences anxiety as an unpleasant affective state that is usually referred to as uneasiness, worry, or apprehension. Whenever a person's needs for control, inclusion, and affection are threatened, anxiety results.

One can differentiate between anxiety and fear. The term *anxiety* is used to describe a threat by an unknown entity or an internal conflict; no specific object can be connected with the condition. Fear (sometimes referred to as *objective anxiety*) is caused by a threat from an identifiable external danger and is considered a reaction to real danger. Primarily, fear and anxiety differ in their causes yet produce similar reactions.

Anxiety as a response is a subjective, individualized experience that cannot be directly observed. It is known only through its effects, which are always communicated. Anxiety as an intervening variable is also an inferred condition. It serves as a factor that stands between the stimulus and a response, but in itself it is unobservable. A person is made anxious when certain goals or values are placed in jeopardy; for example, one may experience such tension when needs for prestige are not met or some personal expectation is not achieved. Anxiety is followed by certain behaviors designed to relieve the situation. In effect anxiety motivates solutions to conditions that produce stress states.

Anxiety may be referred to in terms of the levels or degrees to which it influences a person's actions. Generally, four levels of anxiety are possible: low or mild levels, moderate levels, high or severe levels, and panic levels.[1,4] A mild level of anxiety is common in most daily activities. It serves to motivate the individual to meet demands. When such a level is experienced, the person's perceptual field increases slightly. The individual becomes more alert and sees, hears, and grasps more. Intellectual and cognitive processes remain intact. The individual maintains the ability to relate thoughts and ideas in a coherent manner.

As the anxiety increases to a moderate level, a decrease in awareness occurs. The individual tends to focus on immediate concerns, blocking out peripheral stimuli to some extent. The perceptual field is narrowed as concern for the self increases.

Although the person sees, hears, and grasps less, it is possible to focus attention on specific areas when directed. At this level the individual tends to function with selective inattention.

Should the stress continue, anxiety can rise still higher, reaching a high or severe level. The person's perceptual field is greatly reduced. The individual is only able to focus on a few details, ignoring many other aspects of the situation. Inability to think clearly is noted, and very specific directions are needed for the person to function. The person may use automatic responses or rigid, repetitive maneuvers that do not require much thought. The behaviors seen are aimed toward immediate relief of the anxiety-laden situation.

If the situation continues to intensify, anxiety will rise to the panic level. This level is characterized by severe incapacitation, and there is a general loss of control. The person's sense of judgment is lost, and the individual cannot think clearly or do things even when directed. Contact with the realities of the situation is unstable, and immediate escape from the situation is sought. The individual is incapable of tolerating this panic level of anxiety for an extended period of time. Figure 9-1 illustrates the changes in an individual's field of awareness and interaction with the environment as the level of anxiety changes from a low to a panic level. Consider the following Clinical Example.

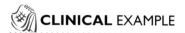

CLINICAL EXAMPLE

Elaine S. was recently promoted to a position that required taking occasional trips within a specific region. She accepted the position, because she thought that she could travel by train to the various places because she did not like to fly. She was petrified of flying. Things went well until she was required to fly to a special meeting for managers. Within 2 weeks of the date of departure, there were noticeable changes in her behavior. She did not notice the "wet floor" signs in the hallway until she tripped over one. She neglected to respond to a greeting from her cousin in the lunchroom. Her weekly reports were sketchy and incomplete, and her secretary had to remind her several times of appointments, including one with the boss. As the date approached it was obvious to her boyfriend that she was a "nervous wreck." She agitatedly went from task to task around the house, never completing anything. She did not notice her boyfriend's presence and even forgot to feed the cat for several days. She kept thinking of the flight and all of the problems that might arise. On the night before the flight she cried uncontrollably and refused to leave her chair. She was immobilized and responded incomprehensibly when her boyfriend arrived to help her to the emergency room. Her anxiety about flying had risen to the point of panic and disorganization.

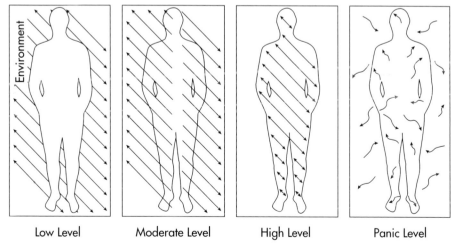

Low Level   Moderate Level   High Level   Panic Level

Fig. 9-1 The individual's perception, range of awareness, and interaction with the environment decrease as the person's anxiety level increases from low- to moderate- to high- and then panic-level anxiety.

CRITICAL THINKING *Question* ················

CRITICAL THINKING *Question* ················

Name three nursing diagnoses that might be indicated in caring for a person with a severe level of anxiety.

··

PSYCHOPHYSIOLOGY OF THE STRESS RESPONSE

The response to frustration, threat, conflict, or anxiety involves specific physiologic and psychologic processes. As soon as a stressor impinges on the individual, sensory motor receptors are stimulated. The signals from the receptors are transmitted through the brain's reticular activating system, which is responsible for selecting and screening out stimuli. Then, through a series of feedback loops, the limbic system (concerned with the emotions), the thalamic and hypothalamic centers (important for autonomic and endocrine responses), and the cortex of the brain are stimulated.[5] The subcortical reactions are interpreted by the cortex as signals of "disease" that serve to heighten the individual's sense of discomfort.

With the complicated life stressors of modern society most persons tend to overlook the bodily reactions accompanying stress.[13] This establishes a negative cycle. The subcortical areas react to stressors by preparing for fight or flight, and the individual consciously or unconsciously resists taking any action. This lack of mobilization is then reinterpreted by the subcortical areas to be indicative of insufficient preparation to attack or flee the situation, and higher levels of physiologic tension ensue.

The physiologic responses that are manifested throughout the body stem primarily from the hypothalamic stimulation of the autonomic and endocrine systems. In particular the sympathetic nervous system responds with a general excitation effect on neural and glandular functions to produce a mass-discharge phenomenon often referred to as the *fight or flight response*. During the stress experience the cardiac output increases and blood flow is diverted from peripheral vessels and the gastrointestinal tract toward the head and trunk. Thus the subjective experiences of clammy hands, a knot in one's stomach, and a racing heart are noted. Other characteristics of this excessive sympathetic nervous system activity include dilated pupils, a tight throat, tense neck and upper back muscles, rapid pulse, rigid pelvis, and contracted flexor muscles in the legs.[6]

The cumulative effect of these responses is the requirement of large amounts of energy for survival; this may be considered to be work. The term used to describe such energy draining reactions is *ergotrophic*. This term means *work generating*, as adapted from the Greek word *ergos*. When an individual's life is such that a great deal of stress is continually being met, the person tends to develop a style of meeting the situations in an ergotrophic manner. The continual demands for energy with little replenishment of reserves have deleterious effects on the body, and these invariably manifest themselves through the development of chronic disorders, often of a psychosomatic nature.

The hypothalamus and its responding sympathetic impulses stimulate the endocrine system through another complex series of feedback mechanisms.[5,10] The sequence is initiated through the stimulation of both the anterior and posterior lobes of the pituitary gland. The posterior lobe by direct neural stimulation secretes vasopressin. Vasopressin, also known as antidiuretic hormone, causes the retention of fluids, sodium, and chloride, which serves to increase the circulating blood volume and blood pressure. The posterior pituitary also has a role in the stimulation of epinephrine secretion from the medullary portion of the adrenal gland.

The anterior lobe of the pituitary gland receives its hypothalamic stimulation through the secretion of hormone-releasing factors transported through the hypothalamic–hypophyseal portal system. This results in the release of gonadotropic hormone, thyrotropic hormone, and adrenocorticotropic hormone. During the stress response gonadotropic hormone influences the alpha cells of the pancreas to secrete glucagon; this assists the body in its preparation to deal with the stress through the initiation of the processes of lipolysis and glycogenolysis in the liver, muscles, and adipose tissues.

Thyrotropic hormone stimulates the thyroid gland to secrete thyroxine. Thyroxine produces an increase in the basal metabolic rate, shallow and rapid respirations, and increased cardiac output, heart rate, and perspiration. It also influences the rate of absorption of food and the secretion of digestive enzymes. The end result may even be a decrease in body weight. Adrenocorticotropic hormone in conjunction with direct sympathetic nervous system innervation serves to stimulate the adrenal gland to produce glucocorticoids, mineralocorticoids, norepinephrine, and epinephrine.

The adrenal gland is divided into cortical (outer) and medullary (inner) portions. The adrenal cortex secretes the antiinflammatory glucocorticoids, including cortisol and cortisone. These hormones influence the depression of the thymus gland, and thus in response to stress there is often a decrease in leukocytes, eosinophils, and the maturation of T cells.

The glycocorticoids also stimulate glycogenolysis (the breakdown of glycogens stored in the liver and muscles). The outcome of this is an increase in the level of serum glucose. In addition, the glycocorticoids are responsible for protein catabolism and lipolysis (the breakdown of fats). The protein catabolism provides free amino acids necessary for metabolic functions, and lipolysis increases the circulating free fatty acids, triglycerides, and cholesterol levels in the blood. Each of these products can potentially be used to provide energy for mobilization.

The adrenal cortex also secretes mineralocorticoids, including deoxycorticosterone and aldosterone, which influence kidney functioning. These hormones affect the excretion of potassium and the retention of sodium and chloride electrolytes. The result is enhanced fluid retention that increases the circulating blood volume.

The influence of adrenocorticotropic hormone and the sympathetic nervous system on the adrenal medulla promotes the secretion of norepinephrine (noradrenalin) and epinephrine (adrenalin). Norepinephrine serves to constrict arterioles, resulting in increased blood pressure and heart rate. It also influences liver metabolism to increase serum glucose and free fatty acid levels. The secretion of norepinephrine has been linked to those emotional reactions reflecting anger, whereas epinephrine has been related to fear.[5,7] The physiologic responses to epinephrine include stimulation of liver glycogenolysis, lipolysis,

gluconeogenesis, and enhanced metabolism of carbohydrates. Associated with these responses are an increase in oxygen consumption, the production of carbon dioxide, and body temperature.

Epinephrine also causes the dilation of the arterioles of the cardiac and skeletal muscles to facilitate the many responses to the stress situation. The constriction of gastrointestinal, anal, and urinary sphincters as well as the dilation of brachial and respiratory musculature are attributed to epinephrine. Figure 9-2 summarizes the interrelated functions of the psychophysiologic response to stress situations.

In the event that a stressor, such as trauma or infection, is localized, a local inflammatory response occurs. This response evolves in three phases characterized by the inflammation, degeneration, and eventual death of cell groups in the directly affected part. The physiologic changes that occur during the inflammatory process include vascular dilation, leukocytosis, and fluid exudation. The vascular changes occur at the site of tissue injury. An increase in blood supply occurs with the dilation of capillaries and arterioles. The speed of local circulation decreases, allowing leukocytes to enter tissue spaces. The number of leukocytes increases, and with the aid of biochemical substances released by the injured tissue they are attracted to the site of injury where they attack the stressor. The body fluids collect at the site (exudate), stimulating antibodies and enzymes while helping to remove destroyed tissue, blood cells, and bacteria. All of these changes produce the classic symptoms of inflammation: redness, swelling, heat, pain, and loss or decrease of function. Selye[13] has referred to these responses as the local adaptation syndrome. If the local adaptation is not effective, a more general response is stimulated.

When a greater tissue area is involved or cellular metabolites and toxins escape from the localized area, a more widespread adaptation response occurs. This broader body response to stress is termed the *general adaptation syndrome.* The general adaptation syndrome is dependent on the response of various body components (see box on p. 227). These body parts all function in conjunction with one another to produce a generalized reaction to attack by a stressor.

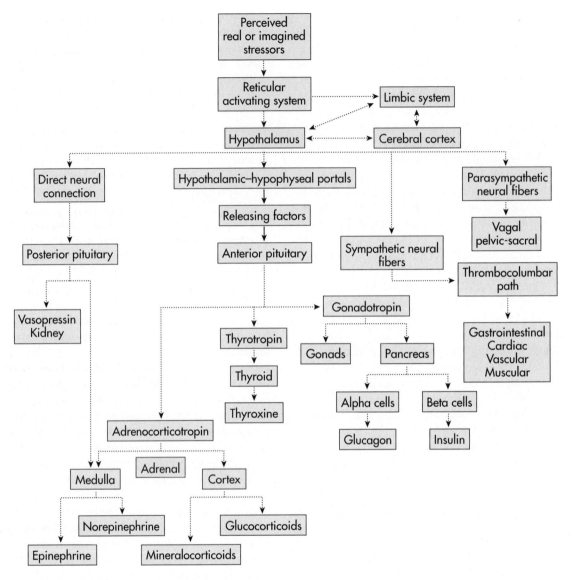

Fig. 9-2 Psychophysiologic responses to stressors.

The responses in the general adaptive syndrome occur in three phases. The initial response is the *alarm reaction.* This represents the body's expression of a call to arms for the defense systems. In this phase the adrenal cells are activated to secrete hormones into the bloodstream, depleting the stores of the gland. The blood becomes more concentrated, and there may even be a loss in body weight. The sympathetic division of the autonomic nervous system is stimulated. The individual becomes alert. Hearing is more acute, pupils dilate, and close vision becomes more acute. Cardiovascular output is increased; at the same time peripheral circulation decreases. The blood flow to the skin, kidney, and other organs not essential for immediate survival decreases. This allows for a greater availability of blood to the brain, heart, and skeletal muscles.

General Adaptation Syndrome Body Responses

• •

- The kidney for regulation of chemical composition of blood and tissues through elimination, as well as its blood pressure regulatory functions
- The nervous system for its reflex action in defense of the organism and its mechanisms for conveying messages throughout the body
- The pituitary and adrenal glands with secretions of hormones for responding to threat and tissue damage
- The thyroid for its hormonal effects on tissue metabolism
- The liver, which regulates concentration of sugar, proteins, and other tissue foods in the blood, as well as for its destruction of surplus corticoid hormones
- The white blood cells, which regulate the serologic immune reactions and allergic hypersensitivity responses in the body (eosinophils and lymphoid cells)
- Connective tissue and blood vessels affecting metabolites circulated, tissue memory of past stress experiences, blood pressure, and hormonal transportation
- The brain for its overall control of regulatory mechanisms, as well as memory of stressful situations and past responses.

From Selye H: *The stress of life,* New York, 1956, McGraw-Hill.

To help stimulate adequate oxygenation for the increased blood volume, the rate and depth of respiration increase. Fluids and electrolytes are retained. Nonessential functions such as excretion and digestion are diminished. Simultaneously metabolism increases to provide the individual with more energy. Muscle tone is increased in preparation for mobilization.

Thus when the person is faced with a threat, a widespread physiologic reaction occurs. The person can then respond in an attempt to cope with the stress state. If the stressor is extremely damaging, continued exposure is incompatible with life. If survival is possible, the person moves into the next phase of the general adaptation syndrome.

The second phase in the general adaptation syndrome is that of *resistance.* In this phase the body attempts to restabilize its processes and resist the demands that are being forced on it. It is in this phase that the person attempts to use various coping strategies to come to terms with the effects of the stressor.

The manifestations of this phase differ greatly from what can be observed in the alarm reaction.

 CULTURAL CONSIDERATIONS

• •

Care should be given to establish cultural norms when evaluating the person for stress and anxiety. Culture will predetermine behaviors that are outside of the "normal" and indicative of a problem. Similarly, a person's perception of an event and the prescribed methods used to deal with the situation are dependent upon cultural context. For example, in many cultures, women are restricted from interactions outside of the home or from conversing with anyone not affiliated with the family. As such, if strangers enter the living area, the level of fear and anxiety escalates. Only if the fear becomes excessive would it be considered pathologic. Similarly, some cultures have rituals associated with life events that would be considered abnormal in another culture. Behaviors should be evaluated in terms of how extreme they are for the cultural expectation. The behaviors would be indicative of a disorder only if they exceed the cultural norms, are manifested at inappropriate times or in inappropriate places, or interfere with functioning as defined by that culture.

• •

The adrenal glands accumulate abundant reserves of secretory granules. The blood becomes less concentrated and approaches the normative volume, and the parasympathetic division of the autonomic nervous system effectively responds to the ongoing adjustments necessary to maintain the individual.

The energy necessary to maintain the level of resistance is eventually lost if exposure to the stressful situation is prolonged. When this happens, the third phase is produced, *exhaustion.* Here extreme responses of the body similar to those of the alarm phase occur. The energy level of the individual is severely compromised. The ability of the body to defend itself against damage is eventually depleted. Regulatory mechanisms no longer function effectively. Organ systems suffer under the chronic assault of the stressor, and dysfunction may occur at the physiologic and cellular levels. Over an extended period of time, exhaustion and even death may occur.

Which specific organs or particular target organ or organs malfunction varies from person to person. It has been hypothesized that there is a biogenetic reason for individuals to have certain weaker systems that are more susceptible to breakdown under the influence of chronic stress. This hereditary nature is supported by the familial tendencies to experience problems such as cardiovascular disease and hypertension. However, this genetic tendency is not a singular causal factor. There are personality and sociocultural variables that also come into play. Learned responses to situations, perceptions, and the repertoire of coping alternatives are also involved in the development of dysfunction and disease.

ADAPTATION

Adaptation to the stress state is influenced by all of the individual's responses interacting together. Adaptation can be thought of as those things a person must do to improve existence under the conditions of the environment. According to Selye[13] actual adaptation occurs at the local level or in the resistance phase of the broader organism. An essential feature of this adaptation is that the individual strives to limit the stress to the smallest area capable of meeting the requirements of the situation. Adaptation is always a special concentration of effort, requiring increased energy utilization. If adaptation is successful, the effects of the stress state are minimized and eventually subdued. If not, exhaustion occurs, eventually to the point of no recovery (death). Figure 9-3 summarizes Selye's approach.

When a person responds to a stressful situation, the resulting behavior is aimed at dealing with or minimizing the real and imagined dangers. Adaptation can be defined as the biologic, psychologic, and sociologic changes that occur as a result of life-stress situations. It involves a complex of processes that bring about and maintain an individual-to-environment relationship that is functional and useful.[2,4] Included in the adaptation process are reflexes, built-in automatic body mechanisms for protection; instincts, deep-seated motivators of behavior patterns; and coping efforts, processes used for meeting the task requirements necessary under difficult circumstances.

Any attempt to master a situation that can be potentially threatening, frustrating, challenging, or gratifying can be called *coping*. The concept of coping includes casual forms of problem solving as well as highly involved or even pathologic efforts. The particular behaviors used to cope with a situation are called the coping strategies. Broadly defined, coping responses are the direct-action tendencies of the individual aimed at the elimination or neutralization of a stressful event, which are task-reality oriented.[11] These responses are mediated by the same variables that influence perception of the stressor, including personality traits, developmental levels, values, past experiences, coping strategies, and available resources. The person appraises the situation, comes to some decision as to what may be done, examines what has worked in the past and what is available now, and then responds.

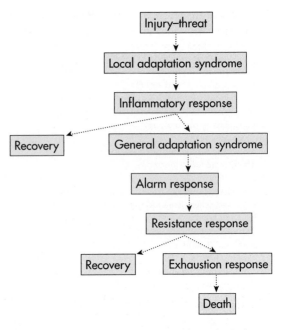

Fig. 9-3 Summary of Selye's approach to physical reactions in response to stress: local and general adaptation syndromes.

This process is quite involved. The individual brings certain personality traits, beliefs, and other dispositional variables to the situation. He must relate to the environmental complex and evident stimuli before he begins to appraise the circumstances. Next, psychologic mediators come into play as he begins a cognitive appraisal of the need to cope. These are mental processes used by the person to evaluate the situation. The individual considers the intensity of the threat, how important it is to him, and what alternatives are available. There is reflection on past experiences and the relative success of those coping strategies previously used. The person must then decide if a particular mode of expression might be useful.

He may elect to use direct actions. These are largely motor responses used to eliminate the threat or gain gratification. Specific responses include attack, flight, and a change in direction. He may also use indirect, intrapsychic processes instead of direct actions. These cognitive modes of conflict resolution include such responses as daydreaming, denial, and fantasies.[2] The behaviors chosen are reflective of the person's needs and experiences. He may or may not be aware of them or of the process involved in their selection.

As long as the intensity, duration, and scope of the stress state are minimal, the coping behaviors tend to be well-thought-out, flexible, and reality-oriented efforts for mastery of the situation. When the stress experience becomes more threatening or more intense, the focus of the coping behaviors becomes narrowed as the person's perceptual field decreases. Then the efforts to maintain balanced functioning become more rigid, less adequate, and less realistic.

One example of this process can be seen with a toddler who enters the hospital for a tonsillectomy. He is at first quiet and reserved, does as his mother tells him, and stays very close to her side. Past experience has taught him that she will care for him and that when he does as she says, she smiles and he feels good. He may relax a bit and play with a toy after he senses that the room is a secure place; he is safe in this room as long as his mother is there. He begins to look around and examine his new environment. He becomes more talkative. He may even make comments about how long they intend to stay there. Generally at this point in time the intensity of his stress state is at a low level.

The extent of involvement (scope) is limited to some psychologic uneasiness in this new situation with many unknown factors. The behaviors are realistic and flexible as he copes. As soon as visiting hours are over, however, the situation changes radically. The child is suddenly alone. His sense of security is shaken, and he becomes more frightened. His mother has left; why can't he go home, too? His entire body tenses, and he may tremble and begin to whimper. All of the other adults in the area say that his mother is gone until tomorrow. This may be heard only as "Mother is gone." The ensuing reactions portray the dilemma. Even though the child did what his mother said to do, she is now gone and he is alone. What alternatives are available? It seems to him that he is powerless. Crying more openly, he wonders if someone will come and comfort him. When the staff tries to console him, he pushes them

away and withdraws to a corner of the bed, rocking and sobbing. The stress experience has become intense; its scope is extensive. The child's behavior is self-oriented, less useful for coping, and rigid. It does not help resolve the stress state, but at his developmental level and with his past experiences, he may see no other alternatives in the situation.

Behavior adaptation

The preceding descriptions of stressful situations imply that some action must be taken to deal with them. Linking stress and coping responses, the *cognitive-field approach* is oriented toward incompatible ways of coping with demands. The incompatible coping tendencies are referred to as *approach* and *avoidance* and can arise from three major kinds of conflicts: approach-approach, avoidance-avoidance, or approach-avoidance. Each of these conflicts may result in frustration: the person is prevented from reaching a desired, attractive goal by a barrier or environmental obstacle.

To illustrate this concept the hypothetic forces operating in approach-avoidance situations can be schematized. In each case an ellipse denotes the person's total environment, a circle represents the person, and a vertical line represents either a barrier to a desired, attractive goal or the thwarting of a motive. Either a plus or a minus sign, a valence, indicates attraction toward or repulsion from the goal. An arrow is used to denote the direction of these forces acting on the individual. Using this framework one can diagram the concept of frustration (Fig. 9-4).

An *approach-approach conflict* arises when two goals are equally attractive at the same time (Fig. 9-5). An example of such a conflict occurs when a person is both hungry and sleepy at the same moment. The way in which this conflict can be settled is either to relinquish one goal and fulfill the other or to satisfy first one goal and then the other. In this example the individual may eat something and then retire or simply choose to go to bed without fulfilling the desire to eat. Such a conflict is fairly easy to resolve in most cases.

The second type of conflict, *avoidance-avoidance*, involves two negative goals. Here each goal is equally unattractive, and the forces acting on the individual are usually away from the goal (Fig. 9-6). An example is when one must decide to have a pelvic examination because of pain and a viscous mucous discharge or to risk a serious infection, complications, and more intense discomfort. Such a conflict tends to cause vacillation, the moving toward and away from both goals. The individual first moves in the direction of one goal, which becomes increasingly repelling. After retreating from that goal, the person moves toward the second goal, which in turn becomes more repelling. There is a tendency to move back and forth without ever making a firm commitment and resolving the conflict. Decision making is greatly hampered in avoidance-avoidance conflicts.

Such frustration frequently produces behavior that is an attempt to leave the situation altogether.

Although this is seldom practical, escape is an alternative whether real or fantasized. The use of fantasy and daydreaming as escape mechanisms is common among all age groups, although it may be seen by some societies as more acceptable in children than in adults. It may be a healthy alternative for the individual if it is not used in excess to escape from reality.

The third type of conflict, *approach-avoidance,* is perhaps the most difficult with which to cope. In the approach-avoidance conflict a person is both repelled and attracted by the same goal object (Fig. 9-7). Frequently such conflicts arise because of internalized motives, such as social norms and values.

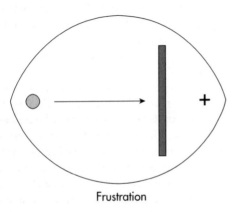

Frustration

Fig. 9-4 Frustration occurs when the individual's attainment of a desired, attractive goal object is blocked by some barrier.

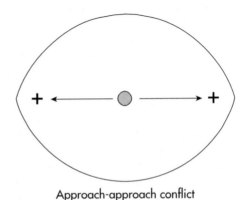

Approach-approach conflict

Fig. 9-5 Approach-approach conflict occurs when the individual is simultaneously attracted toward two equally desired goals.

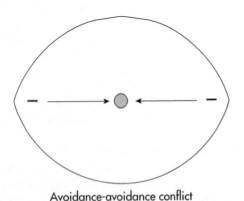

Avoidance-avoidance conflict

Fig. 9-6 Avoidance-avoidance conflict occurs when the individual is simultaneously repelled by two equally unattractive goals.

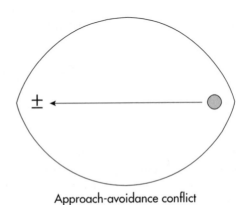

Approach-avoidance conflict

Fig. 9-7 Approach-avoidance conflict occurs when the individual is both repelled and attracted by the same goal.

These create more difficulty when one is attempting to handle the situation than do external barriers. Internalized motives are highly cherished and create great stress when jeopardized. To function the individual has no recourse but to change motives. This involves weakening one of the forces to allow for the accomplishment of the other. For example, such a conflict may arise when a young woman falls in love with an older, married man. She has natural sexual desires and the need for intimacy; at the same time she may disapprove of such relationships and see her desires as immoral. These feelings are congruent with social mores. To function either the desires must be weakened or her present moral ideals must be changed so that she can feel that her behavior is more acceptable. In the meantime she will experience the stress associated with this conflict.

Another example of an approach-avoidance situation can be seen in a young child going to nursery school. The youngster may really enjoy the stories, toys, and playing with the other children. This serves as an attracting force. Still, going to school means leaving his own toys behind and especially being away from his mother. These conflicts make it difficult for the child to want to go to school. It is important for the child to be near his mother, the significant other, and yet it is important for him to go to school like the other children. Resolving this dilemma may involve making school more attractive and therefore more desirable than staying home. This is not an easy task.

These simplified illustrations of conflict become increasingly complex as real-life experiences, internalized motives, and environmental factors all come to bear on the situation. The actions taken to deal with these stress states may be aimed directly at eliminating the threats or be more indirect forms of dealing with the circumstances.

Defense mechanisms

As previously mentioned some of the major indirect forms of behavior used to cope with stressful situations are the defense mechanisms. All defense mechanisms have two characteristics in common: (1) they operate unconsciously so that the person is unaware of what is taking place, and (2) they deny, falsify, or distort reality. The individual uses mental self-deception to protect himself. The particular mechanism used by a person depends on his needs at that point in time. Every person uses some of these coping strategies to an extent. Although the purpose of such defense is maintenance of ego integrity and self-esteem, they are often considered maladaptive, because they tend to ignore reality and hinder somewhat a person's interactions with his environment.

Defense mechanisms are legitimate strategies for adaptation that differ little from other adaptive processes in actual purpose.[1,2,12] These mechanisms may be viewed as adaptive efforts gone wrong, because they sacrifice the interactive processes of the individual with the environment and distort reality. Many processes are involved when defense mechanisms as a group are mentioned. There are at least a dozen separate mechanisms.

Regression The first of these defensive maneuvers, regression, differs from the others in that it is not brought about by the ego, although it does involve maintenance of ego integrity. Regression involves returning to earlier modes of behavior and interests. It is the turning backward of behavior from one stage of development to an earlier one (see Chapter 2). This process can be noted when a child exhibits nocturia after having been successful with staying dry all night when the new baby is brought home from the hospital. The child returns to earlier behavior in an attempt to regain some of the attention that was given whenever the bed was wet. In this way the child is attempting to reestablish feelings of security and love that have been shaken by the new arrival.

Sublimation Sublimation is the process whereby the ego rechannels a drive, modifying its aim or object to a more socially acceptable one. This allows the drive sufficient expression to produce a relief of tension. In so doing the person is able to weaken the force of the instinctual drive by using the energies on another constructive activity. An example of sublimation might be seen when an obese person is forced to undertake a restrictive diet; the inner motives to eat must be rechanneled. The person may take up a hobby, such as painting, whereby still life groupings of fruits or dinner scenes may be duplicated. As such the desire to eat has been sublimated to the desire to paint.

Displacement Displacement is closely linked with sublimation. It involves changing the object by which a drive can be satisfied. This is accomplished unconsciously through the transferral of the feelings, or emotional component, from one object or idea to one that is similar. Such is the case when a person avoids responding angrily to a supervisor and waits until he or she is at home to express the angry feelings. Then the children may be harshly scolded for being too noisy although their behavior is not significantly different from what is usually tolerated. In this case the target of the anger is transferred from the supervisor to the children. Another common example of displacement occurs when a child, having been scolded by a caregiver, vents anger through the destruction of a toy or some household object or by attacking a younger sibling.

Denial Denial is a common and effective defense mechanism. It involves the ego's refusal to allow an awareness of some aspect of reality. The person fails to recognize some of the implications or consequences of a thought, act, or situation. It is as if that consequence did not exist or that situation did not exist. This is often the case when a loved one has died and the spouse continues to speak of the person as if alive. Another example of denial is seen when a paralyzed teenager who had an active sports life plans to return to former activities without considering the limitations of his disability, denying the need for a rehabilitation program. In essence he is denying the incapacitations of his injury and the fact that he may never walk again.

Rationalization Rationalization is a defense mechanism whereby a person seeks to justify actions by stating logical reasons. Socially acceptable explanations are offered for acts or decisions resulting from unconscious or unverbalized impulses. At times these justifications are logical; at others they amount to a series of weak excuses. Whichever form they may take, they serve to protect the self. An example of rationalization might be a student's explanation to her parents of why a grade is low. She might justify the situation, explaining that she failed an exam because she could not find the books in the library. This seems logical; however, she avoids looking at how her behavior contributed to the situation. She does not relate the situation to skipping class, neglecting to do an assignment, failing to go to the library until the night before the exam, and failing to study for the exam.

Repression and suppression The next two defense mechanisms, repression and suppression, are very similar. *Repression* is the involuntary exclusion from awareness of thoughts or impulses that are painful, threatening, or conflicting. These thoughts often threaten the self-concept of the person and the image that he wishes others to have of him. For this reason techniques are used to exclude the related emotions from consciousness. Repression may be considered the primary ego defense that all other defense mechanisms reinforce. As the person develops, many impulses are repressed to allow for maintenance of ego integrity, self-esteem, and general functioning. One of the earliest repressions (according to Freud) occurs when the child witnesses the primal scene. Sexual interactions have strong connotations for the child who has learned through socialization to associate shame with the genitals and nakedness. In most cases the confusion is compounded when the child observes the parents engaged in sexual intercourse. Because of this, such an event becomes deeply hidden from consciousness. There is no choice involved in its exclusion from awareness; this occurs involuntarily as the mental mechanisms function to protect the child.

Suppression is the counterpart of repression on a conscious level and involves the intentional exclusion of thoughts and information from consciousness. Again they are excluded, because they cause discomfort. Suppression is a conscious act of inhibiting unacceptable impulses and painful material. A relatively uncomplicated example might be putting aside the awareness of being ill to be able to go on a long-planned trip. Another example might be a young woman inhibiting thoughts of just how sexually excited she becomes when she and her boyfriend go out on a date. She is consciously controlling the awareness of these thoughts.

Reaction formation Reaction formation is a defensive technique whereby an original attitude or set of feelings is replaced in the consciousness by the opposite attitude or feeling. The mechanism represents going to an opposite extreme in an attempt to overcompensate for unacceptable impulses. One example may be the film censor. This person may present a staunch moral and ethical position in opposition to recognizing the vicarious pleasure derived from pornography. Another example might be a daughter's apparently loving ministrations to her ailing parent when actually the daughter is extremely resentful of being tied down and feeling obligated to care for the patient. The daughter seems to bend over backward to please her parent, all the while negating her own interests. She has replaced the angry, hateful feelings with loving, caring feelings.

Projection Projection is a defense mechanism that occurs when the feelings, wishes, or attitudes of the person are attributed by him to another person (or object). The person feels that it is unacceptable to have these impulses. He seeks to place blame for his inadequacies on someone else; this other person is thought to be responsible for causing his mental anguish. An example of projection is a wife who accuses her husband of running around because she herself has such desires. This thought is somehow uncomfortable for her or incongruent with her self-ideal. Therefore she blames someone else, attributing the impulses to her husband. Projection is also used by children. Such is the case when a child running down the streets with his friends trips and cries out, "Stupid sidewalk!" In so doing the child attributes negative feelings to the environmental object. The sidewalk, not the child's own clumsiness or lack of coordination, is the cause for the fall. In this way he protects his self-esteem and does not feel inadequate.

Introjection Introjection, as a defensive technique, is similar to the developmental process of identification. This is one of the earliest mechanisms used by children. Introjection involves the process whereby a quality or attribute of another person is unconsciously incorporated into the individual's personality. The desirable trait is assimilated into his own self-system ideal. Such is the case when a teenager unconsciously emulates the mannerisms of a favorite teacher. The favored attribute is incorporated and the person's self-concept enhanced. Another example of introjection is the incorporation of certain parental values, such as a neat appearance, into the child's own value system. This helps the child maintain a favorable feeling about himself.

Isolation Isolation, or withdrawal, is the process whereby the link between conscious facts and the related feelings is broken. It is the splitting off of the emotional components from a thought, because they are too painful. This is often seen with people who work in intensive care units, where death occurs frequently. The staff reacts in a fairly cold, clinical manner, failing to express the usual emotional responses elicited by death. To do so would be extremely painful and emotionally draining. Therefore the staff continues to function by negating their own emotions relative to death. Another example would be a young nun's apparently calm report to the authorities that she was raped. Without showing any stress she simply answers questions and relates the circumstances of the event. To acknowledge the fear of death, the negative feelings related to violation of chastity, and the decreased self-esteem would be overwhelming. Therefore the emotional components of the experience are negated at this point in time. In this respect isolation is closely related to repression.

Undoing The last defense mechanism is undoing, which involves an act or communication that partially negates a previous one. The person may treat the experience as if it never occurred. This defense is used to compensate for and neutralize some previous action or wish that the individual feels is unacceptable. Such is the case when after a heated argument with her husband, the wife prepares his favorite meals the next day. In this way she hopes to attenuate the negative feelings and comments she made during the argument. Undoing also can be noted when a child brings his mother a gift in the hope that she will forget how angry she has been with him for coloring on the walls. When he brings her his peace offering, he is being "good." He hopes that perhaps his gift will overshadow his being "bad" by expressing his artistic nature on the walls.

The defense mechanisms described in this chapter are summarized in Table 9-3. They may be used independently or in combination with one another. The individual will use defense mechanisms to varying degrees depending on how successfully they meet his needs. If using defensive maneuvers proves successful in maintaining some degree of functioning, the person is likely to continue using them.[2]

TABLE 9-3   Defense mechanisms

Regression	Returning to earlier modes of behavior and previous interests
Sublimation	Rechanneling of a drive, modifying its aim or object to a more socially acceptable one
Displacement	Transferring the feelings or emotional component from one object or idea to a different object or idea
Denial	Refusing to allow into awareness some aspect of reality that is somehow distressing
Rationalization	Seeking to justify actions by stating logical reasons
Repression	Involuntarily excluding from awareness thoughts or impulses that are painful, threatening, or conflicting
Suppression	Intentional, conscious exclusion of thoughts and information from consciousness
Reaction formation	Replacing an original attitude or set of feelings with the opposite attitude or feelings
Projection	Attributing one's own feelings, wishes, or attitudes to another person or object
Introjection	Unconsciously incorporating into one's personality a quality or attribute of another person
Isolation	Breaking of links between conscious facts and the related feelings or emotional components
Undoing	Partially negating a previous action

Physical reactions

As previously noted, the stress response is manifested in body reactions. When the stress has been of sufficiently extreme intensity for a moderate to extended period of time, the individual's energy stores become depleted. In the physical sense there may even be wasting of muscles, weight loss, and decreased resistance to minor infections. Stress increases one's susceptibility to disease.

Susceptibility may be defined as a lack of adequate resistance to the deleterious effects of some stressor, leading to dysfunction. Susceptibility reflects inadequate coping mechanisms or symbolic expressions in the event of a stressful situation. The end result is cumulative, with the development of chronic disease or psychosomatic disorders, when the extreme levels of internal tension seek expression through the body.[12] This especially occurs when the person has a predisposition, genetic or familial, to some physical vulnerability.

The relationship between emotional stress, personality traits, and the manifestation of certain disorders has been the subject of study.[3,12] Although strong associations have been made between personality characteristics and disease entities, causality has not been established. However, with cognizance of the multifaceted responses to stressful situations one can recognize the potential link between cardiac arrest, hypertension, arte-riosclerosis, vascular disorders, and obesity. A variety of headaches, including migraines, have been identified as having a large component of stress reactivity particular to the differential manifestations of each.[12] Arthritis and cancer have been identified as possibly related to the deficient immunologic responses related to stress reactivity. In support of the various theories related to the psychosomatic nature of such disorders, personality profiles for individuals likely to manifest their stress in such ways have been postulated.[1] Such research may assist in early identification of disease or in preventive measures if and when more data support the direct relationships of these variables.

CRITICAL THINKING *Question* ....

What are some of the different coping methods that might be used to adapt to the situation of receiving a failing mark on a quiz? List five methods, and critically analyze them in terms of the probable outcomes, appropriateness, type of approach, and likelihood in resolving the stressful situation.

STRESS, ADAPTATION, AND NURSING

As the link between stress, adaptability, and preventive health becomes better understood, direct nursing interventions for assisting the client to adjust to ever-changing life situations may become a unique framework for nursing science. A general understanding of stress and adaptation is necessary to carry out the nursing process adequately. One must remember that changes in behavior, whether adaptive or maladaptive, provide cues of increased disequilibrium and the existence of a stress state.

Individuals use a wide variety of coping strategies as they attempt to adapt to threats to their biopsychosocial functioning. Until the situation can be thoroughly investigated the nurse must rely on generalized background knowledge of patterns of daily living and "normal" biopsychosocial limitations. Validation of the meaning of the situation is important, because each individual will respond differently to the same situations. What may prove to be a stressing event for one person may not be for another. Likewise, in the absence of overt cues of an increased stress state the nurse should not assume that the person is functioning at optimal levels. The person may be functioning in the early part of the phase of resistance.

In assessing the stress state, evaluating the stress, and investigating the ensuing behaviors, the nurse can develop her plan of care based on client needs. The nurse must also be concerned with potential stressors, because their effects may be prevented through planned nursing interventions. Through careful observation the nurse can compare the individual's behaviors with previous levels of functioning and with the biopsychosocial norms. After doing this the nurse can infer the person's ability to cope with the existing stress state. With all of this information at hand the nurse can plan care to help solve identified problem areas. In this manner it becomes possible for the nurse to decrease the intensity, duration, and scope of the stress experience, thus promoting the integrative functioning of the person.

Integration of stress theory into nursing practice flows most easily when assessing the effects of a stressor on the person. Information about the subjective impact or meaning of the experience for the person as well as for their significant others adds depth to the individualization of nursing care. Gathering data about the psychophysiologic and sociologic manifestations of stress provides direction for the rest of the nursing process.

Emotional or affective change, including disturbances in feelings and emotional lability, are important factors to assess. Any cognitive alterations such as changes in thought processes, problem solving, judgment, or perception should be noted. Similarly, shifts in activity patterns or level of activity (often expressed as fatigue or lack of energy) provide clues to understanding the impact of the stress state on that person and areas for nursing intervention.

Information related to the physiologic and physical impact of the stress state requires gathering information related to endocrine, neurologic, musculoskeletal, and biochemical imbalances. In addition, reviewing any major disorders or symptoms associated with illnesses frequently identified as having strong psychosomatic components is important.

The nursing care provided is directed toward the reestablishment of prestress state functioning. Nursing actions strive to conserve client energy, maximize existing coping behavior, explore alternatives, and mobilize resources for dealing with stressful experiences. The ultimate goal is alleviation of the stress state.[2] For each individual specific objectives of care are formulated based on the particular nursing diagnosis. The objectives also depend on the characteristics of the stress experience and the individual's adaptive responses. In a more general sense objectives for care can evolve with respect to dealing with stressors, stress experience, behavioral responses, problem-solving processes, and mobilization of resources.

Nursing actions can center around alleviation of the effects of a stressor and protection from exposure to stressors.[15] When an antibiotic is administered, the purpose is to decrease the effects that the causal agent is having on the body by eliminating the agent. Another example occurs when diet exchanges are taught to a diabetic patient. Adherence to the diet restrictions helps in the management of the disease process as well as in limiting consequential complications such as insulin shock.

Other actions are designed to focus on decreasing the intensity, duration, or scope of the stress experience. The nurse might set limits on certain behaviors. Such restrictions can facilitate recuperative processes and decrease the duration of the stress experience. For example, if a person remains in bed during an attack of influenza, there is an increased likelihood that he will regain previous levels of functioning in less time than will the person who tries to maintain a more active routine while ill.

Nursing actions are often designed to assist the individual in problem-solving processes. To cope it is often necessary to seek assistance in the identification of focal problems, existing coping mechanisms, and new alternatives. The nurse gives direction to the client through the provision of specific information and assistance by means of supportive measures. The degree of direct intervention depends on client needs.

If an event is appraised to be more negative or positive by one person than by others in the situation, cognitive distortion has occurred. For example, when a student receives a "D" on an assignment, he may distort it to mean failure for the entire course. In his own thinking process he may go over and over the event. This is called *mental rumination*. He may then begin to talk to himself about it, often using negative labels and self-denigrating comments such as "What a dummy," "I'm so stupid I never do anything right," "Now I've failed for sure," and so on. This mental chatter, which may go on without the person ever being aware of how he is contributing to the negativity, reinforces the cognitive distortion. Often the nurse can assist a person to become aware of his mental chatter and to reestablish a more realistic perspective.[15]

The thought processes are only one part of the response to stress. The actual behaviors used as coping mechanisms provide still another basis for nursing actions. Depending on the circumstances the nurse may intervene directly on behalf of the person. At other times it may be appropriate to alter the client's actions or seek (with the client) to change goals; the nurse can also provide information on alternative behavior and help the person test new coping behavior. In other instances support of existing behavior may be the action of choice, especially when this behavior is effective and constructive.

If the individual is experiencing discomfort and is vacillating between two choices, the nurse might intervene and attempt to help the client make a decision. One example is to assist the person to change a goal to resolve the conflict. On the other hand, if the person

does this of his own initiative, the nurse can provide positive reinforcement and support his efforts.

Nursing actions are also directed toward mobilization of resources. The nurse can help the individual maximize personal resources. This can be done by drawing on past experiences, background knowledge, and biopsychosocial assets. Mobilization of environmental and situational resources is also important. These represent items in the environment that can provide support to the individual's coping attempts and help him conserve energy. A third resource group includes interpersonal resources (i.e., those others in the area who can provide information, ideas, and energy to assist in the resolution of the stress state). The nurse is one example of an interpersonal resource.

CRITICAL THINKING *Question* ....

Using a scale of 1 = low stress and 5 = high stress, ask several nurses in practice to rate the level of stress associated with the profession of nursing. Then ask these nurses how they have chosen to cope with this level of stress. Discuss your reactions to their responses with faculty and classmates.
....

Incorporating the concepts of stress and adaptation into nursing practice can increase the relevance and effectiveness of nursing care. Knowledge of stress theory influences nursing activities ranging from detection and monitoring of signs of biopsychosocial levels of stability to preventive activities for any aspect of the stress experience. Nursing actions can be designed to intervene directly or indirectly in the stress experience of an individual. Use of knowledge and technical skill can prevent, reduce, remove, or balance the stress that the person encounters. Knowledge of the stress and adaptation process provides a method for considering the whole person, variables influencing the situation, and effects of the stressor and stress experience on the person's level of functioning. Such information influences and guides each step in the nursing process.

SUMMARY

Every individual uses energy to maintain life processes, strive to achieve a potential level of development, and meet the demands of daily existence.

Stress can be defined as the energy state of the person when responding to the internal and external demands placed on him. Stress is necessary for existence. Significant features of stress include the intensity, duration, and scope of the stress experience.

The stimulus or agent responsible for producing the stress state is the stressor. The origins of stressors may be internal or external (environmental). Stressors may be of a biologic, psychologic, sociologic, or developmental nature. In describing the stress state one should note the number of stressors, their origin and nature, and the frequency of encounter or exposure. The stress response will be initiated when the situation has been appraised as stressful and its meaning established.

Response to the stress experience is termed *coping, adaptation, adjustment,* or *defense.* The general definition of coping responses is any attempt to master or deal with a situation that can be potentially threatening, frustrating, challenging, or gratifying. The individual responds because of discomfort and emotional disquiet.

Important components in the stress-adaptation reaction are frustration, threat, conflict, and anxiety. *Frustration* is a condition that occurs when a course of action cannot be fulfilled, when goal attainment is blocked or delayed. *Threat* is defined as anticipation of harm of some kind or of an undesirable consequence as a result of tissue needs, drives, and motives. *Conflict* is defined as the simultaneous presence of incompatible tendencies or goals, and makes threat or frustration inevitable. *Anxiety* is a state of uneasiness, worry, or apprehension. It may be in response to threats to self-esteem or when certain goals or values are jeopardized. Anxiety may be of a low or mild, moderate, high or severe, or panic level. At each successive level the behavior noted reflects a decreased perception with an increased disorganization of actions.

To deal with the stress state one may use either direct-action or indirect-action strategies. Direct-action strategies involve commitment to action. Included are preventive preparations against harm, attack on the harmful agent (with or without accompanying anger and aggression), and avoidance of the harmful situation, even through physical escape. If the person lacks alternatives or the impulse to actively cope, inaction and apathy result. In such cases one may adapt through the use of various mental mechanisms.

If energies directed toward accomplishing a desired goal are thwarted because of a barrier, one becomes frustrated. If the barrier is environmental, it is more easily dealt with than if it is internally motivated. If two goals are equally attractive at the same time, an approach-approach conflict results. This type of conflict is resolved either by choosing one goal and giving up the other or by satisfying first one goal and then the other. A second type of conflict, avoidance-avoidance, involves two negatively motivating goals. The individual tends to vacillate between each goal, moving back and forth without ever resolving the conflict; eventually there is a tendency to try to escape or leave the situation. A more difficult conflict to resolve is the approach-avoidance type. In this situation the individual is both repelled and attracted to the same goal object. To resolve the situation one must change motives, weakening one of the forces, to allow accomplishment of the other. These responses all involve direct actions.

When the individual is unable to cope despite the use of direct-action strategies, indirect-action strategies are used. As the level of tension (stress) rises the mental mechanisms used reflect increased disorganization, characterized by the state of internal and external nervousness.

As noted, indirect responses to stressful situations include the defense mechanisms. These are unconscious maneuvers that deny, falsify, or distort reality. They are maladaptive in that they interfere with realistic interactions. The defense mechanisms include regression, sublimation, displacement, denial, rationalization, repression, suppression, reaction formation, projection, introjection, isolation, and undoing.

The individual also responds to stress on a physiologic basis. At the site of tissue injury a local inflammatory response, or local adaptation syndrome, occurs. The body attempts to destroy the stressor at this site. Vascular dilation, leukocytosis, and fluid exudation are noted. This process produces symptoms of inflammation, including redness (erythema), swelling (edema), heat (pyrexia), pain (dolor), and decreased function. If the local response is insufficient, a broader body reaction (the general adaptation syndrome) is activated. The neuroendocrine responses of the body are activated as the person enters the alarm phase of the reaction. The person is ready to mobilize to respond to the stressor. The emotional responses, be they fear or euphoria, stimulate the hypothalamus to emit neural impulses and to secrete hormone-releasing factors that serve to stimulate the pituitary gland. The hormones secreted by the pituitary stimulate the release of glucagon, thyroxine, cortisol, aldosterone, norepinephrine, and epinephrine. These hormones give rise to the direct physiologic expressions of the stress response, serving to mobilize the individual's systems for fight or flight, as described in the accompanying box.

The alarm phase is the first part of the general adaptation syndrome. The second phase, the phase of resistance, represents the individual's attempts to restabilize functioning and adapt to the stress experience. If this phase of the response is extended, the person begins to lose the ability to adapt. Then the third phase of the syndrome is entered, the phase of exhaustion. Here the body no longer has the energy with which to function effectively. Eventually, death ensues. Figure 9-8 summarizes the many adaptational (or maladaptational) responses to stressors.

Knowledge of the concepts and components of stress and adaptation are important to nursing. They provide a framework through which to use human behaviors as cues to the individual's needs for care. Understanding the entire stress experience provides direction and guidance to the nurse relative to her role, goals, mode of action, and clinical practice. Assessment of the person's affective, cognitive, physiologic, and activity behaviors provides the information on which to plan and implement nursing care. Nursing intervention can occur at various points in the stress experience to assist the individual in functioning. It may be appropriate to remove the stressors, take steps to decrease the intensity of tension, or help with reorganization. The nurse may suggest alternative compensatory actions and coping behaviors, clarify experiences, and help in constructive expression of emotions and feelings. In essence the nurse provides resources to assist the individual to reorganize, decreasing the spiraling disorganization that leads to eventual exhaustion. In this manner the person may learn to recognize resources and use coping strategies more effectively in the future.

Emotional, Physiologic, and Behavioral Manifestations of Chronic Stress Reactivity

Emotions

Fear, anger, rage, hate, grief, relief, joy, euphoria, love, passion

Immune responses

Decreased leukocytes
Decreased eosinophils
Immature T cells
Thymus gland atrophy

Endocrine responses

Pituitary secretion of gonadotropin, thyrotropin, adrenocorticotropin, vasopressin
Pancreatic secretion of glucagon and insulin
Thyroid secretion of thyroxine
Adrenal secretions of glucocorticoids, cortisone and cortisol, mineralocorticoids, deoxycorticosterone and aldosterone, norepinephrine, epinephrine

Neuroendocrine behaviors

Pupil dilation, tight throat
Tense neck and back muscles
Rigid pelvis, locked diaphragm
Shallow and rapid respirations
Constricted sphincters
Decreased gastrointestinal functions
Increased cardiac output
Increased pulse and blood pressure
Decreased peripheral blood flow
Cool, clammy hands, perspiration
Contraction of leg flexor muscles
Increased serum levels of glucose, free fatty acids, amino acids, triglycerides, cholesterol, Na^+Cl^-
Increased basal metabolic rate
Increased body temperature
Increased oxygen consumption
Increased carbon dioxide
Excretion of K^+
Protein catabolism
Decreased body weight

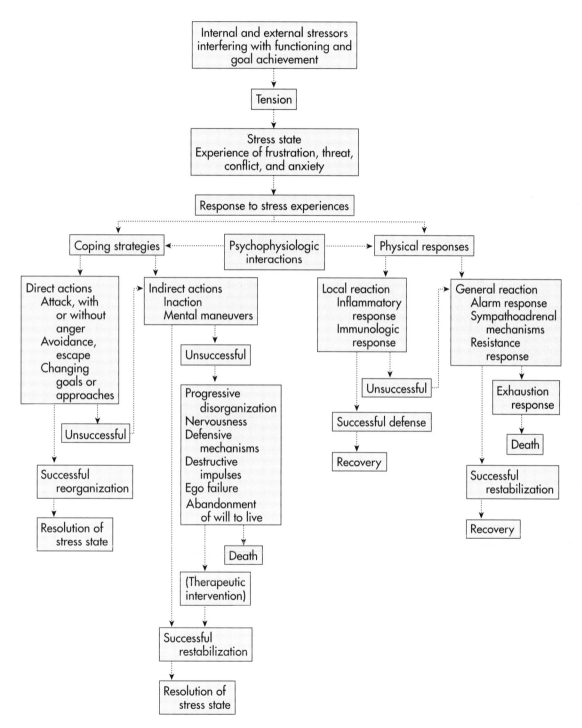

Fig. 9-8 Stress adaptation experience.

DISCUSSION QUESTIONS

1. Compare the different effects and resulting stress states in the following situations:
   a. German measles in a school-age child and German measles in a woman during the first trimester of pregnancy.
   b. An allergic response to poison ivy and an allergic response to a penicillin injection.
2. Identify three specific stressors evident in your life at the present time. Describe them in terms of intensity, duration, and scope.
3. Describe how a person's stress state at a particular point in time influences his or her use of therapeutic and nontherapeutic communications.
4. List four defense mechanisms that you have identified in working with a client. Describe how these either enhanced or hindered the relationship.
5. Describe the situations that illustrate an approach-approach conflict, an avoidance-avoidance conflict, and an approach-avoidance conflict.
6. Identify a current song or movie that emphasizes each of the following concepts: frustration, conflict, and anxiety.
7. Describe a situation with a client where perception would be altered because of an increased level of anxiety. How would you modify your nursing care in this situation?
8. During times of stress, is a person more or less susceptible to infection? Explain your answer.
9. Identify three ways in which a person's stress state influences wound healing.
10. Describe how defense mechanisms can be helpful and how they can be harmful.
11. Name the one thing that determines whether the stress response will occur.
12. Is it possible to experience a stress response without the actual presence of a stressor?
13. Identify two strategies to induce the relaxation response other than those mentioned in this chapter. Describe how these work.
14. Identify when and where you experience the most stress and the greatest relaxation.
15. Describe how the stress response can be altered by changing one's attitudes or perceptions.

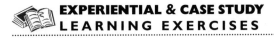

EXPERIENTIAL & CASE STUDY LEARNING EXERCISES

1. The influences of life events on physiologic processes

PURPOSE: To examine how individuals respond to various life events as stressors.

PROCEDURE: This exercise may be carried out in a short time. At the beginning of class announce the following: "OK, all books on the floor, take one sheet of paper and a pen or pencil out; hurry, everyone be quiet . . . now look at your paper; put both hands on desk." (Pause.) "Everyone now take your radial pulse for a period of 60 seconds and record it." After each person palpates and records pulse rate, discussion is to follow and the regular atmosphere reestablished. In addition, announce that at the end of approximately 30 minutes each student is to record another pulse and discussion will follow.

DISCUSSION: The following questions may be posed to the group:

1. Why was this a stressor?
2. Describe the feelings and emotions associated with the exercise.
3. How were the emotions manifested in the body (dry mouth, knot in stomach, sweaty palms, rapid pulse rate, rapid breathing, and so on)?
4. How did these reactions compare with those that occurred when the second pulse rate was recorded?
5. Can you think of other situations when similar stress responses are experienced?
6. Are all the situation-related emotions actually negative or can there be positive experiences that cause similar responses, such as receiving a scholarship award?

2. The positive and negative sides of stress

PURPOSE: To illustrate the importance of perception and appraisal to the identification of a stressor and mediators of stress.

PROCEDURE: Make a list of four of the life events that have been identified as stressors. Ask the students to indicate (a) whether they would label the event as a stressor and why, (b) when would it not be a stressor, and (c) what might mediate the stressful nature of the event.

DISCUSSION: Ask participants to discuss their perceptions about the stressors in small discussion groups. Allow approximately 15 to 20 minutes for the small group discussions. Reconvene the larger group to bring closure to the exercise, emphasizing the individuality of perception and factors that students identify as mediators of stress.

3. Case study: the stress of life

PURPOSE: To apply and synthesize the information on stress and adaptation to a specific case study.

PROCEDURE: Provide the participants with the case study and ask them to be prepared to discuss the questions listed below.

Ms. J. is a 26-year-old graduate nursing student in her first trimester (14 weeks) of a planned pregnancy. She is a full-time student and hopes to complete her education before the baby arrives. She has been married for 4 years and her spouse, though very supportive, has just been laid off from his job in the personnel department of the local hospital. Her extended family live in different parts of the country.

DISCUSSION: Ask participants to:

1. Identify, in each trimester of Ms. J.'s experience, (a) the major stressors, (b) the stress state factors likely to be experienced by the client, and (c) the interrelated biopsychosocial factors.

2. Identify two factors that would mediate the experience for Ms. J.

3. Identify two nursing diagnoses that can be applied to the care of Ms. J. related to stress and anxiety.

4. Identify how the experience would be changed if (a) Ms. J. did not have a supportive spouse, (b) Ms. J. was a 17-year-old high school junior, or (c) there were a potential congenital birth defect to consider.

REFERENCES

1. American Psychiatric Association: *Diagnostic and statistical manual of mental disorders,* ed 4, Washington, DC, 1994, American Psychiatric Association.

2. Benham E: Coping strategies: a psychoeducational approach to post-traumatic symptomatology, *J Psychosoc Nurs Ment Health Serv* 33(6):30, 1995.

3. Benson H, Klipper M: *The relaxation response,* New York, 1993, Wings Books.

4. Burgess A, Roberts A: Levels of stress and crisis precipitants, *Crisis Intervention* 2(1):31, 1995.

5. Carson V, Arnold E: *Mental health nursing: the nurse-patient journey,* Philadelphia 1996, WB Saunders, 137-140.

6. Engler M, Engler M: Assessment of the cardiovascular effects of stress, *J Cardiovasc Nurs* 10(1):51, 1995.

7. Hayes A: Psychiatric nursing: what does biology have to do with it? *Arch Psychiatr Nurs* 9(4):216, 1995.

8. Holmes T, Rahe R: The social readjustment scale, *J Psychosom Res* 11:214, 1967.

9. Huang C: Hardiness and stress: a critical review, *Matern Child Nurs J* 23(3):82, 1995.

10. McCain N, Smith J: Stress and coping in the context of psychoimmunology: a holistic framework for nursing practice and research, *Arch Psychiatr Nurs* 8(4):221, 1994.

11. Rankin E: Stresses and rewards experienced by employed mothers, *Health Care Women Int* 14:257, 1993.

12. Roberts S: Somatization in primary care: the common presentation of psychosocial problems through physical complaints, *Nurse Pract* 19(5):47, 1994.

13. Selye H: *The stress of life,* New York, 1956, McGraw-Hill.

14. Stanford G: The stress response to trauma and critical illness, *Crit Care Nurs Clin North Am* 6(4):693, 1994.

15. Wells-Federman C, Stuart E, Deckro J, et al: The mind-body connection: the psychophysiology of many traditional nursing interventions, *Clin Nurse Spec* 9(1):59, 1995.

Suggested Readings

Badger J: Fourteen tips for managing stress on the job, *Am J Nurs* 95(9):31, 1995.

> *This article presents brief, time-saving strategies that any person can use to reduce the reactivity to stress. The tips can also be useful in health education for clients.*

LaMontagne L, Johnson B, Hepworth J: Evolution of parental stress and coping processes: a framework for critical care practice, *J Pediatr Nurs* 10(4):212, 1995

> *This article presents a conceptual framework for designing coping interventions, based on stress and coping theory, crisis theory, and research on parental stress. The important roles of cognitive appraisal and situational factors are discussed as determinants of adaptation.*

Manderino M, Berkey N: Verbal abuse of staff nurses by physicians, *Image J Nurs Sch* 27(3):244, 1995.

> *This research article applies the transactional model of stress in examining the effects of verbal abuse. The stressful effects of verbal abuse on working relationships and work satisfaction are noted. The importance of the degree of perceived threat and emotional intensity to the degree of long-term negative effects is noted.*

Stiles D: Video display terminal operators: technology's biopsychosocial stressors, *J Am Assoc Occup Health Nurs* 42(11):541, 1994.

> *The roles of the nurse as a member of the multidisciplinary team, in evaluation of the stress of workers, and in designing interventions in the high-tech workplace are discussed. The discussion includes the importance of physical, psychologic, and social support factors related to the workplace.*

CHAPTER

10 *Health Promotion Strategies*

I look to the day when there are no nurses to the sick, but only nurses to the well.

Florence Nightingale, 1893

LEARNING OBJECTIVES

After studying this chapter, the student should be able to:

- Identify factors influencing the recent increased emphasis on health education.
- Compare and contrast various definitions of health and health education.
- Discuss three basic goals of health education.
- Analyze the health belief model and the psycho-educational model as they relate to cognitive and behaviorist theories of learning.
- Describe the steps to be taken and the issues to be considered in developing a health education program.
- Explain the relationship between tertiary prevention and the role of the nurse as an advocate.
- Discuss the impact of consumer activism on the health care system.
- Identify and describe the characteristics of a self-help group.
- Analyze the role of the health care professional relative to a self-help group.
- Describe actions that the nurse may take to reduce the risks of advocacy.
- Define holistic health in terms of biologic, psychologic, sociocultural, and spiritual factors.
- Identify three holistic health promotion strategies.
- Explain the reasons for the shift to community-based care.
- Define *spirituality*.

The primary goal of nursing is to maximize the client's level of functioning. This can also be stated as helping the client attain optimum health or maximizing the potential of the individual. The basic goal is the provision of nursing care that attempts to meet individualized client needs.

According to Edelman and Mandle, health is often equated with a state of wellness.[23] Traditionally, health is defined as the condition of being sound or fit in body, mind, and spirit, free from physical disease, pain, and mental impairment. Health promotion is the process of enabling people to increase control over and improve their health.[21] The nurse's role in health promotion involves various activities. Some of these activities are to advocate, facilitate, consult, deliver services, educate and conduct research. In health promotion, the client is a partner in care.[1]

A focus on health promotion stresses ethical considerations. The nurse is to provide services with respect to the dignity of the client and the uniqueness of the client. Griffith and DiGuiseppi argue for research evidence rather than expert opinion regarding the effectiveness of preventive services to be sure that the benefits outweigh the risks.[32] Currently there are agencies (e.g., the U.S. Prevention Services Task Force) to assess scientific evidence and make recommendations regarding the value and potential risk of different preventive services. Griffith and DiGuiseppi argue that many of the risk factors to health are rooted in behavioral choices.[32] Intervention therefore is health guidance. The authors recommend a shift in control to the client. Clients must assume greater responsibility for their own health.

Chapter 1 listed various dependent and independent nursing functions. Numerous other nursing functions are associated with health promotion. In this chapter several broad areas of independent nursing actions are discussed: health education, crisis intervention, and advocacy. Concepts related to holistic health are explored. The emphasis in holistic health is on prevention, health promotion, and encouraging optimal functioning. Because the current focus is on the client and the family in the community, community-based care is also discussed. Information from Chapter 2 on self-development is revisited, and the concept of health promotion throughout the life span is explored.

HEALTH EDUCATION

Health education is often associated with primary prevention and the maintenance of health. However, health teaching programs can be directed toward ill or recovering clients, such as postoperative health teaching and programs that instruct diabetics in self-care.

Health education as an important nursing function has been stressed in the current literature. Kruger[48] surveyed a stratified, random sample of 1230 staff nurses, nurse administrators, and nurse educators. All three groups of respondents rated the nurses' responsibility for client education as a priority. All groups also chose the nurse as being the primary person responsible for health education, with 97% believing that the nurse's responsibility for health education would increase in the future.

Milde and Heim[54] surveyed faculty and students in two nursing programs regarding present and desired levels of competence in health education. The subjects in this study also responded that health education was an important part of the nurse's role. Faculty and students identified current student competence in health teaching as equal to or less than the desired competence. Students believed that their competence level should be higher than what the nursing faculty considered desirable; nursing faculty considered the students as capable of doing health education but in need of additional practice, particularly in terms of the student's competence to do health teaching with groups of clients. Although both students and faculty were not satisfied with their present level of competence in health education, students perceived themselves as currently functioning at a higher level than faculty perceived their health teaching skills.

CRITICAL THINKING *Question* ················

Tattersall distinguishes between "diseases doctors tell you that you have" and "diseases you know you have."[74] Hypertension and hyperlipidemia are examples of the former; asthma and arthritis are examples of the latter. Quality of life is an important issue, especially in treatment programs for diseases that you are told that you have. It is possible that the treatment can produce negative side effects and thereby decrease the quality of life. Discuss the individual's right to choose treatment. How does the issue of "noncompliance" fit with the idea of client choice?

Higgins[35] surveyed the faculties of 31 Australian schools of nursing. Almost all of the schools indicated that there was preparation of student nurses in health education. The schools often reported having an integrated approach rather than a separate health education course. Higgins concluded that the most notable finding was the variable preparation of nursing students to do health education. Higgins stated that the undergraduate nursing programs using an integrated mode to teach health education skills were the most unlikely to be able to identify specific content, curriculum format, and related clinical experiences to provide their students with health education skills.

Tu et al.[76] described an undergraduate nursing program that provides students with experience in a clinical setting where health education is consistently practiced by nurses who can function as role models for the students. The health education experience includes a review of content material on teaching and learning, as well as content specific to the diabetic self-care program. The clinical experience was 2.5 days of intensive practice in health education, observation of skilled staff, and an individual teaching opportunity. According to the authors, students who participate in this clinical experience demonstrate an increased level of sensitivity to the client's learning needs and are more likely to initiate health education in traditional settings.[11]

Health education has been increasingly emphasized in recent literature. As early as 1918 the National League for Nursing Education stressed the importance of health teaching; however, research on health teaching is a relatively new area. Boyd reviewed the historical precedents and mandates for nursing involvement in health education. Events that had the greatest impact on health education came in the latter part of the 1900s. "In 1950, the Society of Public Health Education was organized ... in 1954 the first health education journal was published."[11] Other events that significantly affected health education listed by Boyd include the following: (1) American Hospital Association presented the *Patient's Bill of Rights* in 1973; (2) National League for Nursing published *Nursing's Role in Patient's Rights* in 1977, which states that clients have a right to information; and (3) Joint Commission for the Accreditation of Hospitals (JCAH) published *Accreditation Manual for Hospitals* in 1981, which mandated requirements for hospital-based client education. This manual included specific instructions regarding the nurse's role. Boyd contends that the strongest legal mandate for nurses' involvement in health education is the Nurse Practice Acts found in all 50 states.[11]

Fernsler and Cannon[25] outline the rationale for health education, particularly cancer health education. Their rationale includes client's rights, professional standards, legal mandates, and health agency requirements. In addition, they discuss the benefits to clients, agencies, and society that health education has provided.

Benefits to the client as a result of health education include varied measures of improved outcome. Client knowledge is most frequently documented in the literature as well as an increased ability to provide self-care and adherence to a therapeutic regimen. For example, a study by Windsor et al.[80] evaluates the cost-effectiveness of health education to increase medical compliance among adults with asthma. The authors conclude that participants in a health education program showed a significantly higher level of adherence to a medical regimen than did those who did not have health education. Reduction in anxiety and less recovery time after surgery are also associated with health education programs, and client and family measures of satisfaction with health care also increase with health education.

Benefits to health care agencies discussed by Fernsler and Cannon[25] include cost-saving benefits, increased client satisfaction, and a reduction in malpractice suits. According to the authors, "health education facilitates open, honest, and sensitive communication, reducing the likelihood of malpractice suits." They believe that health education reduces unrealistic client expectations, which results in decreased litigation.

Bartlett summarized research studies on the cost and benefit of health education. He concluded that regardless of the setting and including managed care or other settings, savings are generally three or four times greater than program costs.[5] No studies reported that health education cost more than it saved.

Definitions

The concepts of health and health education are defined in various ways throughout health education literature. Health education can be narrowly defined as the giving of information. It can also be equated with teaching about illness or what should be done to avoid or recover from an illness. This type of narrow focus is based on the premise that human behavior is shaped largely by rationality and sufficient motivation and that simplistically stated, health represents the absence of illness. Using this basic approach it logically follows that if Client X has been diagnosed as having decreased coronary perfusion (illness) and has received information regarding the pathophysiology of the heart and what can be done to alleviate this problem (health education), Client X will go home and follow the recommended treatment regimen (lose weight, stop smoking, and start an exercise program). Obviously such a narrow approach to the concept of health education will not suffice in many actual cases.

A broader definition of health is a synchronism between the individual and the biologic, psychologic, and social environment.[6] Health education "begins with the recording of factual information to patients but it also includes the interpretation and integration of information in such a manner as to bring about attitude or behavior changes which benefit the person's health status."[71]

A still broader definition of health is based on the premise that health is not an empiric fact or objective phenomenon. Rather it is a human construct that individuals in a given society "invent in accordance with [their] cultural values and social norms."[2]

When health is defined as a culturally bound concept, health is "that state of body and mind well functioning which affords individuals the ability to strive toward their functional objectives and their culturally desired goals.[2] Based on this premise Balog[2] contends that health education should be the dissemination of information concerning what life habits promote the well functioning of the body and mind and encourage the advancement of self-rule and self-care. In Balog's definition of health education, giving information is still a key element; however, the emphasis is placed on individual responsibility within the environment.

Although it is evident that a simplistic concept of health and health education in a multifaceted and complex field is no longer sufficient, there are problems with broad definitions of the same concepts. Balog[2] points out that because the concept of health has no agreed-on boundaries it is difficult to establish a distinctive focus and purpose for the field. The domain of health education has shifted from the teaching of bodily health and disease prevention to teaching about the promotion of physical, psychologic, social, and ecologic well-being. Balog contends that although cultural values affect society's view of well-being, they are not an area for health education. Health education should rather focus on self-rule and self-care or making individuals responsible for their own health care.

Goals

Based on the preceding definitions it is possible to formulate a series of basic goals for health education. They are (1) giving information, (2) behavioral change, and (3) making clients responsible for their own health care. The first basic goal of giving information can be the final goal or an intermediate goal. For instance, numerous research studies evaluate client knowledge about a particular topic. Usually the researcher gives a pretest to determine what the client already knows, then supplies some type of information and ends with a posttest to show that the action taken resulted in increased client knowledge. In this instance client knowledge is the final goal of the health education intervention. In contrast, in the previous discussion of enculturation the final goal is the client being responsible for his own health care; however, an initial goal is to increase client knowledge so that the individual will be able to make decisions about his own health.

Regardless of the complexity of the end behaviors that are desired, in all health education some type of information is given and hopefully learned by the client. This can be theoretic information, such as information regarding a specific illness or medication; information regarding specific behaviors, such as insulin injections; or information regarding complex activities, such as the process of values clarification.

A second basic goal of health education is *behavioral change*. This may be as simple as the learning of a single skill or as complex as the changing of a lifestyle to facilitate health. Because many research studies have concluded that there is minimal correlation between the level of knowledge and behavior, behavioral outcomes are often emphasized as a goal in health education.

A specific form of behavioral change often discussed in health education literature is *compliance*. Compliance refers to the client's ability to follow a

 CULTURAL CONSIDERATIONS

The concept of enculturation has been used to emphasize health education as a process within the environment. According to Nowakowski[58] every interaction a health professional has with a client represents an educational experience. The interaction is part of the client's enculturation or represents one experience involved in growing up and participating in a society. All of the individual's experiences provide an opportunity for the individual to develop intellectual, emotional, and manipulative skills to understand and use appropriate health care knowledge as that knowledge becomes available. A major characteristic of a culture is the way that it chooses to explain pain, suffering, and death. Dimou[20] contends that cultural differences are important in working with clients to gain insight into their thinking, motivation, and explanatory model of what caused their problem. Dimou believes that only if the health worker understands the client's explanatory model will he or she have insight into the client's thinking and a chance to motivate and educate the client.

Shadick[68] states that to implement a health education program the nurse needs to have knowledge regarding the client's health beliefs, values, and practices. In addition, the nurse needs to understand the client's language, level of literacy, and learning style. Shadick also warned that cultural groups are hetereogeneous. She reminds the nurse that generalizations about a particular cultural group are helpful as long as they are not applied to individuals.

prescribed regimen of treatment. For example, Client X has essential hypertension. He is given three medications to take on various daily schedules, a diet and exercise plan to follow, related health information about how to incorporate the treatment plan into his daily lifestyle, and a follow-up appointment. The goal of health education is for the client to follow the prescribed regimen. When Client X returns in 1 month and his blood pressure is within normal limits, his medical consultants deduce that he is following the regimen, the regimen is working, and the health teaching was effective.

The third basic goal of health education is to *make clients responsible for their own health care.* This may be considered the overall objective of all health education based on a broad definition of health education. This goal incorporates the first two goals, because to be responsible for one's own care necessitates a certain level of knowledge and the ability to make behavioral changes that will facilitate health. This goal also includes cultural differences, decision-making skills, and the ability to take responsibility for one's own actions. Figure 10-1 summarizes the goals of health education, arranging the goals in hierarchic order from the general to the specific.

It is important to recognize that in various situations behavioral changes that facilitate health and the cultural and individual value system of the client will not be congruent. For example, Ms. G. is a well-educated young woman who is 30 pounds over-weight. She has knowledge about food, diet, exercise, all of the input necessary to change her behavior. Ms. G. also has the skills needed to change her behavior. She knows how to make a diet plan and how to cook nutritious, low-caloric foods. In the area of values Ms. G. lives in a culture in which overweight women are considered voluptuous. Her husband likes her overweight. She likes herself the way she is. She makes a decision that being overweight is not a problem for her. She is responsible for her own care.

Ryan[67] recommends that the nurse "provide a climate in which clients feel encouraged to discover that which is truly important to them. In other words, they can clarify their own values, choose what they would strive for, and move toward that goal." If the nurse is not aware of Ms. G.'s cultural and individual value system, goals and objectives can be established that are contradictory to the individual's perceived needs. In such situations staff members often become angry or frustrated by their unsuccessful

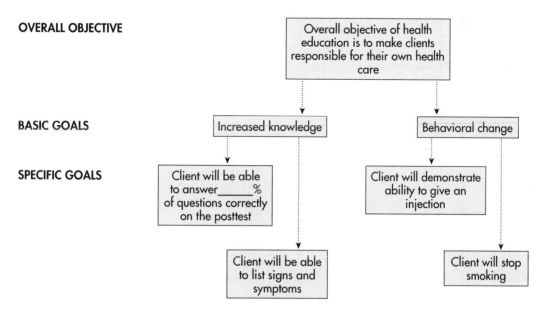

OVERALL OBJECTIVE — Overall objective of health education is to make clients responsible for their own health care

BASIC GOALS — Increased knowledge — Behavioral change

SPECIFIC GOALS — Client will be able to answer_____% of questions correctly on the posttest — Client will demonstrate ability to give an injection

Client will be able to list signs and symptoms — Client will stop smoking

Fig. 10-1 Goals of health education.

attempts "to help." Health goals of the nurse will not meet with success unless they are shared by the client.

Theoretic basis

All of the information presented in the preceding chapters, particularly the content on communication and the behavioral manifestation of communication and on interpersonal relationships, is groundwork for implementing health education. In addition, a number of other theoretic frameworks can be used as a basis for health education. Padilla and Bulcavage[60] review theories used in health education related to prevention and coping/adaptation, and they contend that health education programs "may need to use a multitheory approach to promote health behaviors . . . and to decrease negative responses such as anxiety, distress, pain, and use of damaging alternative treatments."

Health belief model Becker's health belief model was developed specifically for health education. Figure 10-2 is a diagram of the important variables in this model. According to the model individuals will seek preventive health care if they believe that:
1. A particular health problem is serious.
2. They personally are susceptible to this health problem.
3. They can perform certain actions to reduce their chances of contracting the disease.
4. The cost of the preventive actions or medical, financial, or psychosocial costs is perceived as being less than the cost of contracting the disease.[17]

Based on the health belief model, Clark[17] has outlined a number of additional factors that will influence an individual's decision to change their behavior. They are:
1. Belief in the ability of the involved medical personnel and the client's overall relationship with the personnel.
2. Belief in the possible effectiveness of the prescribed regimen.
3. Actual and perceived cost to the client, including time, money, or effort.
4. Number, type, and complexity of new patterns of behavior to be adapted (the more closely the new behavior patterns resemble the current behavior, the easier the change will be).
5. Feasibility of continuing the change over a prolonged period of time.

The basic goal in the health belief model is behavioral change. A person identified as being at risk is given health information or information to change the individual's beliefs. The desired outcome is a change in behavior from those that are characterized as detrimental to those that will facilitate health. King[44] states that beliefs are expressions of what the individual knows; attitudes express the way an individual feels. Information is necessary but often not sufficient in producing attitude or behavioral change. The health belief model is basically a disease model of primary prevention.

Psychoeducational model Another model for health education is the psychoeducational model.

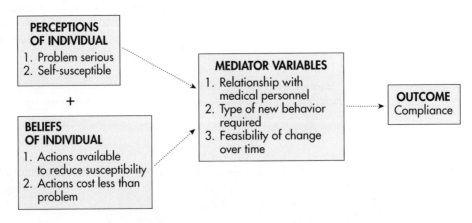

Fig. 10-2 Becker's health belief model.

In contrast to the health belief model, it is based on wellness. Table 10-1 is a comparison of these two models. Payton and Ivey define psychoeducation as "deliberate and planned efforts to teach individuals or groups understanding, skills, or competencies in the area of human relations."[61] Whereas in the health belief model the focus is behavioral change, in the psychoeducational model the focus is attitude and motivation change. The most important goal is for the individual to state and accept responsibility for the individual's own care. According to this model the client is learning a basic way of dealing with life. The individual is learning the processes of values clarification, problem definition, option discovery, action planning, commitment building, and success evaluation. These represent a group of processes that can be applied to a variety of life situations. To point out the differences between these two models for health education Payton and Ivey use an example of a diabetic client. In the health belief model the client is viewed as having the disease called diabetes mellitus; in the psychoeducational model the client is viewed as someone who is eating the wrong food and is not exercising properly. The focus in this latter approach is on what the client can do independently to rebalance his life systems.

Empowerment model There have been articles describing empowerment education, as well as some research based on the empowerment model. Wallerstein and Bernstein[78] describe empowerment as an "effective health education and prevention model for personal and social change." According to these authors, whose work is based on the writings of the Brazilian educator Paulo Freire, powerlessness is linked to disease while empowerment is linked to health. Empowerment is defined as "a social action process that promotes participation of people, organizations and communities in gaining control over their lives in their community and larger society." The steps in empowerment education include:

1. The community members meet in groups and identify their problems.
2. Community members assess the social and historical roots of the identified problem and envision a healthy society.
3. Community members develop strategies to obtain their goals.

Empowerment differs from other theories of health education in many ways. Some of the differences discussed by Wallerstein and Bernstein include the fact that in the empowerment model not only is the emphasis in the clients' (group) identification of the problem, but also that knowledge does not come from experts. Rather, knowledge comes from a collective group experience. Empowerment change strategies are broader. They are directed toward social changes, political changes, or both. For example, Wallerstein and Bernstein describe a typical alcohol/drug abuse prevention program with its emphasis on individual responsibility compared to a health education program based on empowerment in which the goal is to create a healthy environment.

Minkler's review[55] of the history of health education reflects the American emphasis on personal behavior change rather than social change. For example, efforts to decrease cigarette smoking use campaigns focused on individual choice of a healthier behavior rather than social changes to

TABLE 10-1 Comparison of the health belief and psychoeducational models of health education

	PSYCHOEDUCATIONAL MODEL	HEALTH BELIEF MODEL
Goals	Attitude and motivation change	Behavioral change
Client behaviors	State and accept responsibility for own care	Demonstrate change in beliefs or knowledge
	Individual learns processes that can be applied to a variety of situations	
Focus	Client actions to rebalance life	Disease focus

discourage the growing, manufacturing, and distribution of tobacco. The American need to be "in control" was described as an important cultural factor influencing the direction of health education. The broader approach to health education is evident in the World Health Organization "Healthy Cities" projects in Europe; in these projects community members meet and plan strategies to "offset health inequalities" at a community level.

The individual is not solely responsible for health, because the underlying causes for poor health, poverty, stress, and so on do not reside within the individual but within the society. Therefore health education must also target policy makers and controllers of social influence.[6]

Learning theory Several of the preceding models were developed specifically for health education. However, there are numerous general learning theories that can be applied to health education.

Learning theory can be divided into two major groups: behavioral and cognitive theories. One of the main areas of difference between these groups is their description of the nature of the learner. In the behavioral approach the learner is seen as a passive product of the environment. In contrast, the cognitive approach to learning views the learner as active in nature. The learner interacts with the environment, and learning is influenced by innate characteristics of the learner, such as motivation.

Another main area of difference between the behavioral and cognitive approaches is the focus of learning. Behavioral theories of learning are concerned with the description of general laws of learning. The emphasis is on investigating the "sameness in learning" or decreasing variability in performance. In contrast, cognitive approaches to learning focus on the explanation of differences in learning performance. The emphasis is on explaining variability in performance.

An examination of specific research studies points out these differences in the two approaches. In a study conducted by behaviorists Greenspoon and Foreman[31] subjects were asked to draw 3-inch lines while blindfolded. Each subject had 50 trials with 30 seconds between trials. There were five groups each receiving feedback regarding their performance at different times: immediately after drawing the line and 10, 20, and 30 seconds after drawing the line. One group was given no feedback. Feedback was of three types: too short (less than $2^3/4$ inches), too long (over $3^1/4$ inches), and right. Results showed that increasing the delay of feedback decreased the rate of learning and that any feedback was significantly more beneficial than no knowledge of results.

From this study it is clearly evident that the researchers were interested in decreasing the variability in performance. The emphasis was on predicting the subjects' behavior based on the time interval between completion of the motor task and the examiner giving feedback. In application, if an instructor of a simple motor task wanted comparable performance in a group, it would be advantageous to provide subjects with immediate feedback regarding their performance.

An examination of cognitive studies shows that the emphasis is mainly on individual differences. Osherson and Markman[59] investigate the 7-year-old's ability to evaluate contradictions and tautologies in language. They postulate that the differences arise among children because the child takes truth or meaning from the linguistic form. Their emphasis is on explaining individual differences on a growth continuum that reveals changes in cognitive structure. Along the same lines Wilcox and Palermo[79] investigate 18-month-old to 3-year-old children's understanding of the prepositions *in, on,* and *under.* They find that the younger children perform best on incongruent tasks, probably because their interpretation of the situation came more from the situation itself rather than from the linguistic meaning of the words. Once again individual differences across age groups are examined rather than trying to establish general laws of behavior. Table 10-2 is a comparison of the cognitive and behavioral approaches to learning.

Gagné[28] postulates a hierarchic system of learning that incorporates behavioristic and cognitive approaches to learning. The first five stages of learning are behavioristic. They are:

Level 1: Signal learning. This is based on physiologic reflexes and responses that are involuntary to the organism. It is characteristic of some infant learning, especially during the first 4 weeks of life. The number of responses is not increased; rather, the number of stimuli capable of eliciting the response is increased.

TABLE 10-2 **Comparisons of cognitive and behavioral learning theory**

	COGNITIVE APPROACH	BEHAVIORAL APPROACH
Nature of the learner	Active learner	Passive learner
Relationship to environment	Learner interacts with environment	Learner is product of environment
Focus of theory	Examining variability in performance	General laws of learning
Types of learning	Concept learning Rule learning Problem solving	Stimulus-response Motor chaining Verbal associations Multiple discriminations

Level 2: Stimulus-response learning. The organism is demonstrating voluntary behavior, but there is no understanding. The stimulus-response units are isolated bits of information. Infants after 4 weeks of age are capable of this type of learning.

Levels 3 and 4: Levels 3 and 4 are parallel constructs. They are motor chaining and verbal associations. Here a number of stimulus-response units are brought together. Young children demonstrate this type of behavior in learning to walk and in using two-word sentences. Motor learning and rote learning in adults are also forms of this type of learning.

Level 5: Multiple discrimination. In this type of learning the individual is able to take into account a number of variables in making the correct response. Children use this type of learning to classify objects according to their salient physical properties.

The next three levels of Gagné's theory are related to cognitive types of learning tasks. The individual is able to understand and use more information than that originally supplied by the environmental input.

Level 6: Concept learning. The simplest form is learning concrete concepts such as chair, in which examples of the concept can be pointed out. Concepts enable the individual "to identify single instances of classes of objects and object qualities in [the] environment."[28] Defined concepts such as latitude represent a more advanced level of concept learning. Examples of the concept cannot be pointed out; they must be defined. "The learner has acquired a defined concept that he can demonstrate, or show how to use, the definition. In doing this, he is classifying instances of the concept.[28]

Level 7: Rule learning. This type of learning allows the individual to put concepts together and generalize to different situations.

Level 8: Problem solving. This is the highest form of learning. It requires the ability to conceptualize and learn rules for using concepts. Problem solving is the main characteristic of formal operational thought. Gagné believes it is necessary to learn each level before proceeding to the next and that the sequence occurs in an orderly fashion.

Regardless of the approach, behavioral or cognitive, it is possible to extrapolate basic principles of learning and teaching from learning theory that can be used as a basis for health education. Some of these learning principles are:

1. Motivation plays a central role in learning. Any behavior that is rewarded is more likely to occur. Either praise or blame is more effective than is ignoring behavior. There are two types of motivation: intrinsic and extrinsic. A task is said to be intrinsically motivating when the resolution of tension is found in mastering the learning task itself, such as learning about an illness simply to satisfy an internal curiosity. A task is said to be extrinsically motivating when the resolution of tension lies outside the task itself, such as grades or teacher praise. Intrinsic motivation has been shown to increase retention, understanding, and transfer.

2. The probability of success influences learning. Long tasks should not be too easy or too hard. "For success to be experienced as such, there must be the possibility of failure."[8]

3. Goals should be mutually determined by the client and health educator. Goals must be attainable. Participation in the learning plan and goal setting promotes learning. Learning that is teacher controlled can lead to apathetic conformity or open defiance.

4. The individual needs to be ready to learn. Readiness is described as having the biologic and experiential background necessary to accomplish the new task. Some individuals will never be ready for certain learning tasks.

5. Attention is necessary for learning to occur, and attention is often hindered by factors associated with illness, such as pain, stress, medication, and anxiety. Attention is both involuntary and voluntary or directed. Attention is critical to the learning process. Not only must the individual direct attention to stimuli in the environment, competing stimuli must also be inhibited. Directed attention is limited and requires effort; therefore it is subject to fatigue.[16]

6. Practice affects learning in various ways. Practice refers not to doing the same thing over and over again, but rather to "trials that have an experiential character; that is, trials in which the action is varied, even though slightly."[8] Distributive practice is more beneficial than is massed practice. Distributive practice is defined as shorter periods of practice time with other activities in between those periods.

7. Retention refers to the amount of learned material that can be recalled over time. Material that is meaningful is learned easier and retained longer. Forgetting may be purposive. Information that is painful or not congruent with the individual's beliefs may be forgotten. Overlearning does not contribute to retention in the acquisition of meaningful material but may influence the learning of nonmeaningful material.

ESTABLISHING HEALTH EDUCATION PROGRAMS

Assessment

The first step in the establishment of any health education program is the recognition of a need for health education in a particular area. After a need has been recognized and defined, specific content to meet that need can be identified. Zonca[81] calls *need analysis* the first step in establishing a health education program; need analysis may be either informal or formal.

Informal need analysis is the initial step in information gathering. It consists of various unstructured attempts to collect data. Some examples are simply talking with clients and staff that will be involved in the health education, reviewing client charts, and perhaps walking through particular clinical areas to see what type of health education is currently being given.

After an informal need analysis is performed a *formal need analysis* will serve to substantiate initial impressions. Formal need analysis consists primarily of interviews and questionnaires. Interviews are conducted personally by an individual with a single client, families, or small groups of clients. Questionnaires are printed forms given out to the client or staff that they are asked to complete and return. The advantage of a formal need analysis is that it avoids any bias that may enter into the assessment when using informal analysis. The information collected during the informal stage is particularly useful in developing the formal interview schedule and questionnaire. Both interview and questionnaires can be either open-ended, closed, or a combination of the two. An example of an open-ended format would be questions such as "What types of things would you like to know about labor?" An example of a closed format would be "Would you like to know about the types of anesthesia used for labor?" A disadvantage of closed formats is that many questions are needed and often clients do not feel personally involved when they are only called on to make simple yes or no responses. In addition, areas not included on the closed format (which may be important to the client) can be easily overlooked. The open format has the advantage of actively involving the client, but a major disadvantage is that specific areas that the client is potentially interested in may be overlooked. For instance, if a client didn't know that there was a choice in anesthesia during labor, she may never mention anesthesia in an open format.

Another important aspect of assessment is *defining the general characteristics of the population involved*. All data that may be pertinent to the development of a viable teaching plan are included. Factors that could be considered in describing the population are age, gender, educational level, income level, past experiences, and entering knowledge. A specific example of how need analysis could be performed follows:

Nurse A is conducting a need analysis for a prenatal clinic. Nurse A:

1. Identifies the need.
2. Identifies the characteristics of the population involved (in this specific example, parity, marital

status, and percentage of cesarean deliveries would also be general information included).

3. Performs an informal need analysis by walking through the clinic and observing what is currently taught and what questions are being asked, talking to a few clients randomly, and discussing needs identified by other staff who are available.
4. Develops an open-ended interview with other interested staff and conducts interviews with other staff members and a random number of clients.
5. Based on the informal need analysis and the results of the interviews conducted, develops with interested staff a closed questionnaire with an open-ended section at the end and administers questionnaires to a random sampling of the clinic population.

Based on this analysis Nurse A can definitively state the probable areas of interest or need that should be incorporated into the clinic's health education program.

In this example health education is being planned for a small, defined group. The same assessment procedures could be used for other target populations with minor variations. For instance, a prenatal health education program could be established for one client or an entire community. As the number of individuals in the target group decreases, the amount of time needed for assessment and the sources of data collection will also decrease. If Nurse A wanted to formulate a health education program only for Ms. S., a client in the prenatal clinic, Nurse A would not need to interview other clients. Nurse A would consult with the physician and other staff who have contact with Ms. S., Ms. S.'s records, and the client herself. In contrast, if Nurse A wanted to establish a community-wide prenatal health education program, she would need many additional sources of assessment information. As the number of potential program participants increases, the degree of program individuality decreases. The health education program developed for Ms. S. would be specific to her individual needs. A community-wide program, even a program with a great deal of content flexibility, could not be individualized to this degree for each participant.

Planning

After the population is defined and potential need identified, the next phase is planning the health education program. The focus of this phase is how to meet the defined needs or what to teach and how to teach it. Planning requires a basic knowledge of how humans learn.

Learning theory as a theoretic base for health education has already been discussed; however, there are three populations with special learning needs that should be addressed. These populations are adult learners, particularly the aged; the poor; and children.

Adult learners Longitudinal research results suggest that in general, intelligence either remains the same or increases slightly during the adult years.[75] Meaningfulness of content material is more important for the adult learner. Because they are more self-directed, adult learners are more motivated to learn something that they consider important. Another general characteristic of adult learners concerns distraction. Simultaneous activities have a negative effect on adult learners, because they are less capable of ignoring irrelevant information.

In his review of research related to learning and the adult Bischof[9] outlines a number of other characteristics of adult learners:

1. As anxiety decreases, the quality of performance increases.
2. Cautiousness increases with age because adults value accuracy more than speed.
3. Reaction time increases with age because the older adult takes more time to process information.
4. Memory is differentially affected by age. Short-term memory decreases with age, whereas long-term memory is not influenced by age.

Botwinick[10] has suggested a number of ways to help older adults learn more effectively. These include:

1. Slow down the pacing of events.
2. Help clients to organize the material.
3. Give strong emotional support.
4. Employ visual and aural augmentation because the more senses the elderly use the better they learn.
5. Reduce interference.
6. Make the task meaningful or relevant.

The poor Ross[66] has outlined a number of factors that influence health education for the poor. A primary factor is their lack of knowledge regarding health. Ross contends that the poor have a distorted image of health care sources, resulting from a general lack of information about health service sources. This is directly related to their underutilization of health facilities. The poor are the group who need health information the most, have the least amount of health information, and are the least likely to receive such information. Health information that the poor do receive is usually supplied by their neighbors and peers who also are lacking in accurate health information.

The expectations of health professionals are another factor influencing health education for the poor. Health professionals have lower expectations for the poor. These expectations are often based on the stereotyped image of the poor as less educated, passive, alienated, and unable to cope.

A third factor is the time orientation of the poor. This group tends to be more oriented to the present than the future. The formation of health beliefs and the seeking of preventive care are based on a future orientation.

The final factor discussed by Ross is the lack of basic skills that poor people possess. The poor tend to have less of the skills necessary to seek and carry out medical care.

Based on these characteristics of the poor in relationship to health education a number of suggestions can be made to facilitate the giving of health information to the poor. Ross has suggested that the informal communication network within poor communities be used to supply the poor with health education. Specifically, Ross recommends paraprofessional outreach programs in which members of the community are trained as health educators to deliver health education to their own community.

Another recommendation is that health information provided to the poor should be of a nontechnical nature. This is often difficult for health professionals. Many times nontechnical health education results in no health education. Special programs should be developed that will meet this need.

The final recommendation is to increase poor people's contacts with health care providers. Increased contacts will give the poor greater opportunity to learn the skills necessary to be responsible for their own care. Outreach programs are one possibility; another is changing clinic practices. Clinics that serve the poor are often impersonal and busy. Changes in clinic practices that aim to individualize client care may be beneficial.

Children Because parents are primarily responsible for the health of their children, health education for children (particularly very young children) is directed toward the adult caregiver. Health education directed to children themselves is provided mainly by the schools and occasionally by the media and direct-service areas such as hospitals and clinics. Because one fourth of the U.S. population is in schools, this is a major arena for health education for children.

In general health education directed toward the child must take into account the developmental level of the child. (Chapter 2 discusses growth and development.) Most learning tasks for children are associated with the lower levels of Gagné's hierarchy, mentioned earlier in this chapter. The child does not have full intellectual capacity until sometime during adolescence, when he is able to reason and perform other complex mental functions necessary for higher-order learning.

General recommendations for health education for children are:

1. Cognitive learning with the corresponding lecture-oriented teaching method may be beneficial in increasing the child's knowledge regarding health. However, involvement techniques are more beneficial for values clarification and behavioral change. In most settings (particularly schools) the child represents a captive audience. Learning is not facilitated under these circumstances.

2. As with the adult learner information directed toward the child's interests and needs will be more readily learned.

3. The child will have a longer attention span when participating in projects, such as cooking, making posters, and the like, than when called on to listen to a didactic presentation.

4. Particularly as the child progresses into peer-oriented phases of development, peer-led activities are a major vehicle for health education.

5. Play and simulated learning experiences are beneficial, particularly for the young child or when anxiety is high.

An example of a health educative play experience is the use of dolls to prepare the child for surgery. The child can dress as the doctor or nurse, perform the surgery on the doll, and take care of the doll. By doing so the child is able to learn more about the experience than by listening to an adult explanation.

Planning content The next issue in planning concerns the type of content that will be presented. For instance, in the example of Nurse A and the prenatal clinic one of the needs identified is to know what labor feels like. The type of information needed is sensation rather than cognitive information.

Ross[66] discusses three types of information or knowledge: awareness knowledge, principles knowledge, and how-to knowledge. Awareness knowledge is information that attempts to develop recognition or legitimacy for a particular health problem; community media campaigns that attempt to show new parents the importance of using infant seat restraints in cars is an example. "Principles knowledge is more comprehensive, and information in this category would emphasize the functioning principles underlying a health problem."[66] Principles information is more detailed than awareness information and covers the treatments, causes, and characteristics of a health problem. Much of the health education done by nurses involves principles information. Slide-tape presentations, films, and pamphlets also usually contain principles information. However, Ross cautions that "overzealous efforts to educate about an important health issue sometimes result in the inclusion of too much information for the communication medium."

The third type of information is how-to information. This type of information gives clear recommendations for actions to be taken by the client. Ross believes that how-to information is the most important type and includes such things as how to get transportation to the health facility, use medical insurance, and locate health resources. Motor skills learning is also a type of how-to information, such as learning how to administer an injection; learning the motor skills involved in breastfeeding, exercise, coughing, or deep breathing; and any other skills type of information.

Another breakdown of types of knowledge is sensation information versus cognitive information. This dichotomy has received increased attention in recent health education literature, specifically in research studies preparing clients for surgery or intrusive medical tests. For example, Hartfield et al.[33] conducted a study of 20 clients scheduled for barium enema. Half were given sensation information; the other half received cognitive information. Sensation information consisted of a description of what the client would feel and experience during the procedure. In contrast, cognitive information described the actual procedure. The researchers found that clients given sensation information had significantly less anxiety as measured by a standard anxiety scale after the procedure. It was hypothesized that the clients given only cognitive information experienced more anxiety because their expectations regarding the sensations they would feel during the procedure were not congruent with the actual sensations experienced.

Planning goals

One of the most important areas in planning is the development of goals and objectives for the health education program. According to Zonca[81] goals function to delineate the boundaries of the program, describe the philosophic basis of the program, and provide an organizational framework for the actual curriculum or content.

Chapter 1 describes the writing of behavioral goals and objectives in detail. Goals need to be written for the general health education program, as well as specific clients. Client goals are often based on task analysis to describe the component skills necessary to reach a desired behavior. The component skills are sequenced in ascending order of difficulty. The concept of mutuality is stressed in the process of establishing goals. The goals and objectives of health education need to be congruent with those of the client for the health teaching to be effective.

Instructional activities

The next step is selecting the instructional activities that will be used to meet the goals and objectives. Rice and Valdivia[64] present a guide for the design and use of health education materials. Although their guidelines were developed for health workers in Latin America, the principles are valid for all communities. The first principle is to develop educational materials from a community perspective. Specifically, they recommend the development of materials that respect the values of the community, its culture and traditions, and which are relevant to community needs and interests. The authors stress the importance of involving the community in the preparation of materials.

The second guideline is to ensure that the materials are part of a total health education program. Rice and Valdivia emphasize that materials are only part of a program, not the total program. They recommend presenting information through a variety of channels to accommodate the various learning styles of people in the community. For example, if a nurse is preparing health materials for a new baby clinic, it would be best to have posters and pamphlets (visual materials) as well as a video-tape or audio-tape material (auditory information) and perhaps even hands-on demonstrations (kinesthetic information).

The third guideline is that the educational materials must promote the use of services that are readily available. For example, a weight-loss program that promotes the consumption of fresh fruits and vegetables in a geographic area where their supply is limited or their price exorbitant is not only inappropriate but can also make the client resistant regarding any future health education interventions.

The fourth guideline is that all materials should be pretested. This means that representatives of the intended target population have an opportunity to see and work with the materials to ascertain if they are attractive, acceptable, understandable, and persuasive.

The final guideline is that distributed materials must include instructions for their use to be most effective. For example, if an excellent breastfeeding film is developed by the staff and made available to new mothers, it should also include a list of guidelines for the staff who will be showing it. The guidelines may include preknowledge that is necessary before viewing the film, suggested discussion questions to check comprehension after the film, and general discussion questions.

Selecting the medium Part of selecting the instructional activities is deciding on the media to be used. Frantz[27] has outlined a series of considerations to review before deciding on a medium: examine the characteristics of the learner, task, and medium. Many learner characteristics have already been dis-

cussed, and Frantz includes the perception skills of the learners and their level of self-direction as well as their reading ability. Forty-five percent of the U.S. population is unable to read beyond the sixth-grade level. As many as 21 million Americans are functionally illiterate. Dunn et al.[22] recommend the increased use of pictorial cues, audiotapes, storytelling, and other audiovisual supplements in the health education of the illiterate client.

In examining the characteristics of the task Frantz[27] recommends deciding whether the information to be included fits into a cognitive, psychomotor, or affiliative domain. An example of cognitive information is information about the action of the medication, its possible side effects, and any restrictions or special instructions the patient would need to know about. In contrast, the psychomotor domain refers to information pertaining to the actual performance of a task. For instance, doing a series of exercises and performing a breast self-examination are examples of motor learning. Affiliative content is related to the acquisition of values, attitudes, and interests.

In examining the characteristics of the media Frantz[27] uses a chart (Table 10-3) of 76 types of media and various presentation characteristics. The presentation characteristics of media are those variables that affect the way in which the content to be learned is delivered. In using this chart it is possible to ascertain at a glance which particular media will fit a specific group of clients. For example, if Nurse A wants to do a health teaching presentation to a large group of prenatal clinic clients (approximately 100), wants the learner to control the pace to account for the variations in educational level, and wants a fixed sequence of content, the following media are appropriate: printed booklet, programmed instruction, filmstrip, slide, filmstrip cassette, or computer.

Group instruction A popular research question is comparing the effectiveness of group versus individual client health education. In several research studies group health education is as effective as individual instruction. In addition, clients prefer group instruction. Clients often fail to recognize individual instruction as teaching but perceive it as social interaction. Another positive aspect of group instruction is that it requires significantly less time and hence is more efficient.

Mechanical presentations A second popular research question in the area of health education media is examining the effectiveness of mechanical presentations of content. In these studies the client's level of knowledge about some particular topic is first measured. Information on the topic is then presented mechanically, by film, tape, or computer. Finally knowledge of the topic is measured again. If there is an increase in knowledge beyond what is expected by chance, the researchers conclude that the mechanical presentation of content increased the client's level of knowledge on the particular subject under investigation.

Van Reenen[77] discusses the use of interactive videodiscs as the most effective and newest educational technology. The videodisc user is an active participant in the learning process, deciding when and where to interact with the program. The author contends that interactive videodiscs are a better teaching tool for right brain–dominant individuals.

Poston[62] describes how to establish a computer-assisted instructional program (CAI). CAI allows learners to proceed at their own rate and receive immediate feedback. It is particularly well suited to drill and practice, tutorial, and simulations.

Although some intervention is effective when the objective is increased client knowledge, the same results may not be found when effectiveness is measured as behavioral change. No particular format has such overwhelmingly supportive research evidence that it can be proclaimed as the method of choice. Availability must be considered as a primary determinant for the type of media used in health education.

Interaction of treatment and client Some studies have pointed out the interactive effect between treatment and particular client variables. For example, Klos et al.[45] compared the effectiveness of a preoperative treatment pamphlet to individualized nurse preoperative teaching, a combination of both formats, and no treatment. Significant factors that influenced the results were client age and fear levels. The data indicated that clients with high preoperative fear benefited more from a pamphlet approach, while at the same time the pamphlet was detrimental to those clients with low preoperative fear levels. Overall clients who were older or had higher fear levels recovered more slowly than did young or low preoperative fear clients.

Jason et al.[38] compared treatment role-playing groups to discussion groups for decreasing smoking behavior in ninth-grade students. They concluded that both treatments were effective in reducing smoking behavior in early smokers but that neither approach was effective in long-term smokers. The most significant factor was length of smoking behavior. In summary, there are numerous intervening variables in addition to the type of educational format used that may have a more powerful effect on outcome measures.

Media campaigns Some research studies outlined methodology used with larger populations. A study by Hill et al.[36] reported the results of a program to increase breast self-examination in Australian women. The researchers used television to dispel obstacles associated with women not performing breast self-examination, such as a tendency to equate a breast lump with cancer. They distributed literature on breast cancer to all general practitioners in the target area. At the 12-month follow-up they found significantly more women doing breast self-examination in the target area compared with a control area. The authors contend that their program's success was based on two factors. The first was that the media campaign was used to dispel obstacles associated with the desired outcome behavior: breast self-examination. The second was that they enlisted the cooperation of the physicians in the target area.

Another technique that has been used successfully in mass-media campaigns is the single-case example. Jobes et al.[39] believe that the use of nationally known names that are vivid, concrete, and easy to identify with makes the situation described seem more real. Although a nationally recognized name such as Betty Ford may not be representative of a larger population, a discussion of breast cancer focusing on Mrs. Ford's experience can influence the way people process information about the disease. The authors contend that a general campaign citing abstract statistical information does little to produce attitude and behavioral change, because individuals

TABLE 10-3 Types of media and their presentation characteristics

PRESENTATION CHARACTERISTICS	REAL OBJECT	MODEL OF REAL OBJECT	AUDIOTAPE RECORD	PRINTED BOOKLET	PROGRAMMED INSTRUCTION (PRINTED)	CHALKBOARD
Size of audience						
Large (100+)			X	X	X	
Medium (30-100)			X	X	X	X
Small (2-30)	X	X	X	X	X	X
Individual	X	X	X	X	X	X
Sensory stimuli						
Visual	X	X		X	X	X
Audible	X	X	X			
Taste	X	X				
Smell	X	X				
Tactile	X	X				
Learner involvement						
Self-instruction	X	X	X	X	X	
Learner controls pace	X	X	X	X	X	
Learner response required			X	X	X	X
Delivery characteristics						
Motion depicted		X				
Changeable speed of motion		X				
Fixed sequence of content	X	X	X	X	X	X
Flexible sequence of content	X	X				X
Reflects real world	X	X	X			
Content display repeatable	X	X	X	X	X	

From Frantz RA: Selecting media for patient education, *Top Clin Nurs* 2:77, 1980.

actively evaluate and select information. It is easier to identify with someone that individuals perceive to be like them than with abstract statistics.[39]

Peer groups A final methodologic approach to health education discussed in the literature is the use of peer groups. (Peer groups will be discussed more fully in the following section on self-help groups.) In the health education literature the use of peer groups is most often associated with health teaching for children and adolescents.

Implementation

Implementation refers to the actual process of doing the health teaching. After performing an assessment, writing goals, and deciding on nursing actions, how easy will it be to actually implement the program?

Potential for implementation Kolbe and Iverson[47] have outlined a number of program features (see box on p. 260) that will affect its potential for implementation. The first is the relative advantage of the program. This consists of the unique benefits that the particular health education program provides. It considers the economic costs, overall usefulness, and how long it will take to experience the benefits of the program.

The second factor is the program's potential impact on professional relations. This effect can be positive or negative. For example, if one group of

OVERHEAD TRANSPARENCY	FILMSTRIP	SLIDE	16-MM FILM	VIDEOTAPE	FLAT PICTURE	FILMSTRIP CASSETTE	COMPUTER
X	X	X	X	X		X	
X	X	X	X	X	X	X	X
X	X	X	X	X	X	X	X
	X	X	X	X	X	X	X
X	X	X	X	X	X	X	X
			X	X		X	
	X	X	X		X	X	X
	X	X			X	X	X
X	X	X				X	X
X	X	X	X	X		X	
			X				
X	X	X	X	X	X	X	X
X		X			X		
		X	X	X	X	X	
X	X	X	X	X	X	X	X

staff decides to implement a particular program and the content of any aspect of the program is not agreed on by other staff members who have contact with the target population, it will result in a negative professional relationship. This can cause the program to fail, while the same program in a comparable situation with support from all groups involved may be successful.

A third factor is the divisibility of the program. This refers to the extent to which a specific program can be implemented on a limited scale. For example, if a hospital decides to do a preoperative teaching program and begins on only one surgical unit, it will be easier to start, train staff, evaluate, and expand than to start a program on perhaps six surgical units at the same time.

A fourth factor is reversibility. This refers to the ease with which the program can be stopped and everything returned to the preprogram state. Obviously a program that involves massive changes, such as constructing new buildings for a particular health education effort or hiring new staff, will involve more of a capital outlay before it can be shown to be effective. As the number of permanent consequences increases, the likelihood of ever having an opportunity to initiate the program decreases.

Additional factors that affect the program's potential for implementation are complexity, com-

Characteristics of Health Education Programs that Facilitate Implementation

1. Relative advantage

What is the economic cost and overall usefulness of the program compared to the length of time necessary to experience program benefits?

2. Potential impact on professional relations

Do all the groups involved support the program?

3. Divisibility

Can the program be implemented on a limited scale?

4. Reversibility

How easy it is to stop the program?

5. Complexity

How difficult is it to use the program?

6. Compatibility

How congruent is the program with the goals, attitudes, and philosophy of the staff?

7. Communicability

How easy is it to describe and explain the program?

From Kolbe L, Iverson D: Implementing comprehensive health education: educational innovations and social change, *Health Educ Q* 8:57, 1981.

patibility, and communicability. The greater the degree of complexity or difficulty in a particular program, the less likely people are to use it. For instance, earlier a report on a computerized health education program was discussed.[24] This program used a simple, home-style computer rather than a more sophisticated and complex time-sharing computer. Because it was easier to train staff and give directions to client users, the computer programs were more widely used. Compatibility refers to the degree a program is congruent with the goals, philosophy, or attitudes of the people involved. Obviously the more compatible a program is, the greater the likelihood of its success. Communicability is the relative ease of describing and explaining a program. The more easily information about a program can be communicated, the greater the possibility of implementing the program.

In general programs that involve large initial outlays of personnel time and commitment or programs that plan to cover vast areas and are highly complex are the most difficult to implement, particularly if rewards will not be evident for a prolonged period of time. It is more efficient to start with a simple, limited program and, based on the results of that health education program, make adjustments and expansions. For example, Nurse D has identified the need for health education in a pediatric clinic. A program is designed that includes the hiring of a play therapist, refurbishing or building a new space for play therapy, and buying a computer and a television. As the complexity, expense, and commitment needed increase, the possibility of implementing the program decreases. Instead it would be more practical to identify one need that all of the staff agreed on and a limited number of goals and nursing actions to meet that need. After evaluating this limited program additional needs and goals could be added over time.

Evaluation Evaluation is an ongoing process to determine the effectiveness of a particular action or set of actions. Evaluation in health education is similar to evaluation in any other type of nursing care and was described in detail in Chapter 1. Throughout the implementation phase of health education the nurse is receiving from the client or group of clients feedback information that is useful in evaluating the nursing actions.

Because health education is a major goal of nursing, instances of health education must be documented and evaluated. Kuehnel and Rowe[49] identified health education as a nursing goal in their clinical area; however, when client charts were reviewed they found little documentation of any health education nursing activity. In this particular example the director and nursing staff knew that health education was being performed, but they needed a standardized format to document this fact, the client's response to the health education, and the nurse and client's evaluation of the health teaching.

Evaluation of health education serves a dual purpose. First, it communicates to other staff members working with the client what information has been covered and the client's response. Second, it provides a concrete framework for the nurse to critically examine the nursing actions taken in relationship to a particular goal and the effectiveness of those actions. Based on this concrete evaluation the nurse can determine if future goals or actions need modification.

Evaluation is also critical in attempts to create programs that can accommodate the needs of large groups of individuals. For example, the asthma clinic nursing staff have developed a slide/tape presentation on the early symptoms of an asthma attack, what to do, when to call the clinic staff, and specific recommendations regarding general preventive measures to decrease the probability of severe asthma attacks. If clients and staff are asked to informally evaluate this health education program, they may all think it is appropriate and effective. However, if the program is systematically evaluated as to its effectiveness in meeting specified behavioral objectives, the results may not be the same. A number of research studies have pointed out that this is a common occurrence.

The topic of cost-effectiveness has been extremely popular in the last few years of budget cutbacks. Bartlett[5] cautions that health education should not be justified solely as a social investment. This could put health education into a perilous situation, because programs that could not show cost reduction would be abandoned. Bartlett also contends that by advocating health education on a cost-effectiveness basis, a double standard is being condoned. Other medical procedures are approved on the basis of medical necessity, not on necessity plus cost reduction. He suggests that the best argument for health education "is an integral and essential component of high quality health care services."[5]

The steps involved in establishing a health education program are assessment, planning, implementation, and evaluation (see box at right, top).

Obstacles to health education

In designing health education programs Chaisson[14] has outlined a list of commonly made mistakes to avoid (see box at right). First, many health educators want to tell the client what they think they should know rather than what the client wants to know. This is in direct opposition to the learning factor of rele-

vancy that was previously discussed. People learn what they perceive to be important. It is always necessary to assess the client's incoming knowledge level and what the individual client goals are for this experience.

A second pitfall is the failure to individualize educational efforts. Large group presentations, standardized video programs, and other types of media can be effective, but these may require additional input to make them appropriate for a particular client. Programs also need to be at the proper information level for the participant. Health education that is too basic or too advanced provides minimum input for the learner.

A third potential problem identified by Chaisson[14] is a failure to coordinate efforts among various professional groups. If any one group decides to

---

Summary of Steps Involved in Establishing a Health Education Program

1. Assessment
   Do formal and informal need analysis
   Define population
2. Planning
   Identify characteristics of the learner
   Decide on type of content—awareness, principles or how-to knowledge, sensation or cognitive knowledge
   Develop goals and objectives
   Select instructional activities
   Decide on media
3. Implementation
4. Evaluation
   Plan an ongoing and objective process based on goals

Obstacles to Health Education

1. Failure to identify needs of the client
2. Failure to individualize content
3. Failure to coordinate efforts among various professional groups
4. Untrained health educators
5. Providing health education in an incidental rather than in a carefully evaluated manner

initiate an educational program without receiving input from other involved professionals, they will meet with resistance. In addition, if there is not a coordinated effort, many different specialty groups can be giving the client multiple messages, resulting in confusion. For instance, a physical therapist may teach one technique for client transfer, Nurse A another, Nurse B another, and Physician C still another. The client's confusion is predictable.

To coordinate efforts someone needs to be delegated as responsible, deciding who should do the teaching and who should choose what is to be presented. If physical therapists are responsible for teaching transfer activity to a client, it is important that all other staff in contact with the client be made aware of what is being taught. This necessitates communication among a vast number of staff. If other members of the staff are going to offer feedback as well as reinforce and build on what the client has learned, they must be familiar with the content presented. This also necessitates agreement among all professionals regarding what should be taught.

A fourth potential problem is untrained health educators. Other nurse educators have spoken of the importance of incorporating health education throughout nursing school programs. Health education is not only for the spring community health rotation; it is a vital nursing function that is not confined to any nursing specialty area. Appointing specific health educators for a particular area in a clinical setting can be useful, but it can also be problematic. In some situations health education can then become the duty and responsibility of the designated health educator, when in actuality it is the responsibility of all involved. There are many times when a client wants information and may be motivated to learn. These times may not coincide with the availability of the health educator, hence many opportunities for health teaching are lost. The designated health educator can function more efficiently as a resource person, helping the staff plan and evaluate programs (essentially preparing the staff to provide health education). When the health educator functions as a resource more "teachable moments" can be used, and it produces a multiplier effect. One health educator can have personal contact with only a limited number of clients, but a health educator who has prepared a staff to do health teaching can reach a multitude of additional clients through the prepared staff.

The last potential problem area outlined by Chaisson is the provision of health education on an incidental, accidental, or ad hoc basis rather than in a carefully evaluated manner.

Lipetz et al.[52] conducted a survey of faculty members in schools of medicine and nursing. From their results a number of possible impediments to health education in a hospital setting were postulated: (1) structural barriers, (2) the utility of health education, and (3) perception of clients. Sixty-four percent of the physicians and nurses responding stated that lack of time for health education was an obstacle. Other structural barriers identified included brief client hospital stays and the absence of third-party payment for health education. Both of these potential barriers were identified more frequently by the nurses responding than the physicians responding. Lipetz et al. explained these differences in terms of the physicians' and nurses' definitions and views of health education. Nurses defined health education as "an activity which stresses patient-specific assessment, planning, execution and follow-up." As such, it competes with other nursing activities. In contrast, the physicians surveyed defined health education not as a process; rather, each contact with a client is seen as educational. Health education is equated with "informed consent, giving a diagnosis, or giving instructions for medication or self-care." Therefore other tasks are not perceived as competing with health education.

Sixty-eight percent of the physicians who responded to the survey identified lack of effectiveness of health education to change behavior as an obstacle, as did 46% of the nurses who responded. Approximately 50% of the nurses and doctors identified health education's failure to change rates of compliance as a barrier to implementing health education programs.

CRISIS INTERVENTION

Crisis intervention is discussed in detail in Chapter 11. Crisis intervention is an independent nursing action. It is often associated with secondary prevention. The client may be in a state of disequilibrium caused by increased stress. The goal would be to return the client to a state of balance as quickly as possible. Crisis intervention can also be viewed as primary mental health prevention and as tertiary prevention when dealing with clients who have chronic health problems. A unique characteristic of crisis intervention is the emphasis on the here and now.

ADVOCACY

Advocacy for the rights and needs of clients has always been an important aspect of the role of the nurse. Most of the nurses in the past who have gained recognition as leaders and who serve as role models for contemporary nurses were effective advocates. Florence Nightingale fought to obtain the resources she needed to provide adequate nursing care for soldiers who were wounded in the Crimean War. Clara Barton assumed a similar role during the United States Civil War and later during the founding of the American Red Cross. Nurses have served as advocates in civilian settings as well. In New York City during the late nineteenth century, Lillian Wald was instrumental in bringing nursing care to the slums through the establishment of the Henry Street Settlement House and the development of the community health nurse role. At a later time she also became concerned about the health care needs of children and advocated for the placement of nurses in schools. Nurses continue to build on this tradition of advocacy, sometimes pressing for the establishment of innovative health care programs at the community level and frequently seeking new ways to meet the needs of individual clients and their families.

Although the role of advocate is not new to nursing, it has only recently been labeled and defined. This has occurred in the context of the redefinition of the client role from that of a passive recipient of health care services, as exemplified by the term *patient,* to that of an active consumer of services, or *client.* In contrast to the patient, the client demands to be directly involved in health care decisions, informed about alternative approaches to care, and educated about self-care to promote optimal levels of wellness.

Definitions of advocacy

Mitty[56] identifies two sources for examining nursing's advocacy role. They are "the definition of the profession with respect to its social contract with society, and the ethical principles associated with treatment and research." Nurses practice in the context of many expectations, both those of clients and the community and those defined by the profession. To inform nurses about professional expectations and provide a forum for discussion of ethical questions, the American Nurses' Association maintains a Council on Ethics and Human Rights; many health care organizations also have formed ethics committees. Nurses can use these resources when ethical questions arise related to advocacy activities.

Kohnke[46] has defined nurse advocacy as the implementation of the role of informing the client and supporting the client's decision. This may be contrasted with the traditional concept of the lawyer as advocate. In the latter instance the legal advocate represents the client and argues the client's case. This may or may not be part of the nurse advocate's role.

For the purpose of this discussion Kohnke's definition will be used. Therefore the client will be assisted by the advocate to use the health care system most advantageously. The activities to be initiated by the nurse are informing and supporting. The information that is presented in this chapter builds on that which was included in the discussion of the concepts of autonomy and mutuality in Chapter 6.

Models of advocacy

Nursing advocacy covers a range of activities from communicating the wishes of an individual client to social activism promoting the health care rights of groups of clients. Bandman and Bandman[3] have identified three models of client advocacy. The first is a *civil disobedience* model. This is described as a high-risk model for the nurse, who must act in opposition to the established authority structure. It would include the "emancipatory nursing" role identified by Kendall[43] in which nurses assist "oppressed and disenfranchised persons who gain freedom from the people, ideology, or situation that keeps them oppressed." The nurse works from outside the system to push for change.

The second model is the nurse as a *"guerrilla fighter"* within the health care system. This is risky for the nurse and sets up a win-lose situation, which does not lend itself to productive compromise.

Bandman and Bandman[3] point out that the focus in both the civil disobedience and the nurse as guerrilla models is on the nurse, whereas advocacy works best when the client, nurse, and other members of the health care team are united in opposition to the patient's health problems. Therefore the third model, the *legal standing* model, is recommended. Legal standing means that the person has a legitimate right to present views and opinions and that they will be given serious consideration. The nurse works within the health care team as a professional colleague using the strength of competency and knowledge to advocate for the client. This model fits well with Kohnke's definition of nursing advocacy.

Advocacy and tertiary prevention

Advocacy may be an appropriate nursing activity with any client, just as health education or crisis intervention may be needed by anyone with whom the nurse has contact. Most of this analysis focuses on the relationship between advocacy and tertiary prevention. This is because individuals with chronically disabling health problems have long-term contact with the health care system, thereby requiring enhanced ability to deal with the system. However, to illustrate the applicability of advocacy to primary and secondary prevention a Clinical Example of each are presented at right.

It should be noted that Ms. J.'s first attempt at advocacy fell short. Although she informed the client, she did not confirm whether Ms. K. had decided to follow her advice. She completed the process on the next visit when she explored the reason for the client's decision not to follow her advice and provided further information. She was then able to support the client in her new decision to protect her baby from potential injury.

In the second Clinical Example the nurse attempted unsuccessfully to influence a decision maker. However, she perceived that the physician accepted her role as client advocate and was sincerely concerned about the client's welfare. Therefore she did not experience conflict over her role in supporting the client to carry out his decision to leave the hospital.

The preceding examples demonstrate that nurses perform advocacy roles in many health care settings and situations. Tertiary prevention provides a context

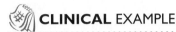

CLINICAL EXAMPLE

Primary prevention: Ms. J. was a pediatric nurse practitioner who provided primary health care in an outpatient clinic. While she was collecting data for her nursing assessment of a newborn baby, she asked Ms. K., the mother, whether the baby rode in an approved car safety seat in the car. Ms. K. replied that she had been given an infant seat by her mother and she used that for the baby when they traveled. Ms. J. explained to Ms. K. that the infant seat was not a safe way for the baby to travel. In addition, there was a state law that required infants to ride restrained in safety seats. She showed Ms. K. an approved seat and demonstrated how to secure the baby in the seat. Ms. K. thanked the nurse and left the clinic. At the next appointment a month later the nurse inquired again about the safety seat. Ms. K. looked embarrassed and then stated that she still used the infant seat for travel. With encouragement from Ms. J. she was able to say that she could not afford to purchase a safety seat. Ms. J. then referred her to a local voluntary agency that loaned safety seats to needy families. On her next visit Ms. K. stated proudly that the baby was now traveling in a safety seat.

in which a multitude of opportunities exist for advocacy. Clients with chronic conditions are usually expected to maintain long-term, periodic contact with health care providers. One frequent outcome of this intensive contact with the system is frustration with the inadequacies and lack of responsiveness that may be experienced by the client. Incidents that seem insignificant to the nurse may represent the most recent events in a long series of minor problems. Anger that is directed toward the nurse in response to a relatively minor incident should not be taken personally. Rather, the nurse should take time to discuss the client's experiences with the system and to assess whether advocacy is needed.

Self-help groups

Some groups of clients and their families have become so concerned about the failure of the system to meet their needs that they have banded together to create their own advocacy organizations, called

CLINICAL EXAMPLE

Secondary prevention: Mr. B. was a 72-year-old man who was admitted to a general hospital medical unit with a medical diagnosis of viral pneumonia. He lived alone and was accompanied by his daughter, Ms. T., who had found him in bed and barely conscious when she arrived for her weekly visit. On admission he was found to be febrile, dehydrated, and hypotensive. Vigorous medical intervention including intravenous fluids and antipyretic medication resulted in stabilization of Mr. B.'s condition. He became alert and oriented. However, he continued to require medication for a persistent cough and fever. He was also weak and needed assistance with activities of daily living.

Ms. T. approached Ms. L., a staff nurse. She told Ms. L. that she wanted to take her father back to his home, believing that he would recover more quickly in a familiar environment. However, his physician objected to this plan and refused to discharge Mr. B. Ms. L. explained the nature of the care that Mr. B. required to his daughter. She said that she was aware that he could not be alone and that she had contacted a home care agency that would be able to provide 24-hour nursing care at a price the family could afford. Based on this information Ms. L. agreed to approach the physician on the family's behalf. After her explanation of the arrangements that could be made, the physician still refused to discharge Mr. B., stating that he was concerned about his own liability if Mr. B. should become worse at home. Mr. B. then decided to sign himself out of the hospital against advice. Ms. L. obtained written permission to release information about his care and provided a copy of the hospital nursing care plan for the use of the home care nursing staff.

self-help groups. Although some self-help groups such as Alcoholics Anonymous have existed for many years, the recent rise of consumer activism has resulted in a proliferation of new groups. In fact the whole network of consumer advocacy groups extends far beyond health care. People have banded together to protest poor construction of houses, inflated costs for repairs of household items, and shoddy workmanship in new cars to name just a few.

The health care system has been a particular target of consumer advocates. In addition, many of the health-oriented self-help groups are focused on chronic conditions and therefore related to tertiary prevention. Although the self-help movement has not welcomed the involvement of health care providers, nurses need to be knowledgeable about these organizations and to explore ways of collaborating with them.

Definition

Kush-Goldberg[50] has defined the self-help group as a "voluntary, small group structure organized by peers who share a common problem, need, or concern and desire to bring about a social or personal change." Similarly, Butler et al.[12a] define it as a "cluster of like-minded or like-afflicted individuals who share experiences and offer each other mutual support and aid." There is a subtle difference in focus between these definitions that may be reflected in the characteristics of actual groups. The Kush-Goldberg definition focuses on an activist, change-oriented group purpose, whereas the Butler et al. definition identifies mutual support within the group as the primary purpose.

Resnick[63] has stated a preference for use of the term *mutual help group,* believing that this more accurately reflects the support derived from the interactive nature of the group process. She describes personal benefits of membership, including inspiration of hope, recognition of the universality of concerns and problems, learning about alternatives, and the opportunity to give and receive help. More general benefits of mutual help groups include an increased public awareness of the illness addressed by the group, fund-raising, and better understanding of coping behaviors by others.

Levy[51] has developed a typology for self-help groups based on the purpose and the composition of the group. His classification system is summarized in Table 10-4. This classification emphasizes the great diversity of types and purposes of self-help groups. The fact that so many of these groups have been organized reinforces the information discussed in Chapter 8 concerning the effectiveness of groups in assisting people to cope with their problems.

Functions A major function of self-help groups is that of advocacy for group members. Provision of

TABLE 10-4   Levy's classification of self-help groups

TYPE	COMPOSITION	PURPOSE	EXAMPLE
I	Individuals who experience problematic behavior	Conduct reorganization or behavioral control	Alcoholics Anonymous, Parents Anonymous, Take Off Pounds Sensibly (TOPS)
II	Individuals who share a common stress-producing status or predicament	Stress reduction by sharing coping strategies and giving mutual support	Make Today Count; Parents Without Partners; Recovery, Inc.
III	Individuals who are labeled as deviant or discriminated against	Maintain or increase self-esteem and gain legitimacy through political action	NOW, Gay Rights, black pride, and power groups
IV	Individuals with no identified problem	Personal growth, self-actualization, enhanced effectiveness	Professional networks, senior citizen activity groups

information about the issue or common concern that stimulated the formation of the group almost always occurs. For example, Alcoholics Anonymous is an excellent resource for information on alcoholism. Many of the self-help groups for people with cancer first reach out to potential members with information about community resources and coping strategies. Some of these groups are Reach for Recovery (breast cancer), Make Today Count, and The Lost Chord (cancer of the larynx). The other component of advocacy and the other major activity of self-help groups is that of support. Whatever the initial reason for the creation of a new group, mutual support and encouragement soon become important factors in the development of cohesiveness, thus ensuring survival of the group. The discovery that other people share the same problems and concerns can be tremendously supportive. Beyond this, group members are able to support each other to address the health care system or the political system and to make their needs known. Success in this arena adds greatly to self-esteem and leads to enhanced ability to cope. One nursing study found that people with serious mental illnesses who were members of a self-help drop-in center were empowered by the experience. *Empowerment* is a process that enables the client to be an active participant in health care by fostering autonomy and choice.[18]

The Clinical Example at right illustrates the value of the self-help group in providing information and support to an individual with a chronic health problem and her family.

The G. family demonstrates one of the problems that consumers often encounter with the health care system leading to the need for the development of self-help groups. Although Ms. G.'s condition was diagnosed and the health care team agreed with their plan to care for her at home, they were not provided with adequate education about her condition. The mounting frustration about the intensity of her demands could have led to her being institutionalized. Fortunately the self-help group was able to provide the information and support that the family needed. Even if the professional health care providers did not present information about additional resources to the G.'s, they should have at least made a referral to the self-help group.

Referral criteria Newton[57] suggests several criteria to be used when considering a referral to a self-help group:
1. The characteristics of group members
2. The group goals
3. The leadership of the group
4. Beneficial characteristics such as acceptance, mutual assistance, or education
5. For whom may it not be beneficial
6. The likelihood of successful continuation of the group

Reasons for establishing Katz and Levin[42] have identified several reasons for the reaction against the

🏵 CLINICAL EXAMPLE

M̲s. G. was a 67-year-old retired nurse who lived with her husband, also retired, and her divorced daughter and two grandchildren, aged 8 and 11 years. Ms. G.'s daughter was also a nurse, working rotating shifts, and leaving her children in the care of their grandparents while she worked. Ms. G. had always been a meticulous person, priding herself on her neat house. The other family members began to notice that she was becoming forgetful. Several of her plants died because she did not water them. On the other hand, she fed the cat three times in an hour. Her appearance deteriorated, her hair was uncombed, and she wore the same clothes day after day.

Because of their concern about this behavioral change Mr. G. took his wife to the family physician, who immediately admitted her to the hospital. On completion of the biopsychosocial assessment it was determined that she had Alzheimer's disease, which is characterized by a chronic progressive deterioration of cognitive functioning. The cause is unknown. The family was very distressed about the bleak outlook for Ms. G. but decided that they wanted to care for her at home.

When she returned home, Ms. G. required constant attention to protect her from injury. She did respond positively to

expressions of love from her family. With patient direction she was able to perform some self-care activities. However, the family members also began to exhibit signs of stress related to the constant responsibility. The children stayed away from home more. Mr. G. and his daughter began to argue frequently.

One day at work the daughter noticed an announcement for a meeting of The Alzheimer's Disease and Related Disorders Association, a self-help group for the families of individuals with Alzheimer's disease. She decided to attend the next meeting. She was very reassured when she heard other group members describe their problems, many of which were similar to her own. She received information about services such as respite care and adult day-care programs that allow families time to be free from the constant demands of the ill member. She persuaded Mr. G. to join the group also. He received a great deal of emotional support from other spouses who were experiencing feelings of loss similar to his own. Because of the consistent support of the group the G. family continued to care for Ms. G. in her own home. They also became very active in speaking out for funding to support research into the cause and treatment of Alzheimer's disease.

---

traditional health care structure that leads to the foundation of self-help groups. These include:

- Depersonalization, overspecialization, and concentration on technology
- Fragmented and episodic rather than comprehensive, continuous care
- Prevalence of chronic rather than acute illness
- Drive for control of one's own life and destiny, leading to consumer empowerment
- Greater understanding by the average person of the relationship between the environment and illness and of the role of stress in illness
- The popularity of alternative therapies such as nutritional therapies, acupuncture, and meditation
- The greater availability of self-help groups
- Increased public awareness about health practices

Consideration of these factors leads to the conclusion that self-help groups have evolved from healthy

cultural trends. Increased concern by consumers for their own health is a positive development and should be supported by health care professionals.

Meeting needs Self-help groups may be formed for reasons similar to those identified earlier. To survive they must meet the needs of their members. Riessman[65] has analyzed the consumer needs that are met by self-help groups. The first is represented by the *helper-therapy principle*, which states that it is the helper who receives the most help. In the self-help group members are called on to be helpful to each other. Especially for people who have been stigmatized or led to believe that they are helpless, it can be a powerful boost to self-esteem to be helpful to someone else. In fact, professional health care providers often report that they made their career choice based on a desire to help others. Riessman also has pointed out that "becoming committed to a position through advocating it seems to be an important dimension associated with the helper role."[65] This principle is widely applied in substance abuse treatment. Drug or alcohol abusers who encourage others to abstain are simultaneously reinforcing their own abstinence.

The second factor identified by Riessman is labeled *consumer intensivity.* A consumer-intensive activity is one in which productivity is dependent on a high level of consumer involvement. Self-help groups are by their very nature highly consumer intensive.

The contrast between the professional and self-help approaches is the third factor, the *aprofessional dimension.* Table 10-5 compares the professional and aprofessional dimensions of helping as conceptualized by Riessman. It should be noted that this representation identifies the extremes of the characteristic behaviors. However, it also describes the way that professional helpers are often viewed by consumers. Nurses need to be sure to keep the dimensions of caring in their professional practice.

Above all Riessman speaks of the value of empowerment for the consumer. The sense of control over one's destiny is particularly important to the individual with a chronic health problem who may have little control over his illness. Self-help groups are totally controlled by the members and are frequently able to make an impact on the larger system by getting it to address members' needs. Collective effort can enhance the individual's sense of power.

Potential problems It can be difficult as self-help groups grow and develop to maintain a balance between the needs of the group members and the demands of operating a complex organization. Some self-help groups have lost their original effectiveness as they have become more involved in creating new groups, developing an organizational structure, and fund-raising. This is particularly so if the expansion involves the employment of a professional staff who are not necessarily members of the target group. Loss of touch with the original goals and decreased accountability to members is a criticism that has been leveled by some at the voluntary agencies and foundations that address health problems. These highly bureaucratic organizations include such well-known groups as the American Cancer Society, the American Heart Association, and the Multiple Sclerosis Society. Critics say that these organizations have deemphasized consumer input and become too formal and impersonal. However, it is hard to be too critical when consideration is also given to the resources that have been amassed by these groups and devoted to research as well as the immediate needs of their constituents. In addition, these large organizations often foster the development of new self-help groups. It appears

TABLE 10-5   Professional and aprofessional dimensions compared

PROFESSIONAL	APROFESSIONAL
Emphasis in knowledge and insight, underlying principles, theory, structure	Emphasis on feeling, effect, concrete, practical
Systematic	Experience, common sense, and intuition are central; folk knowledge
"Objective"—use of distance and perspective, self-awareness, control of transference	Closeness and self-involvement; subjective
Empathy, controlled warmth	Identification
Standardized performance	Extemporaneous, spontaneous (expressions of own personality)
Outsider orientation	Insider orientation; indigenous
Praxis	Practice
Careful, limited use of time; systematic evaluation; curing	Slow, time no issue; informal direct accountability; caring

From Riessman F: How does self-help work? *Soc Pol* 7:41, 1976.

that the consumer receives the best service when the professional health care providers, the large voluntary health advocacy organizations, and self-help groups find ways to work together and combine their efforts in a positive way.

Nurses and self-help groups Where then do nurses interface with self-help groups? Hunka et al.[37] have identified the role of "sponsor." This is a professional person who helps with problem solving and serves as liaison to professional helping resources in the community.

Kush-Goldberg[50] conducted a study to attempt to answer how nurses interfere with self-help groups. Members of a women's self-help health group who were surveyed by the nurse researcher expressed disapproval of the idea that nurses should assume a professional role in the group. However, they reported positive experiences with nurses who had been group members. The investigator concluded that nursing intervention in a self-help group could interfere with the helper-therapy principle and should be avoided. However, she proposed several functions that nurses could perform relative to self-help groups. They include:

1. Acting as resource persons by providing health information, correcting misinformation, teaching specific skills, and helping to identify priorities.
2. Serving as client advocates and consultants regarding the use of health care facilities and professionals.
3. Joining as members and sharing information as a peer. (The nurse in this role must take care not to try to take over.)

Resnick[63] adds the possible nursing contributions of serving as group facilitator, providing training in group leadership, or assisting with specific projects such as the establishment of a telephone hot line.

Although many self-help groups are suspicious of professionals, the nurse who offers assistance sincerely and follows through reliably will probably be accepted. Many health professionals who have personal health problems have joined self-help groups. They are in a uniquely advantageous position to assist clients and families to use the system to their advantage. They also have many opportunities to effect change within the system to make it more responsive to the needs of consumers.

The advocacy role of the nurse

The discussion on self-help groups has pointed out that consumers of the health care system want and need assistance in dealing with the system. If this help is not provided by professionals, clients will find other ways to get it. Although it may be advantageous for consumers to be actively involved in modifying the system to meet their needs, this does not relieve the nurse of the responsibility to be as responsive as possible to the client's needs.

Kohnke[46] has identified a number of interrelated areas of knowledge that are relevant to advocacy. These include "informing and supporting, systems analysis, social ethics, ethics, issues, the medical-industrial complex, social laws, politics, professional education and professional practice."[46] The diversity of these topics emphasizes the complexity of advocacy.

Informing and supporting Informing and supporting are the nursing actions that are central to the advocate role. When carrying out these actions, the nurse will be able to apply theoretic concepts from the other sections of this book. Advocacy should take place within the framework of the nursing process, based on the client's needs, with a statement of the nursing diagnosis and mutually planned goals, implemented with consideration for the client's individuality and evaluated continuously.

Self-knowledge is essential for the nurse-advocate. It is important to be certain at all times that the client's needs are the focus of the plan of care. Without introspection the nurse may inadvertently advocate for the client based on her interpretation of what her own needs would be in the client's situation. Understanding of the client's psychosocial development level and sense of self is also essential for effective advocacy.

Lund[53] has described a situation in which an elderly man who had recently been admitted to a nursing home was refusing his medication. Efforts to persuade him to take medicine and to teach him about it were unsuccessful. However, when a nurse asked him the reason for refusing, he described unpleasant side effects that were interfering with his daily routine. The nurse was able to advocate for the client with the doctor, who agreed to modify the medication orders according to the client's wishes.

The gentleman then took his medicine without any objections.

Informing the client to facilitate decision making requires good communication skills. The nurse must assess the knowledge that the client already has, ascertaining the extent of his knowledge, understanding of the facts he remembers, and the source of the information. It is important to explore whether the client wants any more information. An apparent lack of understanding may represent the client's coping mechanism in response to increased anxiety. Constant validation is necessary so that the nurse is in tune with the client's feelings. Therapeutic relationship concepts should be applied to assist the client to maintain control of the situation by receiving information at a manageable pace. The nurse must be aware of the client's level of stress and plan interventions accordingly.

Stress may be increased for both the client and the nurse when a third party such as a family member or physician does not want information shared with the client. This situation frequently arises when the client's condition is irreversible or terminal. This problem is illustrated by the Clinical Example below.

This situation represents a common ethical dilemma related to advocacy. Both of the B.'s had legitimate needs that were in conflict. At first the health care staff took sides and attempted to advocate the position of either the client or his wife. In reality a positive solution had to meet the needs of both individuals, because they were both profoundly affected by Mr. B.'s injury. An antagonistic attitude toward Ms. B. would risk the loss of Mr. B.'s most significant support person. On the other hand, total evasion of Mr. B.'s concerns would frustrate his need to be in control of his situation and possibly even result in his becoming depressed. This staff resolved the problem in a positive manner by implementing the team model of advocacy. Assigning a staff member to work specifically with Ms. B. was a critical decision. She was then encouraged to discuss her

CLINICAL EXAMPLE

M*r. B. was a 29-year-old police officer who had received a gunshot wound to the back while investigating a domestic dispute. The bullet severed his spinal cord at the level of L1. Following surgery his wound healed rapidly. Mr. B.'s wife refused to believe that he would be paraplegic. She insisted that he would recover if he received the right diet and exercise therapy. Ms. B. brought food and vitamin supplements to the hospital for her husband and insisted that he should not be told his prognosis.*

Very early in the recovery process Mr. B. began to ask the nursing staff whether he would be able to walk again. He said that he had recognized ever since he entered the police academy that he could be seriously injured or killed but that he wanted to be a policeman despite the danger. He added that he was relieved to be alive but wanted to know what his future would be.

The nursing staff was divided concerning the resolution of this problem. Some felt that Ms. B. was right and that Mr. B.'s hopeful attitude would disintegrate if he was confronted with reality. Others believed that Ms. B. was responding to her own need to deny Mr. B.'s illness and

that he would experience less stress if fully informed. Mr. B.'s physician was a person who generally tried to avoid conflict. He was inclined to support the wife, because she expressed her wishes more vehemently than Mr. B.

An interdisciplinary team conference was held to discuss the issue. It was decided that Ms. B.'s need to deal with her feelings about her husband's injury was the major client care problem. The charge nurse on the evening shift had established a trusting relationship with Ms. B., and she was assigned to meet with her each evening she worked to allow Ms. B. to express her feelings and ultimately to accept reality.

Meanwhile Mr. B. was to be encouraged by the physical therapist to whom he related most freely to explore his feelings and to consider his future alternatives. Other staff would support the efforts of the nurse and the physical therapist. The goal was that by the time of Mr. B.'s discharge from the hospital a meeting would take place including Mr. and Ms. B., Ms. B.'s nurse, Mr. B.'s physical therapist, and Mr. B.'s physician, at which time Mr. B.'s prognosis would be discussed.

feelings and received recognition that her husband's loss was hers as well.

The staff in this example agreed on a plan relatively easily. Frequently conflicts of this nature are much more difficult to resolve. Each situation must be addressed individually. However, whatever plan is developed, it is extremely important that all of the individuals involved in the situation be included in the planning process. This includes the interdisciplinary team, client, and significant others. Several discussions may be required and compromise necessary before a decision is reached.

CRITICAL THINKING *Question* ··············

Staff conflicts about providing information to clients create a challenge for the nurse. When the client is terminally ill, individual feelings about death often affect staff beliefs. In addition, family members may request that the client not be told the prognosis. How do the advocacy nursing actions of informing and supporting apply to a situation of this type?

What should be done if a team decision is made but the nurse who is acting as a client advocate disagrees? At this point it is usually wise for the nurse to meet with an objective person who is not directly involved in the conflict. If the nurse is a member of a peer-review group, this would be a good forum to review the situation. A nurse-mentor can be very helpful as a resource when one needs to review a nursing plan. It is important to recognize that the nurse could be responding sympathetically rather than empathetically. Personal experiences and feelings can influence one's view of a situation. A strong emotional response to a decision made by others can be a signal that one needs to examine the reason for that response.

Referral Advocacy can be risky for the nurse. Each nurse must weigh the potential costs of advocating an unpopular position against the advantages that could result from successfully informing the client and supporting his decision. If the nurse objectively assesses that the cost of a potential conflict would be greater than the advantage to be obtained, it is legitimate to decide not to be an advocate. However, if this is the case, it is recommended that this decision and rationale be shared with the client. This additional information could change the decision. If it does not, the client should have the option of seeking another advocate. At times the nurse may refer the client to another health care provider who seems to be better able to represent the client's cause. Referral then becomes an indirect type of advocacy.

Use of referral is illustrated in the Clinical Example below.

Risk reduction Kohnke[46] has suggested ways that the nurse might avoid or at least minimize the risks associated with advocacy. The first is to be well informed. To carry out adequately the responsibility of informing the client, the nurse must possess the necessary knowledge. This requires openness to new ideas and active pursuit of continuing education.

Second, the nurse must resist the temptation to be a rescuer. It may be tempting to make a decision for a client and then urge others to accept that decision. Some clients are very ambivalent about their problems, vacillating between alternative decisions. The nurse needs patience to assist the client to explore the alternatives and make his own decisions.

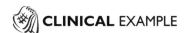 **CLINICAL** EXAMPLE

A *nurse who was bathing a client noticed a rash on his torso. She asked him about the onset and characteristics of the rash. Based on her assessment, including information gathered in the nursing shift report, she suspected that the rash could be related to a medication change. She reported her observation to the client's physician, who disagreed with her assessment. The nurse discussed the situation with the clinical pharmacist. They decided that the pharmacist would inform the client about the medication and its side effects, which included allergic reactions such as rashes. Once informed the client refused the medication. The nurse then supported the client in his right by informing the physician that the client had refused to take his medication. The pharmacist also met with the physician to express his concern that the client could be allergic to the medication and to suggest alternatives. The physician then agreed to prescribe another medication. Thus the nurse carried out part of her advocacy responsibility by enlisting the assistance of another advocate.*

The decision-making process should be a learning experience for the client whether success or failure results. If the nurse makes a decision that fails, the client learns that that nurse is not a good decision maker. If he is responsible for his own inadequate decision, he learns that another solution to that particular problem must be devised.

Similar to the avoidance of rescuing is the caution that nurses not become involved in the interpersonal games of others. One of these games is described in the discussion of transactional analysis in Chapter 5. Games are indirect communication patterns that allow individuals to avoid confronting difficult situations, thus alleviating anxiety. Much pressure may be exerted on the nurse to join the game, with the players thereby continuing to circumvent the problem on a superficial level. However, the basic dilemma continues. The client who rejects authentic communication by playing interpersonal games is unable to acquire the information needed to make a decision and is stuck with the problem. It is the nurse's responsibility to use therapeutic relationship skills to enable the client to accept the needed information. Therefore the development of good communication skills also assists the nurse to avoid risks.

Communication and knowledge of the goals of others also help the nurse to deal effectively with the larger system of which she and the client are a part. A good advocate must be able to support the client's rights effectively. It is possible to hinder the client's efforts by failing to use good interpersonal skills when interacting with other health care providers or the client's significant others. For this reason the nurse must try to approach others objectively and assertively rather than emotionally. Otherwise she risks being labeled as overinvolved or unprofessional. This response is not helpful to the client or the nurse.

Sometimes when a nurse encounters resistance it is because the unmentioned goals of the other person have not been assessed. Assuming that goals regarding a client's care are shared by the family and the rest of the health care team can be dangerous. For instance, a client who is hospitalized for an exacerbation of a chronic illness may look forward to returning home. However, the family may feel that

 CULTURAL CONSIDERATIONS

Successful advocacy with other health care providers also requires sensitivity to the cultural expectations of one's colleagues. Members of other health care disciplines may have expectations of nurses based on their own past experiences or cultural stereotypes. The nurse needs to be aware that these expectations can affect the other person's response, especially if the nurse is assertively pursuing an issue on behalf of a client. Similarly, gender role expectations often influence communications and may affect one's advocacy efforts. Most cultures define roles for men and women. If a nurse of either gender is behaving in a way that seems strange or inappropriate to a co-worker, that person is less likely to understand and accept the nurse's message. It is important to understand that most people are not aware that their response is being affected by cultural influences. Becoming annoyed at the individual's response to oneself only adds another barrier to communication. When a nurse encounters a negative response from a colleague, it can be helpful to learn more about that person and how he or she experienced the nurse's message.

they have exhausted their resources and may instead be exploring a referral to a nursing home. If the nurse neglects to explore the family's goals, she could be received with great resistance on approaching them to discuss arrangements for the client's care at home.

Ethical and legal considerations Ethical and legal considerations are also important for the nurse to consider. Both the client and the larger health care system operate within stated and unstated codes of ethics. Violation of these codes is generally met with suspicion and hostility. In addition, the nurse must be aware of her own ethical position and assess whether the client's decision is one that she can support. For example, a nurse was caring for a terminally ill client who was strongly opposed to any efforts to resuscitate him in the event of cardiac arrest. The nurse was equally committed to the use of all available means to prolong life. She discussed her values conflict concerning this client with the head nurse. Recognizing that both points of view were valid and important to the individual, the head nurse assigned another nurse to that client. Application of the values clarification process presented in Chapter 6 will assist the nurse to become aware of her own ethical positions.

Legal risks should always be considered by the nurse who plans to assume an advocacy role. It is essential to be aware of the parameters of the nurse practice act of the state in which the nurse is licensed. Licensure laws provide guidelines concerning the activities that are expected of the nurse as well as those that are prohibited. In addition, the licensure laws for other disciplines define areas where nurses may not practice. For instance, most nurses may not prescribe medication; however, in many states nurse specialists in advanced practice may. Other laws may establish requirements for client care and in particular define the rights of clients. A nurse who advocates for a client's rights as defined by law is generally operating from a strong position. If the nurse is aware of gaps in the law that hinder advocacy efforts, she should consider taking action to have laws changed or to get a new law passed. Therefore knowledge of the political process can also be of assistance in minimizing the risks of advocacy.

Nurses and clients can join together in the political process to influence the initiation of positive change in the health care system. Coalitions between consumer advocacy organizations (including self-help groups and professional nursing organizations) can be very effective in communicating with legislators and health care policy-makers.

Chalich and Smith[15] have noted that nurses often become politically active when they respond to health issues in their local communities. They have identified a ladder of political involvement. The steps are 1) civic involvement, 2) advocacy, 3) organizing, and 4) long-term power wielding. Nurses' advocacy skills can assist them to move into positions of influence where they can affect the direction of the health care system.

Nurses need to listen carefully to the criticisms of the existing system as stated by individual consumers and groups. They are frequently the same as those that nurses discuss with each other. Collaborative efforts between nurses and consumers are certain to have considerable impact on the health care system. Nurses who are able to think creatively can find powerful allies in consumer groups. It is time to explore and exploit this source of power and pursue positive change in health care delivery.

HOLISTIC HEALTH

The partnerships between consumers and health care providers is especially evident in the arena of collaborative approaches to health care and health promotion. Annually, billions of dollars are spent by consumers for services that can be described as holistic health care. The traditional allopathic medical care system developed around a focus of curing illness and dysfunction; alternative approaches to health promotion, facilitating optimal functioning and prevention, readily fall within the domain of nursing. As such, nursing practice based on a holistic philosophy best meets the needs of the client.

Holistic health is a term used to describe a state of well-being in which each individual's human potential is promoted so the person's unique and unlimited dynamic nature is affirmed.[34] Each person is encouraged to strive for a balanced integration of all aspects of life. The holistic state is more than the absence of illness; it is an ongoing, positive force for experiencing life. There is an associated attitude of self-control, assuredness, and a positive outlook. Emphasis is placed on personally defined, successful adaptation. A realistic, objective outlook is fostered concerning the influences of life stress and available alternatives for adjusting.[72]

The nursing process can facilitate the holistic approach, because health promotion must follow an organized format for data collection, planning, implementing, and evaluating endeavors. It is appropriate to assess stress reactivity, stressors, and usual coping strategies to identify the alternatives that might assist the person to effectively deal with stressors that have been identified.

As the individual becomes familiar with personal responses, adjustment is likely to be more adaptive. The person may be able to alter some situations and directly influence the meanings attached to them. It may be possible to reduce the amount of stress. This shifting about of situations and interactions is called *social engineering.* If attending a weekly dinner at the in-law's house is identified as a stressor, changing the frequency or the location of the event might be useful. Inviting the in-laws to dinner at one's own house can provide an increased sense of security and control analogous to having "the home-team advantage."

Psychotherapeutic modalities may assist in changing the meaning attached to the event. If eating at the in-law's house reactivates unresolved childhood stresses or is identified as a sign of overdependence or disloyalty on the part of one's spouse, the situation will always be somewhat disruptive. Assisting the person to objectively examine value-laden stimuli serves to limit stress reactivity and develop strategies to neutralize its effects. Psychotherapy can facilitate changing of perceptions and reactivity.[13,40]

Of particular importance to holism is the premise that the stress response is incompatible with the relaxation response. The *relaxation response* is an innate, intricate set of psychophysiologic reactions in opposition to those produced by stress.[7] The relaxation response is trophotrophic, energy conserving, and nurturing as opposed to the ergotrophic, energy depleting stress response. Individuals can learn to initiate the relaxation response through the practice of a variety of techniques.

Physical activity and balanced *nutritional habits* minimize the influences of stress metabolites and muscle tensions that accumulate because of stress reactivity.[73] Becoming aware of one's tendencies toward chronic muscular tension and the feelings that are associated with tension and relaxation of muscles are the foundations of techniques such as deep-muscle massage, progressive neuromuscular relaxation, and applied kinesiology. Eventually it is possible to develop skill in identifying which muscles are overly tense and how to relax them. As a result one develops a much greater awareness and appreciation of one's physical attributes.

Learning to control body functions and processes may be assisted through the use of biofeedback techniques. *Biofeedback* uses instrumentation to provide the individual with an immediate indication about the nature of selected internal states and functions to promote conscious control.[29,34] During the training the person practices controlling some type of signal (auditory or visual) that is emitted from the machinery. This signal is related to the person's individual stress reactivity at that moment. Various types of equipment are available to measure muscle responses, temperature, blood flow to digits or limbs, general circulation, cardiac responses, and dermal factors such as perspiration and resistance to impulses. Regardless of the instrumentation the sense of self-mastery that develops is often generalized and serves as a motivating force.

Many individuals feel that they have little control over their lives and that events and other people cause them to feel the way they do. Through the use of cognitive processes the perception of the event can be reformed. The key to this approach is to recognize in a rational way that events can be perceived in many ways, evoking a variety of emotional responses. It is the meaning attached to the event that creates the tension. The person's thoughts about what she wants can result in her feelings. For example, if a nurse thinks "that client absolutely should not act this way," she is likely to experience anger. This thinking suggests that the nurse believes she has control over others' behavior when in fact she does not. However, she does have the ability to control her own behavior and thoughts.

The voluntary altering of distorted, unwanted, or irrational thoughts to produce different emotional reactions and reduce stress is called *cognitive reframing*. To do this the distorted thought is gently challenged, and the possibility of there being other meanings or outcomes is considered. Once the person accepts this possibility he develops a different perspective and is able to see the situation in a more positive, less stressful context.[19,34,72]

For example, the executive who is in the hospital to recuperate from a myocardial infarction may be stressed, because he feels he is responsible for his company and needs to be back at work. His notion of being solely responsible can actually have a negative effect on his recovery. The nurse can compliment him on being "able to respond" (responsible) to the needs of his company and employees. His ability to respond to the employees' need to demonstrate their potential abilities in the day-to-day functioning of the company is superior. It demonstrates a very positive attribute of a wise employer and his sense of responsibility. In doing this the notion of responsibility has been changed by the nurse to the ability to reframe. The focus of the response has been shifted from the employer "doing" to the employer "allowing his employees to do it," thus responding to one aspect of his role. In so doing the perspective of being "super" responsible has been reframed as being able to respond in a superior way without overextending oneself.

One method to assist individuals to enhance their awareness of stress reactivity and patterns of responses is the use of *self-questioning techniques.* Writing the responses to several questions can be enlightening after some brief brainstorming about how one feels and acts when stressed and what might trigger these responses. By answering the questions in the accompanying box the individual's stress profile becomes more apparent. Such self-questioning clarifies the stressor (trigger), the physical and emotional responses, the appraised meaning, and ideas about how to deal with the situation.

A modality often used in conjunction with other techniques is *mental imagery.* The person mentally creates or remembers sights, sounds, feelings, or situations and events associated with the relaxation response. This may be practiced in a relatively unstructured manner, or as in the case of *autogenic training* specific exercises related to body functions, sensations, colors, and shapes may be repeated. *Hatha yoga* uses body positions called *postures* in conjunction with controlled breathing techniques to achieve the effects of relaxation. Imagery and meditative exercises are incorporated into the more advanced positions.[7]

Self-Questioning Technique

What do I usually feel and what happens to my body when I'm stressed?

When does this usually happen?

Where am I and with whom?

What do I react to and how often do I do so?

Is it always the same person, place, thing, and time?

How do I behave after this begins and how would I describe my feelings?

What do I do to express these feelings; do I keep from expressing my true "gut reaction?"

Why do I react to this, what does it mean, what and who does it remind me of?

How would I like to change this?

What alternatives do I have?

Meditation may be used independently for the purpose of quieting psychical and body processes to restore energy resources. Through a passive attitude the person strives either to clear all thoughts from consciousness or hold one, concentrated focus to diminish extraneous energy utilization. The person tends to achieve a hypometabolic state when altered states of consciousness occur.[29]

Just as meditation allows the replenishing of energy, other modalities such as acupressure, applied kinesiology, and healing touch focus on unblocking and rebalancing energy flows throughout the person. This allows for revitalization as energy becomes unbound. The use of therapeutic touch is especially well suited to the nursing field, where touch has historically been used to convey caring while carrying out one's nursing activities. These are but a few of the modalities that can be used to reduce stress reactivity, facilitate relaxation, and promote holism.

The nurse has an important role as a holistic health practitioner in promoting the individual's optimal adaptation and development. Although this is difficult to do within the confines of the traditional medical care system, it can be incorporated into distributive health care centers. With a holistic philosophic approach the person is given the predominant role in dealing with individual stress situations. The nurse serves to assist the individual during the self-management process. In addition, with the emphasis placed on prevention of the debilitating effects of stress reactivity, the goal of promotion of high levels of health becomes more realistic.

Home Health/Community Services

The current health status of the population is challenged by long-term, chronic problems. In addition life expectancy is increasing. Many major health problems are related to lifestyles and personal choice; therefore treatment needs are directed toward an older population suffering with long-term, chronic problems.

Graham and Gleit[30] contend that as the population ages and the number of people with functional deficits increases, the need for home care services also increases. In 1989 there were 8105 home health agencies operating in the United States. This represents a 53% increase from 1986. Often the main objective of home care is client or family education.

Burbach et al.[12] use the Medicare definition of home health care, which is "intermittent skilled nursing care provided under the direction of a physician to an individual who is homebound." Definitions of home health care are often restrictive and confusing. Community health nursing is much broader than this limited definition. Edelman and Mandle[23] define community health nursing as a "synthesis of nursing practice and public health concepts applied to promoting the health of populations."

Graham and Gleit[30] list numerous teaching and training activities that home health nurses often do, but the list is not exhaustive. Many of the independent nursing activities already discussed are also pertinent to home health care. Often the nurse provides information regarding other environmental resources that are available and how to access them.

Forker and Yurchuck[26] call for community-focused, community-based nursing practice in which care relationships focus on community partnerships. Specifically, they ask for nursing education to include reforms that will prepare students for a community-focused practice. Kaiser and Rudolph[41] outline competencies that emerged in an inductive analysis research study. They identify two domains of knowledge and skills that are necessary: role socialization, which includes values and clinical practice; and knowledge skills. Competency behaviors in the socialization domain include recognizing differences in worldviews of the nurse and client and recognizing community systems and functions. Skills necessary include critical thinking, relationship skills, care management, primary care skills, and community focus skills. Outcome measures involve not only health professionals but also community members and consumers of the health services provided.

According to Dines and Cribb,[21] with the shift in the location of services to the community, there has also been a shift in focus from individual to community needs. "Given the indubitable relationship between poverty and ill health, professionals should use their abilities to convince others that health is important and can be improved through social and community programs."

Values in Health Promotion

Within the therapeutic nurse-client relationship, nurses provide clients with a chance to determine what health means to them and an opportunity to negotiate health goals. In this relationship clients have the opportunity to explore their health values. According to Gleit, a "value is learned, arises out of personal experience, forms a basis for behavior, has an internal locus of control, is held over time and is evident in a consistent pattern of behavior."

Authenticity, discussed in Chapter 3, involves exploring one's thoughts, needs, and values. Graham and Gleit[30] state that health values change over time. As new information is added the cognitive and affective quality of values may eventually change. Diet and nutrition at age 20 years may not be a value, but 20 years later nutrition and diet may be viewed by the same client as significantly more important. An individual's definition of health and illness involves values. Personal experiences (e.g., chronic, potentially debilitating conditions such as asthma and arthritis) affect an individual's value of health and definition of health and illness. Whereas a 20-year-old may define health as the absence of illness, a 70-year-old may define health as being able to care for oneself without assistance.

Health Promotion and Stages of Development

Clients' stage of development also influences their values. In Erickson's theory, discussed in Chapter 2, middle age is characterized by increased con-cern for the next generation. Productivity and cre-ativity are personal values associated with generativity. Caring for the next generation and passing along knowledge, hopes, and dreams are also important at this developmental period. Edelman and Mandle[23] discuss health promotion throughout the life span. In the middle adult age, they discuss physical changes, health patterns, and psychosocial changes, particularly those related to coping and stress.

In old age, integrity is the goal. Integrity is defined in terms of acceptance of the life cycle. Values related to the importance of humankind and connectedness to a greater force are also evident, particularly during the latter stages of development. Edelman and Mandle[23] also discuss health promotion with older adults. Physiologic processes, psychologic processes, environmental processes, and social processes are explored. The authors maintain that nurses can assist in health promotion through education, research, and practice.

Spirituality

The concept of spirituality related to health promotion spans the stages of development; however, spirituality is often associated with the mature adult in the quest for generativity and integrity. An independent nursing action is to promote the spiritual well-being of the client. Sherman[69] defines spiritual well-being as a concept that "encompasses inner peace, compassion for others and reverence for life." Smith[70] outlines tools that nurses can use to help clients explore religious or spiritual issues and to identify resources that they can use. Activities listed by Smith include basic questions to help the client focus on spiritual issues. Examples of these questions include "What are your three greatest sources of strength?" and "Do you believe in any kind of existence after this life?" Another technique described by Smith is the journey analogy. Clients are asked to describe their life as a journey. A final technique discussed is asking clients to keep a spiritual journal. In their journals they record their thoughts about religion, spirituality, life, and death.

SUMMARY

Targeted nursing intervention skills can assist clients to meet their needs at all three levels of prevention. Nurses need to develop these skills so they may be used advantageously when appropriate client care situations are encountered.

Health education is useful to all people but is absolutely essential for primary prevention. Cognitive and behavioral education theories may be applied to guide the nurse in developing health education programs. A needs assessment must be conducted so that appropriate program planning can take place. Goals of the program must be developed to meet the identified client needs. They must also be consistent with the system's philosophy and available resources. Programs should be planned to conform to the cognitive level of the learner. Nurses may need to develop special skills to provide health education to targeted populations such as children or the elderly. Program

evaluation should be directed toward measurement of goal accomplishment and client satisfaction with the educational program. Nurses should plan and implement research regarding health education in general and programs that are directed toward specific problems or populations.

Crisis intervention skills are extremely useful to nurses who work with clients who are in need of secondary prevention services. Crisis intervention is discussed in depth in Chapter 11.

Advocacy is a skill that is very useful for tertiary prevention. Frequently clients who are in contact with the health care system over long periods of time become frustrated and perceive a lack of responsiveness to their needs. By informing clients of alternatives and supporting them in their decisions nurses can assist clients to interact with the system more effectively.

Because of dissatisfaction with existing health care programs, consumers and their families have organized self-help groups. By gathering together, people have more impact on the systems and are able to advocate for their needs. Although many of these groups are skeptical about professionals, nurses may be supportive of their efforts and offer professional expertise if it is desired. Nurses who advocate for clients must be knowledgeable about health care systems, the law, ethics, and their own particular area of practice. Planned advocacy can be effective, and the risks inherent in taking a stand can be minimized.

The focus of holistic health nursing is the promotion of optimal client health. Holistic health strategies are designed to increase the client's ability to control body functions and processes.

The client population has changed from hospital-based acute care to chronic health problems and an increased population of adults, middle to old age. This has created an increase in community-based health promotion interventions. Many of these chronic problems involve personal choice; therefore a primary objective is client and family education. Clients are asked to assume more responsibility for their own care. The client's personal values regarding health, health care, and treatment are more important in this model. Values change across the life span.

Finally this chapter explored the concept of spirituality in terms of health promotion.

DISCUSSION QUESTIONS

1. Write your own definition of health education. In what ways can this definition of health education influence your relationships with clients?

2. Identify a theoretic basis for your own definition of health education.

3. Discuss how the goals of health education can change in various client situations.

4. Analyze 1 day in a clinical setting. How many times was there an opportunity to do health education? How often was health teaching actually done? Identify the obstacles that prevented the accomplishment of health education.

5. There are several differences between cognitive and behavioral approaches to learning. Outline various nursing situations in which one approach would be favored over the other and your reasons for this decision.

6. Select a clinical setting in which you would like to do health teaching. Assess the needs of the population selected. Write goals for health education and choose instructional activities to meet the identified goals.

7. Discuss how the needs of adult learners in a general population differ from those of the poor and children.

8. Plan a health education play experience for children in a particular setting.

9. Discuss the various types of information that clients need. In what situations are particular types of information most appropriate?

10. Choose any three health education topics that interest you. Decide on the appropriate instructional activities for each topic. Discuss the reasons for your choice and for not including certain methodologies.

11. Identify ways to concretely demonstrate the effectiveness of a health education program.

12. Describe independent nursing actions associated with various levels of prevention.

13. Discuss the relationship between assertiveness as presented in Chapter 7 and the role of the nurse as an advocate.

14. Select a client with whom you have worked in the clinical setting. Based on that person's nursing diagnoses plan a nursing intervention that incorporates the advocacy activities of informing or supporting.

15. Read an article on advocacy written by a nurse and another written by a member of another health care discipline. Compare and contrast the two approaches.

16. Identify and discuss one way in which a nurse might interact productively with a self-help group.

17. A 28-year-old client with quadriplegia states that he cannot continue to live because of his dissatisfaction with the quality of his life. He refuses to eat. Tube feedings are ordered, and he verbally objects to the feedings. Based on your own value system and your exploration of the laws in your state, discuss your nursing intervention in this situation.

18. Tertiary prevention is the reduction of residual impairment resulting from illness. Discuss the ways in which membership in a self-help group can be a preventive activity.

19. Analyze the relationship between membership in a self-help group and self-concept.

20. What are some of the reasons health-related values change across the life span?

21. How can the concept of spirituality be incorporated into your daily nursing practice?

EXPERIENTIAL & SIMULATED LEARNING EXERCISES

1. Health teaching exercise

PURPOSE: To demonstrate some of the differences and similarities between formal and informal health teaching.

PROCEDURE: Select any common client problem that nurses frequently encounter that requires informal health education or giving information. Define the situation and then ask the students to immediately write the informal health education that they would do in such a situation. Then ask the students to prepare a formal, structured presentation of content appropriate to the same situation, including behavioral goals to measure the effectiveness of the planned intervention.

DISCUSSION:

1. Compare and contrast:
   - Content
   - Format used
   - Effectiveness (related to goal achievement)

2. Are there some teaching methods that lend themselves easily to formal presentations and that are
   easily understood by the lay population (e.g., flip
   charts, modules, slides/tapes)?

2. *Health teaching exercise*

PURPOSE: To identify instructional needs for individuals versus groups of clients.
PROCEDURE: Divide students into small groups. Each
group is given a series of brief client problems from
various categories and developmental levels: child,
adult, poor. An example would be: Judy is a 9-year-old
recently diagnosed as having juvenile diabetes mellitus.
One student is asked to play the role of the nurse and
another the client for each problem. The nurse is
instructed to identify the learning needs of the client
and record them.
DISCUSSION: Focus on the learning needs identified
for the individual client and compare to instructional
needs for a group of clients with similar problems. How
would the teaching plan differ? Also discuss how the
nurse and client perceived and acted out the client
needs and need identification. Which needs present a
stereotype and which are individualized? Discuss ways
to avoid a stereotyped approach to need identification.

3: *Self-help group observation*

PURPOSE: To identify the goals and activities of
selected self-help groups.
PROCEDURE: Prepare a list of self-help groups in the
local community. Each student should select a group
to investigate. If possible, the student should arrange
to attend a group meeting. If not, a group member
should be interviewed. The student should explore the
group's history, goals, membership criteria, activities,
structures, and evaluation of the formal health care
system.
DISCUSSION: In small groups the students present the
data that they have collected concerning their assigned
self-help groups. Based on the information presented
they will be able to discuss the potential role of the
nurse in relationship to the group.

4: *Advocacy role play*

PURPOSE: To practice the advocacy role and receive
feedback about the effectiveness of the intervention.
PROCEDURE: Divide the students into groups of six.
Ask groups of three students to role play the following

situations. Each three-member group should role play
one situation while observed by the other group
members. One student should take the role of the
client, another the nurse, and the third another health
care team member who disagrees with the client. After
interviewing the client the nurse should advocate for
the client's decision with the other professional.
SITUATIONS:
1. A 72-year-old client with impaired mobility related
   to a fractured femur is to be transferred from the
   hospital to a nursing home based on the family's
   wishes. The client prefers to return home.
2. A 35-year-old client with chronic back pain of
   unknown cause requests a referral to an acupunc-
   turist.
3. The parents of a 7-year-old child with leukemia
   refuse a blood transfusion for religious reasons.
   (*Note:* Either the child or the parents may be designated as the clients.)
DISCUSSION: The observers should provide feedback
concerning their impressions of the nurse's success or
failure as an advocate. The following questions should
be addressed:
1. Did the nurse assess the client's position?
2. Did she provide information concerning alternatives?
3. Did she approach the other health care provider
   assertively?
4. Did she seem to be aware of her own values
   related to the situation?
5. Did she focus objectively on the client's need?
   The nurse should also discuss her feelings about the
experience. The client should critique the nurse's interpersonal skills.

5. *Imagery to assist the relaxation response*

PURPOSE: To provide an example of a holistic
modality that can be used to assist in relaxing and
coping.
PROCEDURE: Each person is invited to sit for 5 minutes in a quiet, dimly lit, undistracting setting with his
or her body well supported and limbs uncrossed. Ask
all to close their eyes and picture how they are sitting.
Instruct them that when they have an image of how
they are sitting, they are to focus their attention internally to their muscles and ask themselves if any muscles or other areas feel tight, uncomfortable, or disturbed. Allow them time to focus and suggest that as

each finds a tight area, they signal you with a raised finger. Ask them to create some image of or analogy for the tension, such as a hard lump of clay or a knot in a rope. Then using the image they are to relax the tightness (soften the clay until it is malleable and smooth, or slacken the rope so the twisted knot smooths out, loosens, lengthens). Allow a period of 10 to 15 minutes for the exercise in addition to the 5 minutes of sitting. Follow with discussion.

DISCUSSION: Ask participants to:

1. Describe their imaging for their tension.
2. Describe how they imaged the reduction of the tension.
3. Describe the general sensations of the area before, during, and after the exercise.

Discuss differences in their ability to find an image and work with it..

REFERENCES

1. Assal J: Proceedings of patient education 2000 congress in Geneva, June 1-4, 1994, *Patient Educ Couns* 26:3, 1995.
2. Balog J: The concept of health and the role of health education, *J School Health* 51:461, 1981.
3. Bandman EL, Bandman B: *Nursing ethics through the life span,* ed 2, Norwalk, Conn, 1990, Appleton & Lange.
4. Bartlet E: Cost-benefit analysis of patient education, *Patient Educ Couns* 26:87, 1995.
5. Bartlett EE: Social consumptions of social investment, *Patient Educ Couns* 7:223, 1985.
6. Beck KH: Health education research: the first six years, *Health Ed Res* 6:399, 1991.
7. Benson H, Klipper M: *The relaxation response,* New York, 1993, Wings Books.
8. Bigge ML: *Learning theory for teachers,* ed 4, New York, 1971, Harper & Row.
9. Bischof LJ: *Adult psychology,* New York, 1976, Harper & Row.
10. Botwinick J: *Aging and behavior: a comprehensive integration of research findings,* ed 3, New York, 1984, Springer-Verlag.
11. Boyd M: Policies, guidelines and legal mandates for health teaching. In Whitman N et al, editors: *Teaching in nursing practice: a professional model,* Norwalk, Conn, 1992, Appleton & Lange.
12. Burbach C et al: Issues in home health nursing education, *Home Health Care Nurse* 9:22, 1991.
12a. Butler RN et al: Self-care, self-help and the elderly, *Int J Aging Hum Dev* 10:95, 1979-80.
13. Cacioppo J, Berntson G, Anderson B: Psychophysiological approaches to the evaluation of psychotherapeutic process and outcomes, *Psychol Assess* 3:321, 1991.
14. Chaisson G: Patient education: whose responsibility is it and who should be doing it, *Nurse Admin Q* 4:1, 1980.
15. Chalich T, Smith L: Nursing at the grassroots, *Nurs Health Care* 13:342, 1992.
16. Cimprich B: A theoretical perspective on attention and patient education, *Adv Nurs Sci* 14:39, 1992.
17. Clark M: The utilization of theoretical concepts in patient education, *Nurs Admin Q* 4:55, 1980.
18. Connelly LM et al: A place to be yourself: empowerment from the client's perspective, *Image J Nurs Sch* 25:297, 1993.
19. Cox T: Organizational culture, stress and stress management, *Work Stress* 5:1, 1991.
20. Dimou N: Illness and culture: learning differences, *Patient Educ Couns* 26:153, 1995.
21. Dines A, Cribb A, editors: *Health promotion: concepts and practice,* London, 1993, Blackwell Scientific Publications.
22. Dunn MM et al: Teaching the illiterate client does not have to be a problem, *Fam Commun Health* 8:76, 1985.
23. Edelman C, Mandle C: *Health promotion throughout the lifespan,* ed 4, St Louis, 1998, Mosby.
24. Ellis L, Raines J, Hakanson N: Health education using microcomputers, *Prev Med* 11:212, 1982.
25. Fernsler JI, Cannon CA: The whys of patient education, *Semin Oncol Nurs* 7:79, 1991.
26. Forker J, Yurchuck E: Perspectives on assessment: assessing outcomes of community-based nursing education, *Nurse Educator* 21:15, 1996.
27. Frantz RA: Selecting media for patient education, *Top Clin Nurs* 2:77, 1980.
28. Gagné RM: *Essentials of learning and instruction,* ed 2, Englewood Cliffs, NJ, 1988, Prentice-Hall.
29. Girdano D, Everly G, Dusek D: *Controlling stress and tension: a holistic approach,* ed 3, Englewood Cliffs, NJ, 1990, Prentice-Hall.
30. Graham B, Gleit C: Teaching in selected settings. In Whitman N et al, editors: *Teaching in nursing practice: a professional model,* Norwalk, Conn, 1992, Appleton & Lange.
31. Greenspoon J, Foreman S: Effect of delay of results on learning a motor task, *J Exp Psych* 5 1:226, 1956.
32. Griffith H, DiGuiseppi C: Guidelines for clinical preventive services: essential for nurse practitioners in practice, education and research, *Nurs Prac* 19:25, 1994.
33. Hartfield M, Cason C, Cason G: Effects of information about threatening procedure of patients' expectations and emotional distress, *Nurs Res* 31:202, 1982.
34. Hazell J: Drivers as mediators of stress response, *Trans Anal J* 19:212, 1989.
35. Higgins L: How adequately are nurses prepared for their teaching role? *Austr J Adv Nurs* 8:11, 1991.
36. Hill D, Rossaby J, Gray N: Health education about breast cancer using television and doctor involvement, *Prev Med* 11:43, 1982.
37. Hunka CD, O'Toole AW, O'Toole R: Self-help therapy in Parents Anonymous, *J Psychosoc Nurs Mental Health Serv* 23:25, 1985.
38. Jason L, Mollica M, Ferrone L: Evaluating an early secondary smoking prevention intervention, *Prev Med* 11:96, 1982.
39. Jobes J, Straszak I, de Carafal A: Preventive medicine: getting the message across, *Dimen Health Serv* 12:28, 1981.

40. Johansson N: Effectiveness of a stress management program in reducing anxiety and depression in nursing students, *J Am Coll Health* 40:125, 1991.

41. Kaiser K, Rudolph E: In search of meaning: identifying competencies relevant to evaluation of the community health nurse generalist, *J Nurs Educ* 35:157, 1996.

42. Katz AH, Levin LS: Self-care is not a solipsistic trap: a reply to critics, *Int J Health Serv* 10:329, 1980.

43. Kendall J: Fighting back: promoting emancipatory nursing actions, *Adv Nurs Sci* 15:1, December 1992.

44. King J: The health belief model, *Nurs Times* 80:53, October 1984.

45. Klos D et al: A comparison of two methods of delivering presurgical instructions, *Patient Couns Health Ed* 2:6, 1980.

46. Kohnke MF: *Advocacy: risk and reality,* St Louis, 1982, Mosby.

47. Kolbe L, Iverson D: Implementing comprehensive health education: educational innovations and social change, *Health Ed Q* 8:57, 1981.

48. Kruger S: The patient education role on nursing, *Appl Nurs Res* 4:19, 1991.

49. Kuehnel C, Rowe B: Patient education and the adult, *Super Nurse* 11:15, 1980.

50. Kush-Goldberg C: The health self-help group as an alternative source of health care for women, *Int J Nurs Stud* 16:238, 1979.

51. Levy LH: Self-help groups: types and psychological processes, *J Appl Behav Sci* 12:310, 1976.

52. Lipetz MJ et al: What is wrong with patient education programs? *Nurs Outlook* 38:184, 1990.

53. Lund M: The heart of the matter, *Am J Nurs* 92(4):22, 1992.

54. Milde FK, Heim CL: Competence to provide health education: perception of nursing students and faculty, *J Nurs Educ* 30:397, 1991.

55. Minkler M: Health education, health promotion, and the open society: a historical perspective, *Health Ed Q* 16:17, 1991.

56. Mitty EL: The nurse as advocate: issues in long term care, *Nurs Health Care* 12:520, 1991.

57. Newton G: Self-help groups: can they help? *J Psychosoc Nurs Mental Health Serv* 22:27, July 1984.

58. Nowakowski L: Health promotion: self-care programs for the community, *Top Clin Nurs* 2:21, 1980.

59. Osherson N, Markman E: Language and the ability to evaluate contradictions and tautologies, *Cognition* 3:213, 1975.

60. Padilla GV, Bulcavage LM: Theories used in patient/health education, *Semin Oncol Nurs* 7:87, 1991.

61. Payton O, Ivey A: The role of psychoeducation in allied health practice and education, *J Allied Health* 10:91, 1981.

62. Poston I: How to develop computer assisted instruction programs, *Nurs Health Care* 14:344, 1993.

63. Resnick WM: Nursing and the voluntary association: origin, development and collaboration, *Nurs Clin North Am* 21:515, 1986.

64. Rice M, Valdivia L: A simple guide for design, use and evaluation of educational materials, *Health Ed Q* 18:79, 1991.

65. Riessman F: How does self-help work? *Soc Pol* 7:41, September-October 1976.

66. Ross CK: Factors influencing successful health education, *Health Educ Q* 8:187, 1981.

67. Ryan ER: Viewing health education with in the framework of the consumer's personal value system, *Nurs Forum* 23:60, 1987.

68. Shadick K: Development of a transcultural health education program for the Hmong, *Clin Nurs Spec* 7:48, 1993.

69. Sherman K: *Communication and image in nursing,* Albany, 1994, Delmar Publishers Inc.

70. Smith D: Exploring the religious-spiritual needs of the dying, *Couns Values* 37:71, 1993.

71. Sosin M, Caulum S: Advocacy: a conceptualization for social work practice, *Soc Work* 28:12, 1983.

72. Stachnik T et al: Goal setting, social support and financial incentives in stress management programs: a pilot study of their impact on adherence, *Am J Health Promotion* 5:24, 1990.

73. Sutherland V, Cooper C: Exercise and stress management: fit employees, healthy organizations? *Int J Sport Psychol* 21:202, 1990.

74. Tattersall R: Patient education 2000: take-home message from this congress, *Patient Educ Couns* 26:373, 1995.

75. Troll LE: *Early and middle adulthood,* Monterey, Calif, 1975, Brooks/Cole Publishing.

76. Tu K, Gay JT, McKay J: Undergraduate clinical experience in health education, *J Nurs Ed* 30:235, 1991.

77. Van Reenen J: Technology for health care education, *The Canadian Nurse* 24, 1990.

78. Wallerstein N, Bernstein E: Empowerment education: Freire's ideas adapted to health education, *Health Ed Q* 15:379, 1988.

79. Wilcox S, Palermo DS: "In, on and under" revisited, *Cognition* 3:245, 1975.

80. Windsor RA et al: Evaluation of the efficacy and cost effectiveness of health education methods to increase medication adherence among adults with asthma, *Am J Public Health* 80:1519, 1990.

81. Zonca B: The role of the patient education coordinator, *Super Nurse* 11:21, 1980.

Suggested Readings

Bartlett EE: Historical glimpses of patient education in the United States, *Patient Ed Couns* 8:135, 1986.

> *This comprehensive article traces the historical growth of client education from the formative era through the contemporary period. It includes information on prehistoric health education.*

Batnett J, Clark J, editors: *Research in health promotion and nursing,* London, 1993, MacMillan Press.

> *Excellent comprehensive text that examines the theoretical basis of health promotion and nursing implications. The role of the nurse in health promotion and promoting healthy lifestyles is discussed. Conclusions and results from numerous research studies are presented.*

Boschma G: The meaning of holism in nursing: historical shifts in holistic nursing ideas, *Public Health Nurs* 11 (5):324, 1995.

This article provides a historical overview of the evolution of holistic nursing, from the early part of the twentieth century to the present holistic health nursing model, as well as conceptual analyses.

Butler RN et al: Self-care, self-help and the elderly, *Int J Aging Hum Dev* 10:95, 1979-80.

This article provides a wealth of information about consumer activism in health care. It compares self-help and self-care, reviews relevant literature, and raises research questions. In particular the authors discuss the pertinence of self-care and self-help approaches for the elderly.

Canobbio M, Day M: The role of the clinical specialist in an adult congenital heart disease program, *Nurs Clin North Am,* 29:357, 1994.

This article discusses the role of the clinical nurse specialist, which includes education of the client, family, and nursing staff. The authors also outline selected issues associated with handling chronic illness.

Cassidy C: Social science theory and methods in the study of alternative and complimentary medicine, *J Altern Compl Med* 1(1):19, 1994.

The advanced learner will benefit from this theoretic article that reviews the sociologic and anthropologic foundations of the movement to more holistic-focused complimentary and alternative approaches to traditional allopathic care.

Edelman C, Mandle C: *Health promotion throughout the lifespan,* ed 4, St Louis, 1998, Mosby.

This comprehensive text examines health promotion through the assessment and intervention steps of the nursing process. Health promotion at various stages of the life cycle is explored.

Fortmann S et al: Effect of health education on dietary behavior: the Stanford three community study, *Am J Clin Nutr* 34:2030, 1981.

Report of a 3-year study to change dietary behaviors in two California communities. Encouraging results reported.

Foster C: The use of transactional analysis in patient teaching, *Super Nurse* 12:18, 1981.

Adult-to-adult relationship described as the only economically feasible relationship in modern health care system. Adult-to-adult relationship requires an acceptance of the client's responsibility for his own care.

Frantz RA: Selecting media for patient education, *Top Clin Nurs* 2:77, 1980.

The focus of this article is the selection of the proper media for a particular client. It includes examining the characteristics of the task, media, and learner.

Golland L: How to help patients relax, *Patient Care* 14:138, 1980.

Describes how to teach clients many current relaxation techniques. Includes a discussion of various personality types and the techniques most effective with each type.

Gordon SE: Long-term care sets the stage for student practicums, *Nurs Health Care* 7:85, 1986.

The author describes a clinical experience for registered nurse students that focuses on the advocacy role as a way of teaching change agent and leadership skills. Her frank discussion of successes and problems would be helpful to other faculty who are considering a similar clinical experience for students.

Huckabay L: A strategy for patient teaching, *Nurs Admin Q* 4:47, 1980.

The focus of this article is Glaser's model of instruction.

Hunka CD, O'Toole AW, O'Toole R: Self-help therapy in Parents Anonymous, *J Psychosoc Nurs Ment Health Serv* 23:25, July 1985.

This article reports on a study of the effectiveness of a self-help group, Parents Anonymous, in decreasing the occurrence of child abuse. The authors also describe the role of "sponsor," a professional advisory position that they believe could be filled by a nurse.

Kleiman MA, Mantell JE, Alexander ES: Collaboration and its discontents: the perils of partnership, *J Appl Behav Sci* 12:403, 1976.

The authors document the life history of Can-Cervive, a self-help group developed for people with a medical diagnosis of cancer. In particular they examine the ramifications of efforts at professional involvement in a self-help program.

Kohnke MF: *Advocacy: risk and reality,* St Louis, 1982, Mosby.

This book is unique in its attention to advocacy as an emerging role for nurses. The author analyzes the elements of advocacy at the levels of the client and the health care system. She also discusses the potential risks involved and suggests ways to minimize them.

Lusby RA, Ingman SB: The pros, cons and pitfalls of "self-help" rehabilitation programs, *Soc Sci Med* 13A:113, 1979.

This article provides an excellent documentation of the developmental process of a self-help group. It raises the provocative question, "Must a self-help group be professionalized to compete for resources with traditional programs?" They also discuss issues related to bureaucracies and to charismatic leadership.

McGuire WJ: Behavioral medicine, public health, and communication theories, *Health Ed* 12:8, 1981.

Excellent health education article describing seven steps in creating media campaigns for health education. Contends that people from numerous disciplines, such as epidemiologists, cognitive and social psychologists, and evaluation technicians, must work together to create a successful campaign.

Napalkov N: The role of the World Health Organization in promoting patient education with emphasis on chronic diseases, *Patient Educ Couns* 28:5, 1995.

This article discusses the global public health shift in priorities from infectious disease to noncommunicable diseases. Lifestyle and environmental conditions are often major contributing factors. The role of the individual is emphasized.

Newton G: Self-help groups: can they help? *J Psychosoc Nurs Ment Health Serv* 22:27, July 1984.

This article provides useful criteria to be considered when referring a client to a self-help group. The author also presents several alternative approaches to be considered if the self-help group is determined to be unacceptable.

Price JH: Most frequently cited health education articles, *J School Health* 50:408, 1980.

By using the Social Science Citation Index (SSCI) the author located the major sources of information on health education. Oldest cited articles were in 1966, thus showing how young the field is.

Rankin SH, Stallings KD: *Patient education issues: principles and practices,* ed 2, Philadelphia, 1990, JB Lippincott.

This is an excellent textbook that covers all aspects of health education. It is based on the nursing process. There are chapters on theories of health education, legal and ethical issues in health education, and health education research. There is also a chapter on specific problems encountered in health education, such as ways to motivate clients.

Redman BK: New areas of theory development and practice in patient education, *J Adv Nurs* 10:425, 1985.

The author discusses the social psychology concept of self-efficacy and its relationship to health education. Self-efficacy is the client's belief in his/her ability to perform necessary behavior.

Resnick WM: Nursing and the voluntary association: origin, development, and collaboration, *Nurs Clin North Am* 21:515, 1986.

The author focuses on the roles that the nurse can play in relationship to self-help groups. The discussion is enhanced by the description of the evolution of the Depression and Related Affective Disorders Association (DRADA), assisting the reader to understand the relevance of the principles that are presented.

Sosin M, Caulum S: Advocacy: a conceptualization for social work practice, *Soc Work* 28:12, 1983.

This article is of interest to nurses because it allows comparison with the approach taken to advocacy by another helping profession. The authors present a thought-provoking model for advocacy as conceptualized by social workers.

Steinman R, Traunstein DM: Redefining deviance: the self-help challenge to the human services, *J Appl Behav Sci* 12:347, 1976.

The authors present their research on the characteristics of self-help groups as compared with additional human service agencies. They concluded that self-help groups demonstrate a higher degree of autonomy and solidarity when compared with the professionalism and bureaucracies of traditional agencies.

Syred MJ: The abdication of the role of health educator by hospital nurses, *J Adv Nurs* 6:27, 1981.

Explores use of health belief model as a framework for health education. Basic premise is that health motivation is the key in the health belief model because it is a reflection of deep-seated values interacting with basic drives.

Tilley JD, Gregor FM, Theissen V: The nurse's role in patient education: incongruent perceptions among nurses and patients, *J Adv Nurs* 12:291, 1987.

This is a report of a research study investigating the congruence between nurse and client perception of the nurse's role in health education. Results show that incongruencies exist. The authors call for a clear definition of the role.

CHAPTER

11

Crisis Intervention

....

I tried to pretend I was a fairy princess
Who never had to feel pain or loss or sorrow.
Almost too late I learned that not to feel the bad
  meant not to feel
The sunshine on my flesh, the happiness of life.
I'd rather feel the good and bad
  than nothingness.

Ann Carmel

LEARNING OBJECTIVES

After studying this chapter, the student should be able to:

- Discuss the relationship between crisis intervention, secondary prevention, and stress.
- Identify the factors that contribute to the development of a crisis.
- Give examples of situational and maturational crises and describe appropriate nursing actions.
- Compare and contrast techniques of crisis intervention as proposed by three theorists.
- Discuss the impact of a crisis event on a client's family.
- Identify clinical situations in which crisis intervention may be applied.

Crisis intervention is a primary nursing function. Nurses are constantly confronted with situations that require crisis intervention techniques.

Chapter 9 deals with stress and the individual's response to stressors. Both stress and crisis result in imbalance. Melichar[24] differentiates the stress state from the crisis state. The individual in a state of stress can exist for a relatively long period of time. Stress can be handled to some degree by coping mechanisms. In contrast, a crisis state is a relatively short, self-limited period of time (4 to 6 weeks) and interferes with important life goals.

It is important to understand the concepts associated with stress before discussing crisis content, because crisis builds on stress. Crisis in fact is the result of stress that the individual is not able to cope with and thus alleviate. There is an increased emphasis on methods of dealing with stress and crisis today, because Western industrialized societies produce substantial amounts of stress. Johnson[15] believes that changes in modern society, values, our physical environment, and our personal lives all produce increased levels of stress. Johnson contends that all change, whether it be a positive or negative change, results in psychologic feelings of loss. For instance, when an individual is promoted to a management position, there is a feeling of psychologic loss. It may be loss of the familiar or loss because expectations of others or relationships may change. According to Johnson the basic formula for change is:

$$\text{change} = \text{loss}$$
$$\text{loss} = \text{anger}$$
$$\text{anger (turned inward)} = \text{depression}$$

Table 9-1 in Chapter 9 is a social readjustment rating scale. The table reflects the change produced by various life events such as marriage, birth of a child, or moving. These events are normal occurrences in that they occur regularly in many people's lives. Any compilation of recent United States statistics points out how common these relatively major life events are. For instance, in 1993, 4,039,000 babies were born. In the same year 2,334,000 marriages and 1,187,000 divorces were recorded. Between 1991 and 1992, 247,380,000 people reported a change of residence.[34]

Children's ratings of stressful experiences have also been compiled. Children perceive events such as bad grades, wetting in class, and being sent to the principal as stressful events. They also include events such as the death of a parent, parental fights, and surgery as stress-producing events in their world. All members of society are touched by stress.[15]

The terms *stress* and *crisis* have negative connotations to most people, as if they were things to avoid at any cost. However, there are positive aspects to stress and crisis. Ballou[4] believes that out of the crisis situation there is a potential for further growth. Growth potential increases during a crisis, and intervention at that time may have a greater impact and be more beneficial to the individual. Although stress and crisis produce discomfort, that discomfort may enable the individual to make changes that are beneficial.

CRISIS INTERVENTION

Crisis intervention is related to primary, secondary, and tertiary levels of prevention. Narayan and Joslin[26] state that Lindemann's early work with crisis intervention theory was based on a belief that crisis intervention could prevent mental illness. Therefore crisis intervention was an important aspect of primary prevention.

Crisis intervention is probably most often associated with a secondary level of prevention, shortening the duration of the existing problem with early diagnosis and treatment. Some well-known examples of secondary prevention are suicide prevention centers and crisis hot lines for telephone crisis services.

Crisis intervention is also used in tertiary prevention, such as crisis services for chronic psychiatric clients and crisis intervention anticipatory planning for individuals in long-term, stressful situations.

Nurses are often involved with clients in crisis situations. A few examples are in the newborn nursery working with premature infants or unwanted infants; in well-baby clinics working with a possible hearing-impaired infant or abused children; in the hospital emergency room caring for accident victims, rape victims, and their families; or in community health working with recent single-parent families or families that have recently moved to a new town. Hospitalization itself often creates a crisis situation. Taylor[32] expresses the prevailing attitude toward crisis skills. Although it is generally accepted that the development of full expertise in crisis skills is best achieved at the graduate level, the reality is that on a daily basis nurses are exposed to crisis situations that demand a minimum level of skill.

Because nurses have so many contacts with crisis situations or potential crisis situations it is imperative for nurses to be able to recognize signs of stress, identify the coping mechanisms being used by the individual, assess the degree of success the individual is experiencing using these coping mechanisms, and intervene when necessary.

The concept of crisis intervention explored

"Crisis is defined as a response to external or internal stress which cannot be managed by the usual coping mechanisms of the person stressed."[22] According to Hill[14] three factors lead to crisis:

1. The actual precipitating events causing the crisis
2. The individual's resources available to meet the crisis
3. The individual's definition of the problem

Balancing factors Crisis occurs within a social context and is influenced by both social and individual factors. An example follows:

Ms. K. is an 80-year-old widow living alone. Her pet poodle of 20 years has just died. The poodle dying is an external stress for Ms. K. She is in crisis, because she is unable to cope with this event. Ms. K. does not have external resources available. Her husband and sisters are dead. Her two children live out of state. All of her close friends are either dead or have moved to other areas of the country. Ms. K. perceives her pet's death as the final desertion of all of her close contacts. She refuses to bury the dog or have it removed from her apartment. She is not going out, eating, or sleeping well. She is crying and spending the day sitting in a chair gazing at her dead dog. Ms. K. is in a crisis state.

For another person the same precipitating event may cause sadness or distress but would not lead to a crisis because of social supports available or perception of the event.

Aguilera and Messick[1] refer to these factors, perception of the event and situational supports, as balancing factors. In addition, they discuss coping mechanisms as outlined in Chapter 9 as additional balancing factors. When these balancing factors are present, the individual is able to alleviate the stress and avoid a crisis state.

How an individual perceives an event depends on various factors. Some of these mediating factors are the pattern organization of the individual or his habitual way of responding, the cultural background

🌐 **CULTURAL** CONSIDERATIONS

Weaver and Wodarski[35] discuss the importance of cultural differences in understanding a client's response in a crisis situation. The authors state that culture influences values and beliefs. Culture also affects the client's usual mechanisms for dealing with stress, the nurse-client relationship, and crisis resolution. Consequently, the authors believe that culture helps determine what a client identifies as a problem, what the client believes about the origins of the problem, how the client plans to resolve the problem, and the resources that the client believes are appropriate to assist in solving the problem. Weaver and Wodarski[35] recommend the following guidelines in crisis intervention: (1) be familiar with the client's cultural group; (2) be aware of personal cultural influences and their effect on the nurse-client relationship; and (3) use crisis intervention techniques that are based on a thorough assessment, including a cultural assessment.

of the individual, and various personality factors, such as level of self-esteem, self-concept, and body image.

Phases of crises Aguilera and Messick[1] list four developmental phases in a crisis as described by Caplan[7]:

1. There is an initial rise in tension as habitual problem-solving techniques are tried.
2. There is a lack of success in coping as the stimulus continues and more discomfort is felt.
3. A further increase in tension acts as a powerful internal stimulus and mobilizes internal and external resources. In this stage, emergency problem-solving mechanisms are tried. The problem may be redefined, or there may be resignation and the giving up of certain aspects of the goal as unattainable.
4. If the problem continues and cannot be solved or avoided, tension increases and a major disorganization occurs.

Crisis intervention is a therapeutic treatment to bring about psychologic resolution of the immediate crisis. Crisis intervention is a here-and-now treatment modality focusing on a particular precipitating event. Its goal is to restore the individual to the same level of functioning as before the crisis. In the preceding example intervention would focus on the immediate problem: the death of Ms. K's pet dog.

Types of crises Aguilera and Messick divide crisis into two broad categories: *situational* and *maturational*. Situational crises depend on a stressful external event such as the birth of a premature infant, divorce, rape, or physical illness. Maturational crises are associated with the problems of predictable developmental changes throughout the life cycle.

Lipkin and Cohen[23] discuss various maturational crises. College is an example of a maturational crisis. "The higher rate of suicide among college students is an indication of their inability to cope with the many problems that are present on the campus." Pregnancy is another example of a maturational crisis. "Even the wanted, planned pregnancy leads to some emotional turmoil" according to the authors. Pregnancy represents increased responsibility and unclear role changes. Lipkin and Cohen[23] also discuss homelessness and alternative lifestyles as maturational crises.

The maturational crises are based on Erickson's stages of development discussed in Chapter 2.[2] Baldwin outlines six general types of crisis and suggestions for intervention strategies.[3] His categories are:

1. *Dispositional crisis.* Distress from problems that require nonemotional information or tangible service. Some examples of dispositional crises are providing information to family members about local treatment centers for an alcoholic relative or referring a widow to a discussion group for women who have recently lost a spouse. Baldwin states that at this level many paraprofessionally staffed crisis referral services function well.

   The nurse's role in dealing with dispositional crisis is an example of primary prevention. The nurse makes referrals, provides needed information, or takes some manipulative environmental action to meet the presenting problem. Two potential problems that must be anticipated are (1) the client is making an indirect request for help on another level that he cannot acknowledge directly, or (2) there are serious implications in this crisis situation that may affect the client's later emotional functioning. For instance, Nurse T works in a crisis center. A young woman who is 8 weeks pregnant and new in town asks for a medical referral for an abortion. If this is not explored and the nurse is not attuned to the possibility of future problems, just providing the name of a clinic or medical facility may have deleterious effects for this young woman in the future.

2. *Crises of anticipated life transition.* Baldwin defines this category as "crises that reflect anticipated, but usually normative, life transitions over which the client may or may not have substantial control."[3] Examples are midlife crises, marriage and divorce, career changes, and terminal or chronic illness. Crises of anticipated life transition require cognitive understanding and anticipatory guidance to meet the crisis problem.

3. *Crises resulting from traumatic stress.* These are crises precipitated by external stressors that are unexpected and uncontrolled. Some examples are sudden death of a family member, rape, and sudden loss of a job or status. This category of crisis is similar to the acute stress state described in Chapter 9. The individual's coping responses are inadequate, and new ways of coping need to be explored.

4. *Maturational/developmental crises.* These crises result from attempts to resolve interpersonal problems reflecting struggles with unsolved developmental conflicts. Some examples are crises with the central issue being sexual identity, value conflicts, or responses to authority. These are usually associated with young adults, but they may be seen in older populations as well if the central problem has not been resolved in youth. This type of crisis involves a patterned way of interacting with others over time that produces conflict because it is not socially acceptable or gratifying. The person needs to learn new skills in interpersonal relationships.

5. *Crises reflecting psychopathology.* These are crises in which preexisting psychologic problems are instrumental in producing the current crisis situation. They may require long-term treatment after the initial crisis intervention. Some examples are clients with schizophrenia and severe neuroses. The client usually has poorly developed coping skills and often presents in a crisis situation because of basic personality problems. Part of the crisis intervention is to prepare the client for long-term treatment.

6. *Psychiatric emergencies.* These are "crisis situations in which general functioning has been severely impaired and the individual rendered incompetent or unable to assume personal responsibility."[3] Some examples are suicidal clients, acute psychoses, and alcohol intoxication. The client is in a situation dangerous to himself or others. It is necessary to use available resources to treat the condition effectively.

As the levels in Baldwin's crisis classification progress, there is a need for increased therapeutic skills to handle the crisis; a shift in focus from primary, to secondary, to tertiary levels of prevention; an increased emphasis on precrisis personality as a determinant of present behavior; and an increased probability that referral to long-term treatment will be needed. For instance, in level 1 the nurse does primary prevention. The precrisis personality is basically well developed. There is an external stressor or stressors causing the major problem. The crisis intervention will be sufficient, and there will be no need for long-term treatment. In contrast, in level 6 a nurse specialist is needed to handle the problem. Crisis intervention is basically tertiary prevention for a long-standing personality problem. The precrisis personality is the major cause of the current problem, and the client invariably will need long-term therapy.

Theoretic basis of crisis intervention

The concept of crisis is based on psychoanalytic theory, particularly the work of Erikson discussed in Chapter 2, in which psychosocial development proceeds out of a series of crises or critical periods. The work of Erikson is directly related to the concept of maturational crises.

Two early pioneers in the development of crisis theory were Erich Lindemann and Gerald Caplan. Lindemann's early work focused on the bereavement reaction. He is most often associated with his study of the survivors of the Coconut Grove nightclub fire, in which he described the reactions (immediate and long-term) to the loss of a significant other and made suggestions for professionals working with individuals going through stages of grief. Lindemann believed that the interventions used for grief reactions could be applied to other crisis events. The focus of Lindemann's work became community-wide programs aimed at prevention. In 1946 with Gerald Caplan he established a community-based mental health program, the Wellesley Project. Through his work with Lindemann and on other projects Caplan developed the concept of crisis periods in individual and group development.

Caplan's crisis model is based on the psychophysiologic theory of homeostasis. Basically, Caplan's model of crises views the individual as living in a state of equilibrium with the goal being to maintain that equilibrium. Crisis events occur throughout life and disturb this equilibrium. The crisis is precipitated by an identifiable event that usually occurred less than 2 weeks before the crisis state. The crisis state itself is self-limiting in time and usually runs 4 to 6 weeks. Caplan also believes that a crisis is most accessible to intervention at its peak (Fig. 11-1).

Aguilera and Messick[1] propose a nursing model of crisis similar to Caplan's model. Both are based on the concept of homeostasis. According to Aguilera and Messick a stressful event leads to disequilibrium. The individual feels a need to return to the state of equilibrium. If certain "balancing factors" are present, equilibrium will be regained; if they are absent, a crisis may occur. The balancing factors that help to restore equilibrium are (1) realistic perception of the event, (2) adequate situational supports, and (3) adequate coping mechanisms.

According to Narayan and Joslin,[26] homeostasis "is limited in the range of human behavior and mental life that it explains." The theory of homeostasis explains behavior in terms of drive reduction, gratification of biologic needs, relaxation of tension, and so on. However, this is not adequate to explain higher-order processes such as learning and self-actualization. In addition, Narayan and Joslin argue that homeostasis does not differentiate adaptive from maladaptive behavior. They propose a nursing model for crisis and holistic care based on the concepts of health rather than disease. The concept of crisis in this model is compared with the state of depleted health potential, which is part of the health-illness continuum. Depleted health potential represents a state in which there is an inability to interact with internal and external forces resulting from a temporary to permanent loss of resources. One of the critical components in this model is the individual. The individual is viewed as a purposeful and reactive being. Another critical component in this model is the obstacles to life's goals. These are encountered throughout life in the forms of real or perceived loss. The individual responds to the obstacles using past coping mechanisms and skills to remove them. If the individual is not successful, this leads to increased anxiety. If this anxiety continues to go on, it will eventually lead to disorganization. Narayan and Joslin

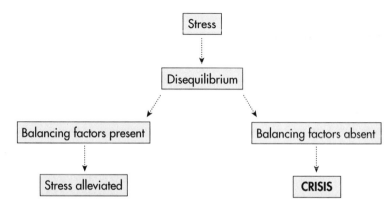

Fig. 11-1 When balancing factors, such as social supports and coping mechanisms, are present, the individual can often alleviate stress and avoid a crisis state.

used the concept of floundering to describe the peak point when intervention is greatly enhanced. Floundering is described as a state in which the individual has too much conflicting information. This nursing model sees crisis as a potentially growth-producing stage of development. The individual's perception of the self and its life purposes is open to new patterns of behavior. In this model the nurse intervenes as a facilitator. The nurse works with the client to develop new behavior based on the client's values and perceptions. The goal is for the client to be able to take care of himself. This model is essentially similar to Caplan's model; however, the view of the client is different. In the latter model the crisis worker is the facilitator moving the client to higher levels of functioning, and the emphasis is on positive aspects of growth. Also, there is increasing emphasis on the client's responsibility for himself. There is no notion of equilibrium. It is based on a health-illness continuum and levels of wellness.

Techniques of crisis intervention

Numerous texts and articles are available describing the techniques of crisis intervention. This section summarizes some of the approaches described in the literature.

Components of crisis intervention Fitzpatrick and Reed[10b] outline five major components of nursing intervention in crisis situations. The first and most important component is the establishment of a therapeutic relationship as described in Chapters 6 and 7. The authors contend that in a crisis situation it is most important to acknowledge this relationship and its importance. Caring and empathy are necessary to communicate to the client the "normality" of the crisis experience, thereby contributing to a positive view of the crisis.

A second major component of crisis intervention as outlined by Fitzpatrick and Reed is competency or "level of knowledge about human behavior that allows one to intervene."[10b] This includes knowledge regarding the characteristics of the various stages of crisis, as well as skills in health education regarding stressful life situations.

The third major component is commitment. Fitzpatrick and Reed define commitment as an acknowledgement of the responsibility of health care profes-

sionals in rendering service to clients. The authors contend that referrals are often done because of a lack of commitment, and they caution that clients in crisis require help in the immediate present.

The fourth component of crisis intervention is the acknowledgement of the client's basic ability to resolve the crisis. Fitzpatrick and Reed believe that "communicating to the client, acknowledgement of his or her vital role in crisis intervention can contribute to a sense of control in interpretation of future stressful events and in resolution of crises."[10b]

The final component is openness. The meaning of a crisis and ways to resolve it depend on the individual's value system and other characteristics of the individual. The nurse needs to be aware of the client's value system, other individual characteristics, how they compare to her own, and be open in allowing the client to choose strategies that are congruent with his individual characteristics, needs, and perceptions.

Steps of crisis intervention Langsley and Kaplan[22] summarize a series of six basic steps in crisis intervention that are generally agreed on:
1. Offer immediate aid.
2. Define the problem, including a differentiation of crisis problems from long-term problems.
3. Have a general focus on the here and now.
4. Use tension reduction techniques, because as tension decreases problem-solving ability increases.
5. Use problem solving to resolve the crisis situation.
6. Educate the client regarding future crises.

Levels of crisis intervention Langsley[21] outlines four levels of crisis intervention based on the needed skills of the crisis worker. Level 1 intervention consists of offering general support. This can be done by health professionals or anyone who wishes to help and can offer emotional support. Level 2 intervention focuses on environmental changes and requires a crisis worker with more skills who can suggest appropriate environmental changes to encourage the resolution of the crisis. Level 3 interventions are called *generic crisis interventions* and require knowledge of psychodynamics, psychopathology, and social systems. Level 4 is termed *individually tailored crisis intervention.* Levels 3 and 4 are similar to the Jacobson dichotomy of generic versus individual approaches to crisis intervention as discussed by Aguilera and Messick.[1]

Generic models of crisis intervention Generic crisis intervention focuses on the process of the crisis itself. A number of patterns of responses to stressful situations are reported in the literature, such as responses to death or the birth of a premature baby. In contrast, individual approaches focus on the interpersonal and intrapsychic processes of the individual in crisis. This type of intervention requires knowledge regarding biopsychosocial processes of the individual and is reserved for highly trained mental health professionals.

One generic model of crisis is proposed by Fink.[10a] He outlines four specific phases of crisis, and Ballou[4] attaches specific nursing actions to each of Fink's four crisis stages. Stage 1 is *shock*. The client may be fearful, confused, and disoriented; feelings of helplessness and anxiety are common. Nursing actions during stage 1 include providing emergency medical care if needed and an opportunity for the client to talk about what has happened. Therapeutic communication skills and relationship skills are what is needed during stage 1, particularly the ability to listen and care.

The second stage outlined by Fink is termed *defensive retreat*. The client uses denial and repression in an attempt to maintain familiar structures. This also allows the client to temporarily retreat from the events causing the crisis. Ballou believes that this stage poses particular problems for the nurse. The nurse does not want to verify unrealistic thinking, but at the same time to confront the client with reality makes the nurse an additional threat to the client, another piece of reality that the self needs to be protected against. Ballou recommends the use of several of the therapeutic communication techniques described in Chapter 5 to communicate to the client the nurse's continued availability and support. The therapeutic communication techniques recommended for clients who are unable to deal with the reality of a current crisis situation include reflection, summarizing, and clarifying. In addition, Ballou believes that during defensive retreat it is helpful to ask the client to explain the consequences of his behavior and acknowledge the client's right to experience his feelings.

The third stage of crisis is *acknowledgement*. In this stage actual therapeutic help can begin if the client starts to face reality. Indications of stress such as increased anxiety, depression, helplessness, and agitation are all possible evidence of acknowledgement. It is during this stage that the nurse helps the client to acquire new skills in handling the crisis. This is done within the context of a healthy relationship by encouraging the client to describe the situation, the client's perception of the crisis, and precipitating events, along with its implications for the client. During this stage the nurse also explores with the client alternative ways of responding and various problem-solving and decision-making techniques. In addition, the nurse may supply information about referrals to the client. The goal is for the nurse to help the client to solve the problem.

Fink's final stage of crisis, stage 4, is *adaptation and change*. During this stage the client implements new behavior to meet the crisis problem. This reorganization of responses gradually decreases anxiety. During this stage Ballou recommends the following interventions:

1. Confronting unrealistic alternatives
2. Helping the client to recognize his autonomy, growth, and problem-solving abilities
3. Supporting the client's goals and decision

Although the stages of crisis are listed sequentially, clients do not progress through this sequence in an orderly fashion. Ballou believes that with effective crisis intervention not only can the client return to the previous level of functioning, he can even progress to a higher level. Hence the crisis situation can be a positive, growth-producing experience rather than a negative, catastrophic experience.

Anticipatory planning Anticipatory planning is a specific therapeutic technique often associated with crisis intervention. Aguilera and Messick[1] discuss anticipatory planning as the final phase in crisis intervention. During this phase the planned actions taken by the client to resolve the crisis are evaluated to see if the goals of the crisis intervention have been met. In this phase future plans are also discussed as the client prepares to meet any similar future crises. Anticipatory planning also asks the client to look at where they enter the crisis intervention service and where they are completing the crisis intervention service. The entering point is a time when the client was completely unable to cope; the exit point is the time when the client has perhaps reached his previous level of functioning if not a higher level. He is now able to cope. This realistic look at the progress the client has made can give the client a sense of accomplishment. Many of the events precipitating the crisis do not go away because of the crisis intervention; rather, the client is helped to identify new ways of meeting the problem. Therefore it can be expected that similar situations may again arise in the future. For example, in the hypothetic case of Ms. K. the basic problem is loss, and although the client may have acquired new skills in dealing with the loss, the loss is nevertheless still there. Anticipatory planning helps the client prepare for situations in the future that may again arise and lead to a crisis situation.

Caplan[7] discusses anticipatory guidance or emotional inoculation as a specific crisis intervention technique that can be used if the crisis can be predicted. For example, a child is scheduled to be admitted to the hospital for corrective orthopedic surgery. Some of the specific actions that the nurse could do to prevent a crisis are:

1. Arouse anticipatory stress by describing what will be experienced before and after surgery.
2. Tell the child about the probable intensity and duration of postoperative pain.
3. Describe what can be done to control this discomfort.
4. Emphasize the normality of fear, confusion, and distress in the situation.
5. Guide the family members in identifying ways that they can help the child before and after surgery.

Caplan states that these interventions will be most effective if they are performed at the time of the scheduled surgery. He encourages interventions with groups of clients and their families so they are able to support each other. In all of the described interventions the central element is to evoke anticipatory distress and then help the individual work out ways to control the expected stress.

Caplan differentiates anticipatory guidance from a second type of crisis intervention that he calls *preventive intervention*. Preventive intervention occurs during a crisis rather than in anticipation of a crisis.

Some of the here-and-now techniques that Caplan describes as preventive interventions are:

1. Helping the client to plan activities to solve the problem
2. Helping the client to focus on the present
3. Encouraging the client to maintain activity and to seek outside help
4. Helping family members to communicate with the client and with each other
5. Emphasizing the normality of the negative feelings associated with a crisis situation

Caplan sees both forms of intervention, anticipatory guidance and preventive intervention, as techniques that focus on the here and now, or current situation, without regard for past experiences or personality development as reasons for current crisis behavior. As such, these methods use the "personal influence of the intervenor to modify current behavior."[7] They do not require advanced skills but are best regarded as offering an "ordinary human helping hand to individuals in crisis."[7]

In addition to these individual methods of intervention Caplan describes various support system methods. In these the focus is on monitoring the social supports available to the individual during periods of increased stress and offering support if needed. Some examples are convening a support group and fostering the development of mutual help organizations. An example of a clinical situation in which the nurse would be involved in support system crisis methods would be that of a nurse working with a new mother, Ms. G., who has just delivered twins and has an 18-month-old baby at home. Nurse A would investigate the balancing factors present and absent. The nurse might need to invite family members to come over and support the individual. If the family is not able to provide the needed support, the nurse might need to find community resources to help. Family members may be so involved in their own personal needs that they are unable to provide support for the individual in crisis. In this example Ms. G. tells the nurse that her mother-in-law will be coming to help. Is this an adequate situational support? To answer this question the nurse must not assume that because a support figure is available that the need for effective support is met. Caplan suggests that the nurse monitor the actual services provided by the support figure.

Families in crisis

A crisis situation not only impacts the client but can have a significant effect on the family of the client. In fact, in numerous situations, such as the critically ill infant, a comatose trauma victim, or an unconscious coronary client, the significant emotional and informational needs of the family should be addressed and not forgotten while providing for the physical needs of the acute-care client. According to Woolley,[36] "crisis theory can provide a framework for preventive, supportive and therapeutic interventions with family members at risk." Kleeman[18] advocates family-focused care based on the recent rise in consumerism that includes clients' and families' rights to knowledge, access, and so on. In addition, families play an important role in the client's treatment, and they can "make a profound difference in recovery or long-term adjustment to disability."[18] One of Caplan's preventive crisis interventions is to help family members communicate with the client and with each other.[7]

The steps in family-oriented crisis intervention, the assessment of the family, planning, implementation, and evaluation, are similar to those used when working with an individual client. Kleeman[18] discusses some areas of differences in dealing with families of clients with trauma. Primarily the open-ended time frame separates trauma crisis from other type of crisis. Additional surgeries and complications all serve to increase the family's level of stress. Moore[25] advocates a quick and accurate assessment and interventions with families in crisis that are based on the nursing process model of assessment, planning, intervention and crisis resolution, and anticipatory planning.

The focus of family crisis intervention is the establishment of an empathic, supportive, and trusting relationship. This can be facilitated by addressing the family's specific concerns. The nurse can assist the family in describing their perceptions of the situation and determining if their perceptions are realistic. If there is distortion, the nurse can help clarify and restate as necessary. Immediate crisis intervention also involves assessment of coping skills, previous experience with similar situations, and supports available. Kleeman[18] describes family behaviors during the immediate crisis period as being extreme, exaggerated, and rapidly changing. The overwhelming input and feelings of powerlessness create behaviors ranging from dependency to distance and distrust. According to Kruger,[20] other behaviors that parents may manifest include anxiety, confusion, psychosomatic symptoms, and guilt. The following nursing actions are helpful during the immediate crisis period:

1. The nurse should encourage the family to share feelings, allowing them to ask questions by providing an environment that is safe and tolerant. Kleeman cautions that the questions often asked by families in crisis are not attempts to seek information but rather are "unanswerable questions" that "reflect their innermost fears." These are not questions that have right or wrong answers or even to which the family expects an answer.

2. The nurse should present a context for what the normal range of expected responses are during an immediate crisis period.

3. The nurse needs to be aware of the family's physical needs. If the family is going to be able to support the client, their needs for adequate rest and nutrition should not be neglected.

4. The nurse needs to maintain a calm, steady, nonreactive presence that is tolerant of the family's reactivity.

5. The nurse can help the family to obtain a clear understanding of the crisis by explaining what has happened and is happening to the client in simple language. During a crisis there is usually information overload, and information often is not processed. Therefore the nurse needs to repeat information to the family. The nurse can also guide family members in their problem solving, giving direction but limiting dependency.

6. The nurse can help link the immediate family with the extended family. This can be done by providing the use of a phone near the critical care unit. It can also be facilitated by having a designated family member who is constantly kept informed of the client's progress. All extended family's requests for information can be channeled to that designated person.

7. Woolley[36] recommends that family members be included in client care as soon as possible. This facilitates the formation of a trusting relationship and allows the family to have a shared sense of purpose rather than being made to feel that they are intruding.

8. A final nursing action is to begin the process of assessment of the family system.

Family assessment includes obtaining information about various areas of family functioning, including coping skills, support systems, stressors, and interpersonal relationships. In addition, Johnson and Mattson[16] state that family assessment should include cultural background of the family, educational level, religious preference, and the family's socioeconomic status.

Coping skills To assess coping skills the nurse determines the family's usual way of responding to stressors. The nurse can assess coping skills directly and indirectly. Direct assessment may include asking the family if anything like this has ever happened to them before, how they responded to the situation, and how successful were they in their efforts. Woolley[36] states that indirect assessment involves carefully observing the emotional behavior of the family to determine the success or failure of their coping strategies. When strategies are successful, the family will demonstrate positive affect, exhibiting joy, relief, and contentment. "However, if the strategies have proved unsuccessful then negative-toned affects such as depression, hopelessness, helplessness and anxiety are observed."[36]

Support systems The nurse assesses the support systems available by determining if there is an extended family or network of friends available to help with the tasks of daily living that must continue during the crisis. The amount and the types of these daily-living tasks represent the demands on the family system. They include such things as child care, meal preparation, bill payment, care of pets, and managing business requirements. The nurse needs to determine the balance between the demands on the system and the system supports available. For instance, a mother, Ms. W., with small children whose husband is hospitalized following an automobile accident and resultant severe head trauma may be concerned with child care, finances, and care of the home and pets. If Ms. W. has an invalid mother in a nursing home, has only lived in the area a short period of time, and has no close friendships or knowledge of the area resources, the support system available may be inadequate to deal with the physical needs of this family. Ms. W.'s mother may be an adequate or superior emotional support for her daughter even though she is unable to provide for their physical needs.

The assessment of a support system should include an evaluation of the family culture and patterns. Kleeman[18] contends that "the more open these connections are and the more available these relationship networks are, the more anxiety will be diffused in the present generation."

Interpersonal family relationships The nurse needs to assess how the family functions, as well as their roles, routines, rituals, and customs. Research indicates that families who have established routines and rituals are able to deal with a crisis situation more effectively. It is suggested that these routine patterns of behavior provide the family with a feeling of security. The nurse also needs to assess the way that family members relate to each other and communicate. Satir's communication patterns discussed in Chapter 4 are based on her work with families. The dysfunctional communication patterns of placating, blaming, computing, and distracting are ways to deal with increased stress. According to Kleeman[18] "the more clearly that individual family members can see themselves functioning within the family unit (that is, independent or interdependent,

CRITICAL THINKING *Question* . . . .

Because most families in the United States no longer live in multigenerational homes, experience with the gradual decline and death of family elders is limited. Shapiro and Koocher[30] believe that "our children have lost exposure to the full circle of life." Hence society, which has rituals and social rules for greetings, birthdays, graduations, and other important life events, lacks established rituals and rules for communicating with the dying.

Do you believe that this is an accurate depiction of current American culture? Explain your response.

autonomous when appropriate, decisive, able to hold different opinion than others in the family), the more functional their response will be to crisis."

The final stage in crisis intervention, anticipatory planning, is also appropriate for families in crisis. During this stage the actions taken by the family are evaluated to see if goals have been met, and future plans are discussed. Woolley[36] states that this final phase varies according to the client's prognosis and may take the form of bereavement counseling. She also contends that follow-up support may be "equally as important as support during the crisis." Referrals to a self-help group, aftercare program, support group, or the like are very important. Lack of intervention during this period has been connected to increased family difficulties and marital discord.

Application of crisis intervention techniques

Aguilera and Messick[1] discuss a number of situational crises that have been previously studied, noting the common behavior patterns associated with each crisis. These authors contend that knowledge of expected courses of behavior in certain stressful situations can be helpful in planning for prevention as well as intervention in a crisis. The stimuli that may lead to a crisis, such as a premature birth, produce disequilibrium or increased stress. Whether a crisis situation will occur depends on the other factors involved, the client's perception of the situation, and the individual resources available to meet the situation.

Situational crises

Various situational crises will be discussed. Included will be crisis associated with death and dying, crisis associated with life-threatening illness such as cancer, and the application of crisis techniques in dealing with the pain and disability of chronic illness.

Death and dying Kubler-Ross described five stages of grief that persons go through when they are told that they have a fatal illness. The first stage is shock and denial. In this stage, the client cannot grasp what has happened. Gray states that the shock and denial may be accompanied by physiologic reactions, including pallor, sweating, rapid heart rate, restlessness, and confusion. Smith[31] states that because Kubler-Ross listed denial as the first stage, it

is often perceived as an immature response. He contends that clients have a right to choose the coping strategy most beneficial to them. The nurse's role is to support the client's choice. Frisch and Kelley[11] contend that although some people may see hope as an indicator of denial, others see hope as essential to the maintenance of emotional well-being.

The second stage described by Kubler-Ross is anger, followed by a stage of bargaining. The fourth stage is depression. In this stage, the client rarely speaks and discourages visitors. Kubler-Ross states that during the stage of depression, the client needs time to grieve. The final stage is acceptance. The client is neither happy nor sad.

According to Timmermans,[33] nursing intervention with the dying client should be broadly defined to include physical, social, religious, and psychologic care to obtain as high a level of comfort as possible. The goal is the humanization of death. Nursing care involves the minimizing of physical discomfort. Nursing intervention also includes mediation between family and client, and client and religious representatives. A goal is to help the client achieve or maintain integrity rather than despair. Kemp[17] states that helping a client achieve or maintain integrity requires not only physical, social, and psychologic care, but also spiritual care. Spiritual care is "being present in the face of suffering."[17] Nursing actions associated with spiritual care include listening, diagnosing distress of the human spirit, and affirming the importance of spiritual concerns. The concept of spirituality is discussed further in Chapter 10.

Shapiro and Koocher[30] recommend additional nursing interventions with the dying client. They believe that an open, nonjudgmental attitude is important. They state that the nurse should be aware of cues that the client wants to discuss dying. They contend that broad questions such as "Have you been thinking about dying?" or "How old do you think you will live to be?" enable clients to think about and discuss their reactions.

Glazer and Landreth[13] discuss the dying child. The child's concept of death and dying depends on the child's level of cognitive development. Young children under 2 years of age do not understand the concept of dying. The preschool-age child often uses magical thinking, hence death may not be seen as final. The early school-age child, age approximately 7 to 11 years, views death as specific, concrete, and irrevocable. It is only the formal operational level of cognitive development, which usually occurs after age 12 years, that permits a child to understand the reality of death and integrate death into a view of life. Children communicate through play. During play, children are able to transfer anxiety, fears, and guilt to objects. According to Glazer and Landreth,[13] nursing interventions with the dying child should include helping the child focus on appreciating the moment, not preparing for the future. The nurse also needs to be able to listen and understand the child's questions. The question "Am I going to die?" may mean "Is someone going to stay with me?" A final nursing intervention is to provide a warm, accepting, and safe environment. Beaudoin[5] states that it is vital to provide environmental support to the caregivers who work with terminally ill clients. Most nurses report that caring for the terminally ill is depressing or discouraging at times.

Constantino[8a] reports the results of a study on levels of depression and social adjustment for widows who receive bereavement crisis intervention compared with those who do not. Bereavement crisis intervention consisted primarily of social interaction with a group of recent widows, including 4 weeks of planned social events. Widows in the bereavement crisis intervention group had a significant increase in socialization after the group experience. Depression significantly increased in the control group and significantly decreased in the bereavement crisis intervention group. Constantino[8a] recommends bereavement crisis intervention as a treatment modality for widowhood that should be incorporated into nursing curricula. She also recommends the formation of community mental health programs based on the bereavement crisis intervention approach for widows.

Life-threatening illness A recent diagnosis of cancer, human immunodeficiency virus type 1 (HIV-1), acquired immunodeficiency syndrome (AIDS), or any other potentially life-threatening illness is a crisis-producing event. Andersen[2] researched adaptive strategies of clients recently diagnosed with cancer. She found that the magnitude of the disease was a critical variable in predicting outcomes. Crisis intervention strategies had the most positive benefit for high-morbidity clients, those with a possible but unlikely 1-year survival. Crisis intervention included emotional support, information about the disease and treatment, and practice using behavioral coping strategies, for example, role playing.

Ettinger and Heiney[10] discussed age-specific problems for teenagers diagnosed with cancer. According to the authors, these teens had both a maturational crisis and a situational crisis at the same time. Adolescent concerns included loss of control and family relationship problems, because parents often became extremely protective of the adolescent. Poor peer relationships and social isolation were also frequent areas of concern.

The severity and unpredictability of AIDS make it a severe physical and emotional crisis for clients and their families. The large number of people diagnosed with AIDS or HIV-1 presents a major challenge to caregivers. Christ et al.[8] discuss possible client reactions to the crisis that occurs after confirmation of HIV status is received. The authors outline the crisis intervention strategies appropriate for clients diagnosed with AIDS or any other severe progressive illness. The authors encourage nurses to help clients selectively disclose their diagnosis. This allows the client to plan for changes in their responsibilities and to increase their social support system. Because rejection is a possibility, the nurse needs to help the client identify sources of support. A second intervention is to help clients become task focused. Helping the client to plan a flexible work schedule when possible often creates a greater feeling of personal control. A third intervention is to evaluate the need for additional specialized services. Some clients may need financial or psychologic assistance.

Schulz and Masek[29] used crisis intervention theory in their work with clients diagnosed with a chronic illness. The goals of their interventions were for clients to increase their ability to cope with specific expected stressors and to maximize clients' level of functioning. Schulz and Masek[29] outline crisis intervention strategies for dealing with pain associated with chronic illness. The first strategy is to normalize the experience. This reassures clients that the concerns and fears that they feel are

CASE STUDY: *Crisis Intervention*

Melichar's[24] description of a child's temper tantrums producing a family crisis is a good example of how crisis theory can be applied to a variety of situations. Melichar uses the steps in the nursing process as a framework for her description of the interventions of the nurse. In the first phase, data collection, the nurse assesses the reason for the client's seeking help at this time (the precipitating event). The nurse also assesses the family's perception of the problem and the resources available to meet the problem. In this case the family identified the problem as their inability to handle their 5-year-old's temper tantrums. Their daughter had been having temper tantrums since age 2, but in the last 6 months the parents were no longer able to cope with them. Their previous method of dealing with this problem was to put their daughter in her room during her tantrums. The family had recently moved over 1000 miles away from their extended families. They now lived in smaller quarters and were no longer able to use their habitual coping mechanism. The child's tantrums were increasing in frequency and severity, thus leading to the present crisis in which the mother was afraid that she would physically harm the child.

Phase 2 of the nursing process is the formulation of the nursing diagnosis. Melichar identifies two nursing problems based on the nurse's assessment of the situation: (1) the parent's inability to cope with the child's temper tantrums and (2) the parent's fear of loss of control resulting in harm to the child.

Phases 3 and 4 of the nursing process are planning and intervention. In this situation the nurse formulated with the parents new techniques to control their child's tantrums. Specific interventions included a 2- to 5-minute time-out period, consistent handling of temper tantrums, and a behavior modification program to reward the child's appropriate behavior.

Phase 5 of the nursing process is evaluation. In this case study the nurse met with the parents 2 months after the initial meetings. The immediate crisis had been resolved, and the parents had learned a more effective way to deal with their child's behavior. Melichar stresses anticipatory planning as part of the nurse's intervention after the immediate stress has been reduced so that the client can review the progress that has been made and realistic plans formed to avoid a recurrence of the crisis in the future.

This case study points out the values of crisis intervention techniques for situations that are relatively common but still capable of initiating a crisis. Brennan[6] reports a case study in which crisis intervention techniques are used to prevent a crisis. The precipitating event is a move to a new town. The mother has an 18-month-old son and lives in a home needing extensive repairs. She knows no one and is having difficulty handling her son. She blames him for her inability to meet new people, work, or fix the house. She visits a family physician to discuss her feelings of depression, and he recognizes the potential crisis and involves a number of community agencies to help the family successfully relocate in the new town.

---

normal. In addition, it is important to emphasize the complex nature of pain and the importance of viewing it from a biopsychosocial perspective. Client concerns often focus on isolation and abandonment, especially for the child who may no longer be able to attend school. There are also significant concerns about vulnerability and death. A key intervention is often to increase the client's level of activity. Another intervention is to provide education about the functional nature of pain and how this function is lost in chronic pain. Behavioral

relaxation strategies are often useful in helping the client manage pain. Another intervention recommended by Schulz and Masek[29] is to elicit from the client a personal illness narrative. This is the client's explanatory model of disease. This model can influence the course of an illness and the client's motivation to follow a treatment plan. The narrative is based largely on the client's culture, pattern organization, and past experiences. The nurse tries to help the client restate the narrative to be more adaptive and health promoting.

Maturational crises

Aguilera and Messick[1] apply crisis intervention techniques to maturational crises from infancy through old age, and Gaston[12] discusses midlife crisis and relates it to cultural beliefs about death. According to Gaston denial of death is the central issue in midlife crisis. Western culture does not incorporate death. Religions speak of reincarnation and life after death. Hospitals segregate the dying, while language supports elaborate euphemisms to prevent even saying the word *dead*. Gaston outlines major changes that occur in midlife, such as aging, an increased concern with health, and marital turmoil that can also contribute to midlife crisis. Factors that could help the individual handle midlife changes are often absent. For example, by denying death the individual's perception of the problem is distorted, and marital turmoil and role changes often leave the individual without the needed situational supports. A crisis then ensues.

Crisis intervention techniques can help the individual to understand the problem and find new supports or reestablish existing situational ones. Gaston believes that Kubler-Ross' stages of dying are common defense mechanisms used by individuals faced with a midlife crisis. The final stage according to Kubler-Ross is the acceptance of death. The nurse needs to help the individual in midlife crisis work through the stages of dying to come to an acceptance of death, a resolution of the crisis, and into generativity.

CRITICAL THINKING *Question* · · · · · · · · · · · · · · · ·

Regan[28] outlines a creative teaching strategy to help students learn how to apply crisis intervention theory. The faculty "puts the students in a crisis" by announcing without warning a major calamity that places the students' education in jeopardy and may lead to the school's closure. After this brief personal encounter with a crisis the students are asked to discuss their feelings and actions.

Do you think that this is a legitimate and ethical strategy to teach students about crisis? How do you think you would respond in a similar situation?

· ·

SUMMARY

Crisis theory and crisis intervention techniques are applicable to a wide variety of situations. Langsley[21] lists a number of general groups for whom crisis techniques are useful. They include acutely and chronically ill psychiatric clients, aged people, minorities, disaster victims, and other special populations who operate under high levels of stress, such as policemen. In addition, crisis techniques can also be used in many general nursing situations. Kroner[19] discusses the use of crisis intervention skills in caring for confused and disoriented clients as well as steps to prevent a potential crisis situation when clients are hospitalized. Pisarcik[27] deals with ways to handle hospitalized clients who are violent or aggressive.

Cooper[9] applied crisis intervention techniques working with the staff of a psychiatric unit. Crisis techniques were used to alleviate the impact of client suicide or client assault on the staff. Cooper followed the model of "critical incident stress debriefing" used in the military. It includes a description of the grieving process, stress management techniques, and information regarding community resources available.

Hospitalization or illness is always capable of producing a crisis. Crisis intervention skills are extremely useful to nurses. Crises can also be related to unanticipated life events, normal developmental experiences, or situational circumstances. The crisis situation creates a sense of vulnerability for the client and provides an opportunity for personal growth. An individual who is assisted to handle a crisis effectively may learn new and more effective coping skills. Crisis intervention is directed toward assisting the individual to reach the previous or a higher level of functioning. The crisis intervention process is very similar to the nursing process. Assessment includes exploration of the crisis situation, the client's coping skills, and the availability of supportive resources. The individual is then assisted to mobilize existing resources or to develop new ones where none exist. Rapid and intensive intervention is required because the crisis state is time-limited. Nurses frequently encounter people who are in crisis and need to develop the skills required to be of help to them.

⚕ DISCUSSION QUESTIONS

1. Identify examples of crisis situations in your life. Compare and contrast these to stress situations in your life.

2. Discuss how crisis theory and crisis intervention techniques can be incorporated into daily nursing practice.

3. Relate the steps in the nursing process to the process of crisis intervention.

4. Compare and contrast situational with maturational crises.

5. Identify a potential crisis situation in a clinical setting and outline possible nursing interventions. Discuss this identified situation in relationship to Baldwin's categories of crises.

6. Discuss the positive aspects of crisis.

7. Discuss the role of the family in a crisis situation.

📖 EXPERIENTIAL & SIMULATED LEARNING EXERCISES

1. Perception of potential crisis situations

PURPOSE: To identify various reactions to potential crisis situations and techniques to reduce tension.

PROCEDURE: Assign students to small groups of 5 to 10 participants and give each an identification number. Ask each student to write down a potential crisis situation from any source and place the assigned number on the top of the paper. Then ask them to pass their situations to the person on their left, so that the next person can read the crisis situation and write down on another piece of paper his or her response to the crisis. Continue to pass and write down responses until all members have responded to each situation. At the conclusion each member should have his or her own situation and responses to all the other crises.

DISCUSSION: Read one situation and share the responses to this situation. Discuss why the responses differ in terms of perception and the factors that influence perception, such as pattern organization, cultural background, personality factors, and situational supports. For each crisis situation ask the group to identify at least one tension reduction technique that could be used.

2. Crisis plan development

PURPOSE: To develop possible nursing interventions for a crisis situation.

PROCEDURE: Divide students into small groups. Each group should select a recorder. Provide each group with the description of a potential crisis situation. Examples include those described in the text—a diagnosis of AIDS or cancer, death of a loved one, or chronic pain. Other examples are rape, earthquakes, fire, or any maturational crisis. Students can be given basic information and are instructed to develop the specifics of their crisis participants. They should be instructed to identify potential stressors, balancing factors, and the role of the family. Using a crisis intervention model, each group should develop a possible nursing care plan for the client.

DISCUSSION: Group recorders share with the total group their basic assessment information given by the faculty, potential stressors identified, balancing factors, role of the client's family, and their plan of care. What are the similarities and differences across groups? How did the client's family and culture influence the choice of potential interventions?

Small groups can also be given complete assessment data of a client in a crisis situation. This would include stressors, balancing factors, culture, and other pertinent information. Why is it significantly easier to develop a plan of care with complete assessment data? Is it important to be able to develop a plan of care without complete assessment data? Why?

REFERENCES

1. Aguilera DC, Messick JM: *Crisis intervention: theory and methodology,* ed 8, St Louis, 1998, Mosby.
2. Andersen B: Psychological interventions for cancer patients to enhance the quality of life, *J Consult Clin Psychol* 60(4):552, 1992.
3. Baldwin BA: A paradigm for the classification of emotional crises: implications for crisis intervention, *Am J Orthopsychiatry* 48:538, 1978.
4. Ballou M: Crisis intervention and the hospital nurse, *J Nurs Care* 13:15, 1980.
5. Beaudoin S: Caring and surviving: coping with patient death, *Can Nurse* 86:19, 1990.
6. Brennan PJ: A family close to crisis, *Nurs Times* 77:1390, 1981.
7. Caplan G: Recent developments in crisis intervention and in the promotion of support services. In Kessoer M, Goldston S, editors: *A decade of progress in primary prevention,* Hanover, NH, 1986, University Press of New England.

8. Christ G, Moynihan R, Gallo-Silver L: Human immun-odeficiency virus and crisis intervention: a task-focused approach. In Roberts AR, editor: *Perspectives in crisis intervention and prevention,* Englewood Cliffs, NJ, 1991, Prentice Hall.

8a. Constantino RE: Bereavement crisis intervention for widows in grief and mourning, *Nurs Res* 30:351, 1981.

9. Cooper C: Psychiatric stress debriefing: alleviating the impact of patient suicide and assault, *J Psychosoc Nurs Ment Health Serv* 33:21, 1995.

10. Ettinger R, Heiney S: Cancer in adolescents and young adults: psychosocial concerns, coping strategies and interventions, *Cancer* 14(1):3276, 1993.

10a. Fink S: Crisis and motivation: a theoretical model, *Arch Phys Med Rehab* 48:592, 1967.

10b. Fitzpatrick JJ, Reed PG: Stress in the crisis experience: nursing interventions, *Occup Health Nurs* 28:19, 1980.

11. Frisch N, Kelley J: *Healing life's crises: a guide for nurses,* Albany, NY, 1996, Delmar.

12. Gaston SK: Death and the midlife crisis, *J Psychosoc Nurs Ment Health Serv* 18:31, 1980.

13. Glazer H, Landreth G: A developmental concept of dying in a child's life, *J Humanistic Educ Dev* 31(3):98, 1993.

14. Hill RL: Generic features of families under stress, *Soc Case* 39:139, 1958.

15. Johnson JW: More about stress and some management techniques, *J School Health* 51:36, 1981.

16. Johnson L, Mattson S: Communication: the key to crisis prevention in pediatric death, *Crit Care Nurse* 12:23, 1992.

17. Kemp C: *Terminal illness: a guide to nursing care,* Philadelphia, 1995, JB Lippincott.

18. Kleeman KM: Families in crisis due to multiple trauma, *Crit Care Nurs Clin North Am* 1:23, 1991.

19. Kroner K: Dealing with the confused patient, *Nursing 79* 9:72, 1979.

20. Kruger S: Parents in crisis: helping them cope with a seriously ill child, *J Pediatr Nurs* 7:133, 1992.

21. Langsley DG: Crisis intervention: an update, *Curr Psych Ther* 20:19, 1981.

22. Langsley DG, Kaplan DM: *The treatment of families in crisis,* New York, 1968, Grune & Stratton.

23. Lipkin GB, Cohen RG: *Effective approaches to patient's behavior,* ed 5, New York, 1992, Springer-Verlag.

24. Melichar MM: Using crisis theory to help parents cope with a child's temper tantrums, *MCN* 5:181, 1980.

25. Moore AC: Crisis intervention: a care plan for families of hospitalized children, *Pediatr Nurs* 15:234, 1989.

26. Narayan SM, Joslin DJ: Crisis theory and intervention: a critique of the medical model and proposal of a holistic nursing model, *Adv Nurs Sci* 2:27, 1980.

27. Pisarcik GK: Psychiatric emergencies and crisis intervention, *Nurs Clin* 16:85, 1981.

28. Regan J: Teaching crisis creatively, *Nurse Educator* 7:18, 1982.

29. Schulz M, Masek B: Medical crisis intervention with children and adolescents with chronic pain, *Professional Psychology* 27(2):121, 1996.

30. Shapiro D, Koocher G: Goals and practical considerations in out-patient medical crisis intervention, *Professional Psychology* 27(2):109, 1996.

31. Smith D: The terminally ill patient's right to be in denial, *Omega* 27(2):115, 1993.

32. Taylor LS: Policemen and nursing students, *J Psychosoc Nurs Ment Health Serv* 23:26, 1985.

33. Timmermans S: The paradox of nursing terminal patients in a Belgian general hospital, *Omega* 27(4):281, 1993.

34. U.S. Department of Commerce: *Statistical abstracts of the US,* ed 103, Washington, DC, 1995, Bureau of the Census.

35. Weaver H, Wodarski J: Cultural issues in crisis intervention: guidelines for culturally competent practice, *Family Therapy* 22:213, 1995.

36. Woolley N: Crisis theory: a paradigm of effective intervention with families of critically ill people, *J Adv Nurs* 15:1402, 1990.

Suggested Readings

Aguilera DC, Messick JM: *Crisis intervention: theory and methodology,* ed 8, St Louis, 1998, Mosby.

> *Comprehensive textbook that includes situational and maturational crises and burnout syndrome. Discusses various types of specific crisis situations in terms of assessment, planning, intervention, and anticipatory planning.*

Anderson MD: Care for the worried well, *Issues Ment Health Nurs* 2:15, 1980.

> *Interesting look at one group of clients, the worried well. Described as people with no biologic base for physiologic illness but who nonetheless perceive themselves as ill. Author relates this group to crisis theory.*

Caplan G: *Principles of preventive psychiatry,* New York, 1964, Basic Books.

> *A classic discourse on the developmental phases in a crisis. Primary, secondary, and tertiary prevention of mental health problems are explained using a public health model.*

Kleeman KM: Families in crisis due to multiple trauma, *Crit Care Nurs Clin North Am* 1:23, 1989.

> *This article discusses the crisis intervention role of the trauma nurse with a focus on the family of the injured client. The author gives a detailed list of questions the nurse can use to assess the family's level of functioning in four areas: level of chronic anxiety, emotional relationship, communication, and multigenerational heritage and patterns.*

Langsley DG: Crisis intervention: an update, *Curr Psych Ther* 20:19, 1981.

> *Comprehensive discussion of developments in crisis therapy.*

Lusby RA, Ingman SB: The pros, cons and pitfalls of "self-help" rehabilitation programs, *Soc Sci Med* 13A:113, 1979.

> *This article provides an excellent documentation of the developmental process of a self-help group. It raises the provocative question, "Must a self-help group be professionalized to compete for resources with traditional programs?" Also discusses issues related to bureaucracies and to charismatic leadership.*

Narayan SM, Joslin DJ: Crisis theory and intervention: a critique of the medical model and proposal of a holistic nursing model, *Adv Nurs Sci* 2:27, 1980.

> *This paper presents crisis theory in terms of a holistic health nursing model with an emphasis on the growth-producing aspects of crisis.*

CHAPTER

12 *Comprehensive Case Study*

No one could ever know: the warmth, the joy,
   the wonder
When I feel this baby move.
I know the pains of labor and of growth.
I know the worry and fear of the unknown.
Will this baby, kicking hard, heart beating
Be the answer to a dream, or
Is this another cross to bear?
No one could ever know.

Ann Carmel

LEARNING OBJECTIVES

After studying this chapter, the student should be able to:

- Describe the value of using process recordings of nurse-client interactions.
- Discuss the advantages and disadvantages of the various methods of recording interactions.
- Identify the components of a nursing care plan.
- Recognize the importance of supervision for the nurse.
- Develop a case study for a client with whom the nurse is working.

Chapter 1 of this text presented theoretic material regarding the nursing process, the format used by the nurse in dealing with client problems. The following chapters dealt with content related to the therapeutic use of the nursing process.

Chapters 2 and 3 examined theories related to the growth of the individual's personality and concepts used to assess the individual's perception of the self. Not only the client but also the nurse is proceeding through stages of growth and development. This requires the nurse to have an awareness of her own perceptions of self in addition to an awareness of how these perceptions influence nurse-client interactions.

After this exploration of the self, Chapters 4, 5, 6, and 7 delineated content related to the nurse-client relationship. Included are the abstract concepts of relationships, formation of the relationship, role of the nurse in establishing and maintaining the relationship, and the behavioral manifestation of the relationship-communication. Communication not only reveals the relationship between two or more individuals, it is also a means of assessing the participants' perception of their selves. What each individual brings into the relationship, the pattern organization of each self, is demonstrated in their communication. Chapter 8 presented information on group theory, roles, and relationships within a group setting.

Chapter 9 dealt with the concept of stress. Within the context of a therapeutic relationship the nurse assesses and directs actions toward stabilizing the stress state of a client. The stress that a client is experiencing and his adaptation to this stress produces nursing problems. In addition, how to identify the stress state of the client and of the nurse was described.

Chapter 10 outlined specific nursing actions that promote health within a community health framework of primary, secondary, and tertiary prevention. Chapter 11 provided information about dealing with crises.

This chapter presents a compilation of previously discussed theoretic information applied to a specific case study. It is hoped that this application will move previously abstract material into the realm of concrete reality. Before this case study is presented the procedures of recording and analyzing data gathered from the client are reviewed. Three methods and various formats are explored:

the process recording, the nursing care plan, and the supervision process.

PROCESS RECORDING

As the name implies, *process recordings* are recordings (written, audio, or audio-video) of the nurse-client interaction. They serve as tools to assist the nurse in compiling information to assess the needs of the client and to identify nursing problems. In addition, they are an excellent means for the nurse to achieve self-growth and develop self-awareness.

The nurse may use a variety of methods to record interactions. Mechanical devices such as tape recorders and videotapes may be used, or handwritten notes (in a general outline form or as actual verbatim notes) may be taken during the meeting with the client. In addition, the nurse may choose to wait until after the interaction to record in writing what transpired. Each method has certain inherent advantages and disadvantages. In general mechanical devices allow the nurse freedom to concentrate on the interaction with the client. It is not necessary to write, listen, and talk or to remember all of the verbal and nonverbal communication; rather, it is possible to focus on the process of the relationship. Mechanical devices are also effective in providing feedback for one or both participants in the relationship. In particular, videotaping is an excellent tool for evaluating nurse-client interactions.

In addition, mechanical devices provide an opportunity for numerous replays not available in live observation. Mechanical devices do present problems, however. There is always the possibility of mechanical failure, and in the case of videotaping a third person is necessary to operate the equipment. Often the addition of an extraneous "machine" is initially distracting and may hinder the relationship. Another important consideration is the feasibility of using such devices. Financially it can be very expensive. Also agency policies are often prohibitive. Agencies may require written consent from clients for mechanical recording.

In comparison handwritten recordings of the interaction are less expensive and do not require mechanical devices. They also allow the nurse to record not only what is actually occurring but also her perceptions and feelings regarding the content. However, they usually require more time and energy and if written in the presence of the client can distract the nurse from the relationship. To decrease distortions of what is actually said they also require a great deal of skill in learning how to write without looking. Table 12-1 presents a summary chart of the advantages and disadvantages of each method.

When deciding which method or methods to use, the nurse must take into account not only the advantages and disadvantages of each but also individual preferences—both her own and those of the client. This decision is frequently based on the nurse's comfort and skill in the use of a particular method. Often, however, the nurse must choose an alternative method in view of the preferences of the client and the constraints of the situation. At times it is desirable to use more than one method to provide a comprehensive recording of all aspects of the interaction. For example, a tape recorder could be used to record the verbal level, and general notes with specific nonverbal communication could be written simultaneously. Regardless of the method some form of recording of the communication between the nurse and client is an excellent database for assessment of the relationship. Whatever format is used, the most important aspects are objective and comprehensive recording and a detailed analysis of the process.

In this chapter's case study the student has taken postinteraction notes. The verbatim recordings of her verbal and nonverbal communication and that of the client are presented. The student's analysis of the verbatim material is presented opposite the recordings. In addition, the student has supplied the context for the interactions. This has been termed the *preinteraction,* and it includes a description of her thoughts and feelings before the meeting with the client, the physical setting, a physical description of the client, and the student's goals for the interaction.

TABLE 12-1 **Advantages and disadvantages of methods of recording nurse-client interactions**

ADVANTAGES	DISADVANTAGES
Videotape	**Videotape**
Provides excellent opportunity to see, record, and analyze both nonverbal and verbal levels of communication.	Mechanical devices are necessary.
	Mechanical failure can occur.
Participants are not distracted by writing.	At least one other person is necessary to operate equipment.
Can be preserved for comparison with future interactions.	Often distracting to participants, at least initially.
Can provide participants with audiovisual feedback of their responses.	Transcriptions are time consuming.
Possible to see and hear entire interaction for review and supervision.	Unless more than one monitor is available, comparison is time consuming.
Possible to replay segments for comparison, analysis, and supervision.	
Tape recording	**Tape recording**
Complete verbatim conversation is available.	Mechanical devices are necessary.
Participants are not distracted by writing.	Mechanical failure can occur.
Can be preserved for comparison with future interactions.	Often distracting to participants, at least initially.
Can provide participants with audio feedback of their responses.	Transcriptions are time consuming.
Possible to hear entire interaction for review and supervision.	Unless more than one tape recorder is available comparison is time consuming.
Possible to replay segments for comparison, analysis, and supervision.	Nonverbal communication is not available.
	With cassette-tape recorder it is often necessary to disrupt interaction to turn tape over.
Verbatim notes	**Verbatim notes**
Possible to record thoughts and feelings during interaction.	Difficult to concentrate on interaction until technique of writing without looking is mastered.
Messages recorded as said rather than as what was intended.	Often distracting to participants, at least initially.
Possible to quickly review specific areas for comparison, analysis, and supervision.	Requires greater skill in recording.
Both verbal and nonverbal levels can be recorded.	Segments of the interacton are usually missing or incomplete.
No mechanical devices to distract participants.	
General outline notes	**General outline notes**
Possible to record thoughts and feelings during the interaction.	Often distracting to participants, at least initially.
Possible to quickly review specific areas for comparison, analysis, and supervision.	Necessary to fill in general outline with specific data at a later time.
Both verbal and nonverbal levels can be recorded.	Often actual messages are distorted by intended messages.
No mechanical devices to distract.	
Requires less skill than verbatim notes.	
Decreases amount of energy needed for writing during interaction, hence increases energy available for communication with client.	

Continued

TABLE 12-1   **Advantages and disadvantages of methods of recording nurse-client interactions—cont'd**

ADVANTAGES	DISADVANTAGES
Postinteraction notes	**Postinteraction notes**
No distractions during interaction.	Relies entirely on memory.
Possible to focus attention entirely on communication process.	Often actual messages are distorted by intended messages.
Possible to record information at one's convenience.	Often tends to be a more haphazard notation and analysis unless one is well organized.

NURSING CARE PLAN

The purpose of nursing care plans is to outline the nursing problems identified and the corresponding client needs. They are used to record expected outcomes in terms of nurse-client goals and the relevant nursing actions that will be implemented to meet those goals. This will assist the client in his adaptation to stress. Care plans also include evaluation of the success of the nursing process and possible modifications of goals and actions. The format used for nursing care plans varies. Often it involves only problem identification and nursing actions. At other times it may be a detailed assessment of the behaviors observed; problems identified, priority of the problem and rationale for the selection of priorities; nurse-client expected outcomes and goals; and nursing actions and their corresponding theoretic rationale. Evaluation of the problems, goals, and actions is then based on newly assessed data. Table 12-2 is an example of a detailed and comprehensive care plan format.

Observable behaviors can be differentiated as subjective and objective data. Subjective data refer to anything that is reported by the client, and objective data refer to those behaviors observed by the nurse. Examples of objective data are the results of laboratory tests, a physical examination, and actual behaviors of the client such as crying, laughing, and posture.

Abbreviated forms of the nursing care plan are used for communication between personnel working with the same client at various times. It is important to record data in a concise manner to save time and

energy and be useful. A 10-page care plan on each client would not be feasible or desirable, because the writing and reading of such a care plan would not be an efficient use of time. However, shortened care plan formats must avoid vague generalities. They need to describe individualized nursing care based on a thorough assessment. It is also necessary that they be revised daily or as the needs of the client change. In certain long-term treatment areas or community health agencies this may not be for weeks or even months.

Detailed nursing care plans are often used as learning tools. Recording behaviors and the related problems and needs that are identified reveals the nurse's thought processes. It helps point out errors in logical decision making. All of the components of the detailed care plan are thought through and used on abbreviated forms, but they are not put down in writing. The process is similar to learning to drive a car. In the beginning it is necessary to actively think about each step—putting the car in neutral, checking the emergency brake, depressing the clutch, turning the key, and so on. After repeated performances of this sequence, it is no longer necessary to actively concentrate on each step unless a problem arises, such as the car does not start. The behaviors are then not effective in accomplishing the goal, and one must concentrate on each step of the procedure, attempting to logically deduce what has happened.

The same is true in the nursing process. After repeated situations it is no longer necessary to write down that in working with a suspicious, battered child, forming trust is the first priority rather than

TABLE 12-2 Detailed care plan

BIOPSYCHOSOCIAL BEHAVIORS	NURSING DIAGNOSIS	PRIORITY	RATIONALE	EXPECTED OUTCOMES	NURSING ORDERS/ ACTIONS	RATIONALE	EVALUATION
Objective data: Sits away from other students. Eats meals by himself. Doesn't talk unless asked specific questions. Subjective data: "I like to draw." "I like to play basketball."	Withdrawal related to change of environment evidenced by classroom behavior.	3	Preadolescents need peer group involvement. Does not have any siblings at home. Entered new school in middle of year.	Expected outcome: Client will initiate age-appropriate activities with peers. Long-term goal: Client will participate in a group activity for 30 minutes each school day. Short-term goal: Client will obtain information about community basketball league.	Nursing order: Basketball with at least one other student twice weekly. Nursing actions: The nurse will arrange a basketball game with one other student in the gym twice a week. The nurse will play in the beginning. The nurse will introduce another student at the end of the first week.	Textbook source.	Nursing actions were appropriate, because client stated that he liked to play basketball. They were adequate to accomplish the goal; client played basketball for 30 minutes twice the first week. Actions were therefore effective. Nurse had to play only the first day; after that two students played by themselves. Actions were therefore efficient. Will not be able to use gym next week. Will need alternatives. Not comprehensive or flexible enough. Modifications: Speak with teacher about including student in group art projects.

helping the child keep up with school work. Including a textbook rationale for nursing actions does not facilitate staff communication or continuity of care, but it does help the learner separate nursing actions based on scientific theory from illogical decision making.

As stated in Chapter 1 problem-oriented medical records (POMR) are being used more widely today to save staff members from repetitive writing of data and provide an orderly arrangement of client records. The care plan format in this chapter's case study is based on POMR and nurse-client goals, and an evaluation of the nursing actions, problems, and expected outcomes has been added.

SUPERVISION

The process of supervision is recommended as a mode of validating the progress of the helping relationship. Although supervision is crucial for novices, it is of great importance for experienced practitioners as well. It is never possible to be completely objective in a helping relationship, but objectivity should be a goal. Supervision can facilitate examination of one's own behaviors and responses to a client.

If supervision is to be useful, it is essential that one be open with the supervisor. This can be difficult if the supervisor is also responsible for evaluating one's performance. However, most people in supervisory positions react positively when students or personnel request feedback for the purpose of professional growth. Openness to criticism indicates maturity and self-confidence, which are important attributes of the helping person.

Supervision can be done individually or in groups. Platt-Koch,[2] among the first authors to describe clinical supervision, described four methods of supervision:

1. Case material discussion. The supervisee reports verbally from memory or uses process recording notes to present a case to the supervisor and sometimes to peers. The interaction is analyzed in terms of what was and was not addressed. Alternative approaches are considered.

2. Conjoint interviewing. The supervisor participates in nurse-client sessions. It is possible to role-model communication techniques and observe the supervisee's approaches. This is helpful if a problem cannot be well enough defined to address it in a case discussion.

3. Direct observation techniques. The supervisor uses an unobtrusive way to gain direct experience of the nurse-client relationship without participating and thus influencing it. This includes one-way mirror observation, audiotaping, and videotaping.

4. Peer group supervision. Preferably this involves a group of nurses who are clinically and administratively equals and provide each other with supervision regarding their clinical practice.

Group supervision may also involve a supervisor and a number of individuals requesting validation and assistance. Within the group the emphasis is again placed on the nurse-client relationship. This can be accomplished by individuals presenting their clients and receiving feedback from the supervisor and other group members. This is similar to individual supervision, but it is done within a group setting.

Another approach to group supervision is to present a problem area that commonly occurs in helping relationships or a problem that a number of individuals within the group are presently experiencing, such as difficulty in establishing trust. Participants then contribute examples from their own experiences and attempt to apply the concepts to their own interactions.

Regardless of the approach supervision requires that participants prepare thoroughly for the sessions, bring all necessary data, and most important, contribute openly and freely to the discussion. Careful preparation is useful, because often during supervision previous areas of concern are forgotten. It is also advisable to take notes during and immediately following supervision to follow through with recommendations made. It must be remembered that supervision takes place for the benefit of the client and nurse, or it becomes a meaningless

CASE STUDY

The following case study shows the relationship between the theory presented in the preceding chapters and an actual clinical situation in which a student nurse goes through the process of establishing a relationship. The concepts related to self, communication, relationship, and stress are correlated with specific situations and should thereby increase the reader's understanding and ability to apply these concepts to the reader's own experiences. Most important, the growth process of the student nurse and her increasing self-awareness can be examined, not by abstract statements or short examples but by viewing each step in this lengthy and evolving process.*

In the following case study much emphasis is placed on the thoughts and feelings of the nurse. For many years this type of approach was associated only with psychiatric nursing. However, all nursing care requires involvement in situations that may arouse feelings. Because feelings are related to actions their importance in all areas of nursing cannot be negated.

The student nurse, M.B., is a 26-year-old woman. She is a junior in a 4-year baccalaureate nursing program. This is her first clinical year. Her personal history includes the following information: M.B. is single and currently engaged to be married after graduation from college. She is the only daughter in her family and has older and younger brothers. Her parents are Scottish and describe themselves as liberal Roman Catholics. She lives in an apartment close to the campus with two other nursing students. Scholastically M.B. is an average student who is highly motivated but who usually prefers not to study. She works part-time as a nursing assistant in the hospital near her apartment.

M.B.'s nursing program includes the requirement of following one client over a 6-month period. During this time the students are to establish a long-term relationship, identify nursing problems, institute actions, and evaluate the care given to the client. Most important, they are to recognize their own strengths and weaknesses in working with clients. Group supervision is provided for the students throughout the 6 months. In addition, individual supervision is available when necessary.

M.B. chose to select her client for long-term study from the obstetric clinic, because she was interested in this specialty area. Background information that M.B. obtained from the hospital record before meeting the client is shown below.

exercise.

CLIENT: Connie V.	AGE: 22	EDUCATION: High School
		OCCUPATION: Clerk
HUSBAND: Joseph V.	AGE: 23	EDUCATION: High School
		OCCUPATION: Salesperson

CURRENT LIVING ENVIRONMENT:
   Rent lower-middle class row house in Italian neighborhood
RELIGION: Roman Catholic
RACE: Caucasian

CHILDREN: Lisa	AGE: 3	EDUCATION: To start nursery school in the fall

RELATIVES: Paternal grandparents (live 6 blocks away)
REASON FOR REFERRAL: Pregnancy
PAST MEDICAL HISTORY:
   Tonsillectomy at age 6
   Broken leg at age 17
PREVIOUS PREGNANCY:
Full-term pregnancy; delivered with spinal anesthesia, vaginal delivery, episiotomy; no complications;
   delivered at University Hospital
HEIGHT: 5 ft 5 in   WEIGHT: 140 lb
MENSES: Onset age, 12 years; every 28 days

---

*In analyzing this growth process we have chosen the three methods previously discussed: the process recording, the care plan, and supervision. The process recording is of the postinteraction type. The care plan is an abbreviated format, and the supervision process is alluded to by the inclusion of the supervisor's remarks throughout. To relate concepts previously discussed to the nursing process the supervisor's comments have been expanded to include a discussion of theoretic material. This material is in brackets following the supervisor's state-
Continued

CASE STUDY: *First Meeting*

ments. No attempt is made to refer the reader to specific pages within the text. For further explanation of content the index should be used.

PREINTERACTION

SETTING: Obstetric clinic

NURSE: Somewhat anxious, because I wasn't quite sure if I had sufficient information available to answer client's questions.

CLIENT: Sitting by herself in the last row of seats. She was knitting.

GOALS: Nurse will:

1. Initiate a relationship with client.
2. Establish a contract.
3. Assess client's level of wellness.
4. Identify possible health stressors and plan appropriate nursing actions.

Supervisor's Comments:

1. Describe the setting. What did it look like? Was the room crowded or empty? How was the furniture arranged?
   [Communication and the nurse-client relationship occur within a particular context. A description of

the setting establishes the tone for what follows and will often influence what occurs. For instance, in a noisy, crowded area it is more difficult to establish a contract with a client, because there are so many other stimuli intruding on the client's receptors.]

2. Describe your feelings: What was your reaction to the setting? What kind of day had you had? What were your fears, anxieties, and hopes for this interaction? What were your initial impressions of the client? What prompted you to select her?
   [The nurse must be able to focus on her own feelings and thoughts, because they will often influence the course of the relationship. For instance, initial student-client interactions may take on the nature of approach-avoidance situations where both participants are somewhat hesitant because of the unknown aspects of the situation.]

3. Another nursing goal that should be included is the assessment of the client's preparation for labor, delivery, and postpartum. The reason for the client's clinic visit—pregnancy—enables the nurse to identify specific areas of focus in addition to her general assessment of the client's level of wellness. Although the importance of complete data collection and assess-

VERBATIM	STUDENT ASSESSMENT	SUPERVISOR'S COMMENTS
ment cannot be overlooked, it is equally important to focus on the reason the client has sought health care.		Did you give the client an opportunity to respond here?
NURSE: Hello, you're Ms. C.V.? My name is M.B. I am a student nurse here. Do you mind if I sit down and talk with you while you are waiting?	Smiling is a social behavior that encouraged me to continue.	The client's verbal and nonverbal communication are congruent. The message is "I will talk with you."
CLIENT: No. It is usually a long wait. (Smiling.) What is your name again?	I should have further explained my purpose in talking with the client.	How were you feeling here? Was your body sending you messages that might have cued you to your own anxiety level at this point? Such cues include sweaty palms, unsteady hands, and a dry mouth.
NURSE: I'm M.B. This is your second baby?		

VERBATIM	STUDENT ASSESSMENT	SUPERVISOR'S COMMENTS
(I sat down next to client.)		How secure did you feel in your role? Often one's own confusion about purpose and actions prevents one from presenting a clear picture to the client.
CLIENT: Yes. My mother-in-law is watching Lisa, who's 3.		You did not respond to the client's remark. Why did you change the subject?
NURSE: What are you knitting?		
CLIENT: I love to knit. This is going to be a baby sweater. (She held up the blue yarn.)	Responding to the object nonverbal; the yarn was blue.	Good example of validation.
NURSE: You want to have a boy?		Remember to include your nonverbal communication and that of the client. (There are numerous problems in interpreting the meaning of verbal communication. Nonverbal communication may assist in establishing meaning or in defining the context in which the verbal behavior occurred.)
CLIENT: Yes, a girl and a boy. That is what I've always wanted—two children.		
	I am asking too many questions.	What were you feeling that could have caused this behavior? You have also changed the topic again. Were you feeling anxious?
NURSE: Have you been to the clinic before?		(The student's recognition that something is wrong is an important first step. The supervisor's remarks attempt to help the student explore possible causes for this nontherapeutic behavior.)
CLIENT:		

Continued

CASE STUDY: *First Meeting—cont'd*

VERBATIM	STUDENT ASSESSMENT	SUPERVISOR'S COMMENTS
Yes, I came here when I had Lisa.		Perhaps a more open-ended comment would have facilitated communication here; for example, "Would you like to tell me a little about your experiences and feelings with that pregnancy?"
NURSE: Do you have any questions about the clinic procedure?		You seem to be using the distracting pattern of communication, and the client seems to be following your lead. She responded to your question about clinic procedures with her perception of the clinic walls.
CLIENT: No. They've done some remodeling here, I see. I think the pastel colors and pretty pictures are very nice.		(The distracting pattern of communication attempts to ignore threats to the self with irrelevant communication. Tension also tends to increase when this communication pattern is used.)
NURSE: How many weeks pregnant are you? **CLIENT:** Well, I've missed two periods. So I guess about 2 months or so. **NURSE:** Have you had a pregnancy test?	I am asking too many questions, but I didn't know what else to say. My anxiety level is high.	You need to review your therapeutic communication techniques. You seem to be on a fact-finding mission instead of allowing the client to take the lead. What was the cause of your anxiety? How has your anxiety level influenced your behavior? (It is important for the student to recognize that her anxiety influences both her behavior and the client's. After the student's characteristic mode of responding to anxiety is revealed she can begin to concentrate on more effective ways of dealing with the uncomfortable feelings.)

VERBATIM	STUDENT ASSESSMENT	SUPERVISOR'S COMMENTS
CLIENT: No, but I've always been regular, so when I miss a period, it can only mean one thing.		
NURSE: Do you have any other symptoms. . . similar to those of your first pregnancy?		Your use of the term *symptom* connotes the idea of illness.
CLIENT: Well, I have to go to the bathroom more often, and I'm tired. I could sleep for days, I think.		
NURSE: That could be a problem with a 3-year-old.	Therapeutic communication technique: exploring a possible stressor.	Good example of reflecting back to the patient something you have inferred from her communication, thereby asking her to validate your inference.
CLIENT: Yes, when I come home from work, I'm too tired to even cook. My mother-in-law is a real gem. She even makes dinner some nights so my husband and Lisa have something to eat.		
NURSE: Where are you working?		Why the sudden change of subject? You could have empathized more, then picked up on her work. (Sudden topic changes can be caused by faulty listening skills. Instead of hearing the total message the listener picks up on key words in a response and immediately begins to formulate the next statement. Failure to listen has a deleterious effect on the relationship through the loss of information and by negating the worth of the client's statements.)

Continued

CASE STYDY: *First Meeting—cont'd*

VERBATIM	STUDENT ASSESSMENT	SUPERVISOR'S COMMENTS
CLIENT:		
I work at the Fidelity Company as a clerk. It's horrible. Just sitting there filing and pushing paper.		
NURSE:		
I hate to do that also. I couldn't do it for more than an hour.	Did I cut her off? Should I have pursued her feelings more? I was being more sympathetic than empathic.	Yes, you seem to be communicating based on your own needs rather than those of your client. Perhaps you could have reflected back what you felt the client was saying; for example, "It must be hard to be pregnant, work, and be a wife and mother."
(Silence for about a minute.)	I was feeling uncomfortable.	Any nonverbal communication during this silence? Recording nonverbal communication may help you determine if this was a therapeutic use of silence.
		(Silence can be used therapeutically by nonverbally communicating interest to the client.)
NURSE:		
You've already been weighed and had your blood pressure taken?	Doing something would have made me feel better.	Try to analyze your own feelings.
		(As one's anxiety increases, perception is altered and responses tend to become more self-centered. It is only after an understanding and acceptance of the self has been established that one can acknowledge the uniqueness and differences within a client.)
CLIENT:		
Yes.		
NURSE:		
What was your first pregnancy like?		
CLIENT:		
Not very difficult. I really enjoyed being pregnant. I was working then, but I quit in my third month. The nausea and vomiting were pretty bad, so I was missing a lot of work anyway.		

. . . .

VERBATIM	STUDENT ASSESSMENT	SUPERVISOR'S COMMENTS
NURSE:		
How much weight did you gain?	Exploring a possible problem area: she appears to be slightly overweight.	True, but again you have failed to follow the lead of the client. It may have been more beneficial to explore one of the topics that she introduced—morning sickness, and quitting work.
CLIENT:		
Oh, I wasn't very good with a diet. Sitting home all day I gained 55 lb, but after Lisa was born I didn't have any trouble losing the extra weight. Taking care of a baby is a full-time job.	She seems to be feeling guilty. She sounds rather defensive.	You should have validated this inference. You might also have asked if she intends to continue working.
NURSE:		
What types of foods do you usually eat?	Assessing her eating patterns.	You might also have further assessed her understanding of the implications of excessive weight gain.
CLIENT:		
Oh, I like just about everything. Joe likes his pasta, but I'm more a meat-and-potatoes type of person.	She didn't give a very descriptive answer. I need to pursue this in more detail at a later time.	Could this be related to the way you phrased your question?
NURSE:		
Do you know about the food pyramid and what you should be eating because you're pregnant?		The use of the word *should* sounds judgmental, as if you know what is right. Judgmental statements tell the client that to maintain a relationship with you, she needs to think as you do.
CLIENT:		
I had a nutrition course in high school, so I know about including vegetables, meats, and breads.		

Continued

CASE STUDY: *First Meeting—cont'd*

VERBATIM	STUDENT ASSESSMENT	SUPERVISOR'S COMMENTS
NURSE: That's good. So many pregnant women aren't aware of the effects of their diet on the unborn child.	Giving positive reinforcement.	"That's good" is a judgmental statement. You don't want the client to feel that she needs to please you. This is an area of contradiction that needs further exploration. If the client knows about nutrition, why did she gain so much weight? (Premature positive reinforcement may inhibit exploration of areas that the client wants to discuss by indicating a lack of interest in further discussion on the part of the nurse.)
CLIENT: Yes. There was a special on TV not too long ago about Americans being overweight yet undernourished.		
NURSE: That's so true. We have so much food, but so much of it has few if any nutrients.	Therapeutic communication technique of acknowledgement.	

Then Ms. V. was called into an examining room. I went with her and helped her. The physician's pelvic examination confirmed a pregnancy; he asked her if she had any questions and said she should return in a month. I stayed with her and helped her get dressed. I felt more relaxed while I was involved with some technical skills. I guess I'm still not very comfortable just talking with clients.

NURSE: Do you have any questions, Ms. V.?		
CLIENT: No.		
NURSE: I'd like to talk with you next month when you come in again. If you think of anything you want to ask or if you have any problems, maybe we can talk about them.	Establishing a contract.	In establishing a contract you need to also discuss confidentiality, the duration of the relationship, and role expectations. (Contracts include all the obligations that participants will meet. Verbally stating them helps clarify exactly what types of behavior are relevant within the relationship.)

VERBATIM	STUDENT ASSESSMENT	SUPERVISOR'S COMMENTS
CLIENT: That would be nice. Thanks for staying with me. It really helps pass the time. I hate to wait. It always seems such a waste of time.	This indicates some trust. The patient has agreed to a future contract and seems grateful for my attention.	You could have shared your feelings also; for example, "I enjoyed talking with you too."
NURSE: Do you understand about your prescription?		
CLIENT: Yes. I took vitamins with Lisa. They're about the only pills I ever take.		
NURSE: You need to be very careful of what medications you take during pregnancy. Lots of things can hurt the baby. You should *always* consult a doctor before you take anything, especially when you're pregnant.	Therapeutic communication: giving the client information.	Perhaps, but you sound like a parent giving directions to a child. (Giving information is an adult-to-adult transaction.)
CLIENT: I haven't taken any pills in ages, and I know I shouldn't use *anything* when I'm pregnant.		You should try to spend some time thinking about your own reactions and your goals before your next interaction. If you feel more comfortable with yourself and your role within the relationship, you may be better able to access the client's total health needs.
NURSE: Good-bye. I'll see you next month.		

NURSING CARE PLAN
Nursing Diagnosis:
Altered nutrition potential for more than body requirements, related to the increased food intake during pregnancy evidenced by excessive weight gain during last pregnancy. This is the only nursing diagnosis that I have identified and is a mutually identified problem.

Subjective:
Client stated that:
1. She likes meat and potatoes.
2. Husband likes pasta.
3. She knows "food pyramid" and has taken a high-school nutrition course.

Continued

CASE STUDY: *First Meeting—cont'd*

4. Mother-in-law does some cooking for client's family.

5. She doesn't think she is presently overweight.

Objective:

Client gained 55 lb during last pregnancy. Present height: 5 ft 5 in; weight: 140 lb.

Assessment:

Client needs to control her weight during pregnancy.

Expected Outcomes:

Long-Term Goal: Client's weight will not exceed 180 lb during 9 months of pregnancy.

Short-Term Goal: Client's weight will remain at 140 lb during the first trimester.

Planned Nursing Actions:

1. Implement health education regarding low-calorie diet if client starts to gain weight.

2. With client, plan diet appropriate to her lifestyle.

Supervisor's Comments: Your identification of the problem, assessment, and goals is appropriate; however, your nursing actions are vague. What diet plan do you intend to use? It needs to take into account the nutritional needs related to pregnancy. Based on your initial assessment of the client's needs and background information you should be able to construct a structured health teaching plan individualized for this client. You also need to include evaluation in your care plan.

Summary of First Meeting:

In this initial meeting the dynamics of an individual's growth, use of communication to build a relationship, and influence of stress on that relationship are manifested. The nurse is attempting to assess the individual needs of a particular client while simultaneously assessing her own performance in a new situation. Two areas of interest are brought out in this initial meeting: (1) common problem areas for beginning students, and (2) the role of the supervisor in dealing with these problems.

The two problem areas common to most beginning students are inadequate interpersonal skills and role confusion. In this interaction the student's lack of skills in using therapeutic communication techniques as well as the difficulty encountered in the specifics of forming a helping relationship are evident. In addition, lack of skills in observing the situation and her use of self in the relationship are depicted. The student finds it difficult to record nonverbal communication and report her feelings at the time of the interaction, let alone relate those feelings to her behavior and that of the client.

Role confusion is partially a result of inadequate skills. In this meeting it is evident that the student's purpose is unclear. Most beginning students find it difficult to relate to a client without physical duties to perform. The purpose of the relationship needs to be constantly repeated. The student must be reminded that her role includes not only the assessment of a particular client's reactions to pregnancy but also how the nurse's thoughts, feelings, perceptions, and behavior influence the nursing process. As a result of the lack of skills and role confusion, stress is produced in varying degrees. Manifestations of stress—for instance, topic changes and inability to tolerate silences—are evident.

The second area of interest brought out in this initial interaction is the role of the supervisor, particularly how the supervisor deals with the problems of lack of skills and role confusion. The supervisor attempts to deal with the student's problems in various ways. The supervisor presents alternative possibilities to the student (e.g., "What would happen if you did this instead?"). In this way the supervisor serves as a role model in the use of skills that the student has not developed. A second method used by the supervisor is questioning. The supervisor asks for additional data regarding the use of self, nonverbal communication, and the context of the behavior. This helps the student to focus on more important aspects of the relationship and encourages the development of observational and recording skills. The final method used by the supervisor in this interaction is providing feedback. The supervisor validates inferences drawn by the student (e.g., "Yes, I think that is happening.") and also provides reinforcement when behavior approaches the desired goals.

It is evident in this interaction that the nurse is not only developing a relationship with a specific client but is simultaneously developing a relationship with the supervisor. In this initial phase the supervisor provides increased input and direction while attempting to foster the student's individual growth and independence.

CASE STUDY: *Second Meeting*

PREINTERACTION

CLIENT: Arrived approximately 5 minutes late for her appointment. She was smiling and appeared slightly anxious. She was wearing a blue maternity dress and a white shawl that she later said she had made. She was also wearing support hose and 3-inch heels.

GOALS: Nurse will:

1. Weigh client, and if client has gained weight, discuss with client her present eating patterns and plan with her a 2000-calorie diet with 64 g protein daily. (Health teaching plan follows.)
2. Complete assessment of the client including preparation for labor, delivery, and postpartum, and identify other possible problem areas.

3. Establish a contract, discussing confidentiality, roles, and termination date.

HEALTH TEACHING PLAN FOR WEIGHT CONTROL DURING PREGNANCY:

LEARNING OUTCOMES: At the conclusion of the teaching, the client will:

1. Correctly identify the foods necessary in a 2000-calorie diet.
2. List protein sources.
3. Identify nutrients that are necessary during pregnancy.

Teaching plan:

Content

1. Description of 2000-calorie diet

2. Role of protein and protein requirements during pregnancy
3. Vitamins A and C, calcium, and iron needs during pregnancy

Instructional activities

1. Chart of basic food groups with sample 2000-calorie diet meal plans
2. Ask client to name foods that are high in protein

3. Ask client to name food source for each

Supervisor's Comments:

1. Your goals are behavioral and well written.
2. What behaviors led you to infer that the client was anxious?
3. The health teaching plan needs to be more specific. Focus on the individual needs of this client. For instance, client stated that she liked meat and potatoes. What necessary nutrients will be excluded in a meat-and-potato diet? Also you should include an evaluation section. For example, if you ask the client to name protein food sources, the evaluation would read that client names at least 10 protein food sources in addition to meat.

(When students initially do health teaching, their plans need to be more detailed and comprehensive. In the actual teaching situation students usually do not have the same degree of flexibility or content mastery as an experienced health educator. They need comprehensive plans to prepare them for many possible contingencies. Teaching content, as in this example, is very often based on what a student was taught about a particular subject. In many cases this is not appropriate for client needs. For example, 64 g of protein may have meaning to a nursing student but may be too technical for the client. It may be more appropriate to discuss protein requirements with a client in terms of actual number of eggs, ounces of meat, or glasses of milk.)

Continued

CASE STUDY: *Second Meeting—cont'd*

VERBATIM	STUDENT ASSESSMENT	SUPERVISOR'S COMMENTS
NURSE: (Smiling) Hello, Ms. V. How are you today?	She looked well and happy to see me.	What object nonverbal communication did you see here? (Object nonverbal communication includes the intentional and nonintentional use of material things.)
CLIENT: Oh, I'm doing fine. You're the student nurse I talked with last time, aren't you?	She remembered me; that was encouraging.	
NURSE: Yes, I'm M.B. How have you been since your last clinic appointment?		The repetition of your name indicates that you were sensitive to the fact that she could have forgotten it after only one meeting.
CLIENT: Oh, everything is about the same, except that now I look like I belong here. (She smiled and patted her abdomen gently.)	Congruency of verbal and nonverbal communication. She seems pleased by her pregnancy. I should have validated this inference.	I agree. Perhaps a question such as "You seem pleased by your pregnancy?" may have validated this inference. (Reflecting awareness of the client's feeling completes the process of empathy by allowing the client to validate the accuracy of the nurse's perception. This facilitates the growth of trust and allows for the tension level to diminish, promoting a more comfortable atmosphere.)
NURSE: Would you come back to the office so I can weigh you and take your blood pressure? (We walked to the back of the clinic.)		
CLIENT: (Frowning.) This is the worst part, getting on the scale. (She removed her shoes to be weighed. She hadn't gained any weight since her last visit.)	I was glad that the client had not gained any weight. I should have responded to her successful weight control.	You might have explored why the client felt that this was the worst part. Maybe you should add this action—giving positive reinforcement—to your care plan.
NURSE: Did you bring a urine specimen with you?		

VERBATIM	STUDENT ASSESSMENT	SUPERVISOR'S COMMENTS
CLIENT: Yes. Here it is.	I tested the urine for sugar and acetone. It was negative for both.	
NURSE: The doctor isn't ready to see you yet. Would you like to return to the waiting area and talk some more?	Giving the client the initiative, allowing her to decide if she wanted to talk to me (mutuality). I felt confident that she would agree.	
CLIENT: That would be nice. I didn't even remember my knitting. I was in such a hurry to get here, and I thought I'd be late. (Smiling.) I should have known by now that you always have to wait. (We found a quiet corner in the waiting room. I moved my chair to sit at a 45-degree angle from Ms. V. so that I could see her better.)	By not remembering her knitting she may have unconsciously remembered that I would be here.

I wanted to observe her nonverbal communication. I didn't want to get too close and invade her personal space. | It would have been helpful to have validated this inference.

Good application of theory. Finding a quiet place decreases environmental distractions, thereby increasing the possibility of effective communication. |
CLIENT: Is all your nursing experience in this clinic?	I felt that the client was demonstrating an interest in me and mutuality.	This is also part of the process of building trust. She may be asking the question, "How experienced are you?"
NURSE: No. We rotate through many different areas. Rather than seeing everyone only once or twice, we're trying to follow one patient in a clinical area for a length of time this semester.	I felt that the client was trying to define our roles within the relationship and was beginning to see me as "person" rather than as "nurse."	How did this make you feel? (Role confusion may result when one's perceived role in a relationship is questioned. In such an event anxiety tends to be aroused, with the concomitant physiologic responses.)
CLIENT: That seems to be a nice idea. (She begins to play with the straps on her purse and looks away.)	Could be an outward sign of anxiety. I thought about asking her if she was anxious, but I didn't think I could handle her response. Basically I was afraid of rejection.	You are showing a good deal of insight into your own behavior.

Continued

CASE STUDY: *Second Meeting—cont'd*

VERBATIM	STUDENT ASSESSMENT	SUPERVISOR'S COMMENTS
NURSE:		
I would like to talk with you each time you come to the clinic. Answer any questions you may have . . . try to be useful to you. (I began to play with the edge of my uniform.) I will discuss this experience with my instructor and my clinical group.	Contract formation—something I should have done last time. I began to feel anxious. I noticed my voice trailing off at the end.	You have not mentioned termination. (Definition of the circumstances of termination is an integral part of the establishment of the contract. It provides security by defining the limits of the relationship.)
CLIENT:		
(Smiling.) That's nice.	An empty platitude. I really don't know how she feels about this.	The contract that you presented seems one sided. Could this be the reason for the interpersonal anxiety? How could you have handled this differently?
(Silence—approximately 3 minutes. No eye contact.)	Seemed like an awkward silence. I felt slightly uncomfortable.	(Interpersonal anxiety can occur in situations where roles are unclear. Because the contract presented did not sufficiently explain what was expected from the client, anxiety will be produced.)
		Any nonverbal communication during this silence? Is the intensity of the situation changing and affecting your behaviors?
		(Intensity refers to the magnitude of the stressor. As stress becomes more intense, reflections of this change may be observed in the nonverbal communication.)

Then the client was called into the examining room, and I went with her. The height of the fundus was compatible with the gestational age of the fetus. The fetal heart rate was audible.

VERBATIM	STUDENT ASSESSMENT	SUPERVISOR'S COMMENTS
CLIENT:		
(Dressing and smiling broadly.) It's certainly great to hear that little heart beating. He's really alive and well! My husband and I are looking forward to this baby so much.	I felt happy to hear the heart beat too.	Would you assess this client to be in Erikson's stage of intimacy versus isolation or generativity versus self-absorption?
		(Erikson's stages of development progress with each stage building on the previous stage. The client's statement regarding her husband can be seen as a reflection of a mature relationship; the concern for the next generation, the unborn child, reflects generativity.)

VERBATIM	STUDENT ASSESSMENT	SUPERVISOR'S COMMENTS
NURSE: It certainly is. I notice you said "he."	Last month she also said she wanted a boy; may be a possible stressor if the new baby is a girl.	You did not mention your nonverbal response. Did you also smile and show her that you empathically shared her joy?
CLIENT: Of course. We already have a girl. (She smiled and laughed softly.) Do you know if they offer natural childbirth here?	Trust is beginning to develop. She's asking me for information. Roles are becoming clearer.	
NURSE: What do you mean by "natural childbirth?"	Trying to obtain her denotative and connotative meanings for the term *natural childbirth.*	Your communication skills seem to be drawing her out more. This is also a good basis for mutual planning.
CLIENT: You know, courses in breathing so that you don't need anesthesia, and you watch the baby being born and your husband can be there. (She talked on rapidly about how a friend at work had told her about natural childbirth and her sister-in-law had said she was crazy if that's what she wanted and so on.)		
NURSE: They have childbirth education classes here. We can look at a brochure in the waiting room to see if it's what you want. There are other groups in the city that teach Lamaze breathing exercises. Is your husband interested also?	Therapeutic communication: giving information. I felt I was really beginning to help her and also carrying out the advocacy role of supporting her decision to have natural childbirth.	
CLIENT: He listens to my sister-in-law, and she said I was crazy, but I don't think he really understands.	If husband's goals are not congruent with those of client, could be a possible stressor.	

Continued

CASE STUDY: *Second Meeting—cont'd*

VERBATIM	STUDENT ASSESSMENT	SUPERVISOR'S COMMENTS
NURSE: How does that make you feel?	Therapeutic communication: focusing on the client's feelings.	Good. (It is only after the client is able to recognize feelings as part of her self-system that she will be able to examine her behaviors and their relationship to the feelings expressed.)
CLIENT: Well, Beth is older, and she has had four children. I used to get very angry and feel that my husband didn't care. Sometimes I would sulk for days, but now I realize that he respects Beth and her opinion and experience, and if I can support my case (smiling), he usually agrees with me. He's really a logical person. I'm probably more emotional. I get excited and sometimes tearful when I think of the two of us having a baby together, watching and working together. He thinks of my comfort and safety and that of the baby.	She seems to be rationalizing. That she is able to express her feelings shows trust.	Rationalization is one method to relieve conflict. The client seems aware of her communication patterns with her husband. They seem to communicate on an adult-to-adult level. (It is important to clarify exactly what the client is discussing here. Is she really interested in prepared childbirth, or does she only want her husband present during labor and delivery? By relating this discussion to her previous childbirth experience it may be possible to help her determine exactly what she disliked about her first experience and how she would like this experience to be different.)
NURSE: Prepared childbirth seems very important to you. Can you think of anything that might help him understand?	Responding to the client's feelings?	Empathic response. (Empathic in that the student seems to have entered the life of another and perceived accurately that person's feelings and their meanings.) Mutual planning with the client increases the chances of goal success. (Goals based on the client's individual needs and those that have been defined by the client as important have the greatest chance of being met, whereas goals based on the nurse's perceptions or textbook goals fail to incorporate the needs and desires of the individual client.)

VERBATIM	STUDENT ASSESSMENT	SUPERVISOR'S COMMENTS
CLIENT: I'm sure if he went to the classes . . . but I'm not sure how to get him there. Maybe if somebody who knows more about it could explain . . . but I don't know who or when.		Judging from the client's hesitation this seems to be an area of unresolved tension or conflict. (Ongoing tension of moderate intensity may be manifested in chronic physical dysfunction. It is important to maintain an awareness of this possibility.)
NURSE: Maybe I could talk to him about the classes and answer some of his questions.	Acting as an advocate by offering to inform Mr. V. about natural childbirth.	How can this be related to crisis theory?
CLIENT: (Knitting her brows and holding eye contact.) I'd like that, but he can't come here during the day.	Indicates hope that I can assist her to arrange a fulfilling birth experience.	(Birth of a baby is a life event that produces change and increases stress for the individuals involved. The balancing factors that determine whether it becomes a crisis include perception of the event and situational supports.) This action is also supportive of Ms. V.'s decision by assisting her to enlist her husband's active involvement in the situation.
NURSE: I could visit you at home if you like?		It's good that you worded this as a question. Giving the client the responsibility to make the decision says that you realize that she is an adult capable of solving her own problems. Your role is to facilitate her problem solving.
CLIENT: (Smiling broadly.) Oh, yes, two against one. That sounds like a good idea.		
NURSE: I would be coming to give information.	I didn't want her to think I was going to form a coalition with her against her husband.	Further clarification of the limits of the contract.

Continued

CASE STUDY: *Second Meeting—cont'd*

We went into the waiting room and found brochures on the prepared childbirth classes. Ms. V. decided to take them home and talk to her husband about them. I also told Ms. V. that there was a nutrition course on Wednesday mornings and a prenatal exercise program on Tuesdays and Wednesdays. She said she could not attend either, because she was still working.

VERBATIM	STUDENT ASSESSMENT	SUPERVISOR'S COMMENTS
NURSE:		
We'll meet again in 4 weeks for your next appointment and talk about the prepared childbirth classes.		Good—reviewing the contract with mutual goal setting for the next visit.
CLIENT:		
Hopefully my husband will consent to come with me. It's something I really want.		

NURSING CARE PLAN

Nursing Diagnosis 1:

Altered nutrition: potential for more than body requirements, related to the increased food intake during pregnancy, evidenced by excessive weight gain during last pregnancy—priority 2

Subjective:

Client stated, "Getting weighed is worst part" of clinic visit.

Objective:

Weight 140 lb.

Assessment:

Client has had no weight gain in last 4 weeks.

Expected outcomes:

Long-Term Goal: Client's weight will not exceed 180 lb during 9 months of pregnancy.

Short-Term Goal: Client's weight gain will not exceed 2 lb per week during the second trimester.

Planned Nursing Actions:

1. Continue to weigh client at each clinic visit.
2. Give positive reinforcement for maintaining weight within limits set.
3. Plan with client a 2000-calorie diet with 64 g protein daily if weight gain exceeds goal.
4. Explore client's feelings about weight, self-concept, and body image.

Evaluation:

Goals are being met. Teaching plan not initiated. Addition of positive reinforcement for maintaining weight.

Nursing Diagnosis 2:

Family coping: potential for growth, related to marital conflict about natural childbirth, evidenced by client's report of husband's skepticism—priority 1

Subjective:

Client stated that she is interested in natural childbirth and husband is opposed because sister-in-law says she is "crazy."

Objective:

Client has not experienced natural childbirth previously.

Assessment:

Client needs to feel a sense of self-esteem and autonomy in decision making with husband about method of childbirth.

Expected Outcomes

Long-Term Goal: Client will use whatever childbirth method she chooses.

Short-Term Goals:

1. Client will state positive and negative aspects of previous childbirth experience and will relate previous experience to expectations for this labor and delivery.
2. Client and spouse will reach a mutually agreeable decision by the sixth month regarding the type of childbirth to be experienced. Client will state that she is pleased with this decision.

Planned Nursing Actions:

1. Meet with husband and client to discuss types of childbirth.
2. Assess their knowledge of natural childbirth and previous childbirth experience.
3. Offer them information regarding types of childbirth that they are interested in.
4. Facilitate their discussion of childbirth by helping to clarify feelings, presenting facts, answering questions, and relating to previous experience.
5. Support their decision-making process.

Evaluation:

Did not intervene yet. Goals and actions are appropriate.

Supervisor's Comments:

1. Your problem identification reflects a thorough assessment of the biopsychosocial aspects of this client.
2. You should give the rationale for the priorities you have established. Priority can be related to description of stress state (intensity, duration, or scope of stress experience).
3. Your evaluation of problems, expected outcomes, and actions have improved.

Summary of Second Meeting:

In this second meeting the development of interpersonal skills and defining of the nurse-client roles within the relationship are depicted. The student shows an increasing awareness of her use of self within the relationship. For instance, she could not validate her inference that the client was anxious, because she was afraid of rejection. In such circumstances the student begins to see how her own feelings and thoughts affect her behavior and in turn the behavior of the client. In addition, the student demonstrates a growing ability to focus on the nonverbal communication as well as the verbal statements of herself and the client. This ability clarifies and adds depth to the meaning of the interaction for both the student and the supervisor. Although there is still a need during this meeting to accomplish goals regarding contract formation that should have been included in the first interaction, roles are becoming more clearly outlined. As role definition occurs the client and nurse emerge as individuals. Autonomy, mutuality, and trust begin to emerge as the relationship progresses out of the orientation phase. As goals are identified (in this case information and decisions regarding prepared childbirth and weight control) the relationship progresses to the maintenance phase.

The role of the supervisor also changes in this interaction. Primarily the supervisor reinforces the student's skill development. However, there are still occasions in which the supervisor uses the techniques of questioning, focusing, and presenting alternatives.

CASE STUDY: *Third Meeting*

During the meeting the student discussed Ms. V.'s previous labor and delivery and how the client expected this labor to differ. Ms. V. stated that she wanted her husband to be with her "this time" and that she had felt "so alone" delivering her 3-year-old. Also, the student asked about the reactions of Ms. V. and her husband to the prepared childbirth brochures. Ms. V. stated that although she wanted to attend the classes, her husband still insisted that the idea was "silly." She was certain that his stubbornness was influenced by her sister-in-law's vigorous, anti-natural childbirth campaign. Ms. V. was very verbal regarding her dislike of her sister-in-law, especially her sister-in-law's "know everything" attitude. The student helped Ms. V. express her anger toward her sister-in-law and her disappointment with her husband's reaction. Ms. V. invited the nurse to come to her home to discuss prepared childbirth classes with her husband. Although the nurse supported the client's desire to involve her husband, she verbalized that the client might want to attend the classes alone if her husband was still adamant or have someone else act as her labor coach. Together the nurse and Ms. V. explored possible alternative labor coaches available. Ms. V. decided that if her husband still refused when the classes began and because there was no one else available that she would like to have as a labor coach, she would ask the childbirth group at the hospital to assign one of the volunteer labor coaches. Ms. V. had gained 12 lb in the last month. She attributed this weight gain to feeling bored at work. Together Ms. V. and the nurse planned a sample diet for the following week.

NURSING CARE PLAN
Nursing Diagnosis 1:

Short-term goal was not met. Client gained 12 lb in last 4 weeks. Implemented nursing actions. Mutually planned with client a 2000-calorie diet with 64 g protein. Need to further assess client's feelings about work and their effect on her eating patterns.

Nursing Diagnosis 2:

Marital conflict continues. Importance of prepared childbirth for this client explored in relationship to previous labor and delivery experience and expectations for future experience. Client does not want to be alone during labor and delivery. Appointment made to discuss childbirth process with client and husband. Introduced possibility of client attending classes without husband. Client decided to use someone else as labor coach if necessary.

CASE STUDY: *Fourth Meeting*

PREINTERACTION

SETTING: Living room of the V.'s. The room was small and contained a couch, two chairs, two tables, and a television. Furniture arms were frayed. Tables appeared new—no scratches. Plants were everywhere—I counted 15. There were probably more. Everything was in place—no dust or toys. It was very clean and tidy.

NURSE: I was terribly nervous. My stomach ached, and my head pounded as I approached the house. It was a small row house in the middle of the block. I was already late, because I wasn't able to find a place to park and didn't know the neighborhood at all. I was worried about meeting her husband and began to have self-doubts about implementing my nursing actions.

CLIENT: Ms. V. greeted me with a smile; she was wearing jeans and a blue blouse. She looked very pregnant and somewhat tired—her eyes were dark and hair uncombed. Later she said she had cleaned as soon as she got home from work, because the "house was such a mess." Mr. V. was not at home. He was having dinner with his parents who lived six blocks away and was expected home with Lisa any minute.

GOALS: Nurse will:
1. Assess family interactions and facilitate communication and decision making.
2. Answer any questions Ms. V. and her husband might have regarding the classes and delivery.
3. Share information gathered on prenatal classes with them.

HEALTH TEACHING PLAN:
Learning Outcomes:

At the conclusion of the teaching, the clients will be able to:
1. Define prepared childbirth.
2. Identify the types of childbirth preparation classes available to them.
3. Compare and contrast the philosophies and methodologies of programs available.
4. Compare information on concrete issues such as cost, location, time.
5. Decide on a program that most fits their needs.

CONTENT	INSTRUCTIONAL ACTIVITIES	EVALUATION
Define prepared childbirth. Dispel any myths or misconceptions that clients may have regarding prepared childbirth.	Ask clients what the term means to them.	How close are clients' perceptions to reality?
Identify programs available within community: 1. Hospital classes 2. Childbirth Education Association 3. Lamaze classes	Give clients outline sheet with three types available with times, prices, and philosophies.	
Discuss differences among programs available: 1. Philosophy 2. Methodology 3. Cost 4. Locations 5. Times	Ask clients: What they would like to be the outcome of attending classes? What program do they think would be most beneficial to them?	How well do the available programs fit the needs of the clients? Decide on a program and register for it.

Continued

CASE STUDY: *Fourth Meeting—cont'd*

SUPERVISOR'S COMMENTS:

1. Your objective recording of the client's appearance validates the inferences you made.

2. Your ability to assess your own feelings of inadequacy is a start in identifying your needs for self-growth.

VERBATIM	STUDENT ASSESSMENT	SUPERVISOR'S COMMENTS
MS. V.:		
Did you have any trouble finding our house?	Caring. Client didn't want me to get lost, or perhaps she was curious as to why I was late.	Be aware that any change in the environment or context of the nurse-client relationship may have a significant effect on the nature of the interactions.
NURSE:		
No, but a parking place, yes. I'm sorry that I'm late.	I realized I felt more relaxed once I saw her.	What internal feedback were you using to identify feelings of relaxation?
MS. V.:		
That's fine. My husband and Lisa are still at Mom's. We had dinner there. I wanted to put this place in order. . . . Sit down. (She pointed to a red, overstuffed chair in the corner.) Would you like something to drink?	She may have felt some role confusion—needs to be hostess in her house. This was hard for me, too. I felt more like a guest than a nurse.	Going into another's home versus meeting on "our" territory often causes such feeling initially.
NURSE:		
(Sitting down in the chair.) No, thank you.		
MS. V.:		
(Sitting on sofa opposite me.) I can't wait until I can be a full-time mother. (She sighed loudly and pushed her hair back from her face.)	Pushing her hair back is a recurrent behavior pattern with the client.	Can you assign any meaning to this and validate it?
NURSE:		
When do you plan to stop working? (I moved to the edge of the chair.)	I felt lost in that big chair.	
MS. V.:		
(Laughing.) Hopefully tomorrow. I wish tomorrow, but probably not for a few weeks or months. My husband thinks I should work up until I deliver. (Frowning.) Beth did with her first two.	Again her negative feelings toward her sister-in-law were evident.	

VERBATIM	STUDENT ASSESSMENT	SUPERVISOR'S COMMENTS
NURSE: Your husband thinks that you should do what your sister-in-law does?	Validation.	
MS. V.: Yes. (She got up to close the curtain and then returned to the sofa.) I'd like to stay home and take care of Lisa—the way a mother should—instead of sending her to Mom's every day. (She paused and looked at the large plant across from her.) That rubber tree is giving me so much trouble. Do you know anything about rubber trees?	I felt that by closing the curtain she was trying to say that this is a private conversation. Demonstrates trust in being able to share her feelings with me. She was becoming anxious talking about her feelings regarding her husband's family; therefore she changed the topic. She also seems to feel guilty about neglecting her daughter.	It would be appropriate to clarify her self-ideal regarding her mothering role. (If a person's self-concept does not conform to one's self-ideal, low self-esteem will be experienced.) Asking about the rubber tree might be an indirect way of saying, "Can you help me with my problems?"
NURSE: No. I'm not much with plants, but it appears that you have a green thumb. (I looked at the abundance of plants in the room.)	I couldn't decide if I should pursue her feelings regarding work and her husband's family.	You might have tried to focus back on this topic. If she refused, then you would know that she was not ready to discuss this at this time. Also remember that the client will bring up an important area again.
MS. V.: I guess it's a good thing that Lisa isn't here very much, or she would probably ruin most of my plants.		She seems to be rationalizing. (Maintenance of ego integrity is attempted by stating logical reasons to justify behavior.)
NURSE: She's home in the evening and on weekends, isn't she? (I held eye contact with her.)		You are not responding to her feelings. You failed to be empathic here.
MS. V.: Yes. She visits here pretty regularly. (She smiled slightly and looked down.)	The word *visit* sounded so distant. I could empathically sense her sadness.	(This is an example of how a verbal message, here the word *visit*, obtains its particular significance within the context of the situation.)

Continued

CASE STUDY: *Fourth Meeting—cont'd*

VERBATIM	STUDENT ASSESSMENT	SUPERVISOR'S COMMENTS
NURSE: It sounds like you miss your daughter very much.	Therapeutic communication technique: seeking consensual validation. More than missing her child is involved; the client is also feeling guilty and probably angry at her husband and sister-in-law.	Do you feel comfortable discussing these feelings with her? How might you help her deal with her anger? You seem to be avoiding it. (Anger has the potential of being frightening to the participants in a relationship because of the destructive aspects of this emotion; therefore many times nurses do not feel comfortable discussing anger. Anger needs to be dealt with individually by first validating that the client is angry. Next the nurse needs to discuss with the client ways to express this anger constructively.)
MS. V.: I remember when I was a child. My parents were always busy, always working. They had babysitters and more babysitters. There was one that for a while I was sure was my real mother. I called her Nana. That's what Lisa calls Joe's mother—Nana. (She said this softly, and for a moment I thought I saw tears in her eyes.)	Seems as though the client's past experiences with multiple mothering figures has affected her perception. My own mother never worked, but I could feel the client's sense of loss and identification with Lisa.	How does this relate to theory regarding the importance of the maternal-child relationship? What were your feelings and reactions to the perceived tears? (The nurse first needs to deal with her feelings regarding crying. Statements that encourage a client to stop crying—for instance, "Everything will be fine"—are inappropriate, because they often make the client feel more uncomfortable. It is more helpful to acknowledge that crying is acceptable and then to stay with the client until she has regained control. Acceptance of the client's right to cry builds trust in the nurse.)
NURSE: You would really prefer to be home with Lisa.	I sensed (wanted to validate) that she was struggling with her self-ideal versus reality.	
MS. V.: Yes, and this new little one will give me a chance to stay home and be a really good mother. (She patted her abdomen softly.)	Self-concept. Touching her abdomen is also a recurrent behavior.	How would you evaluate her self-concept? Remember, when parents have positive self-concepts, their children do also.

VERBATIM	STUDENT ASSESSMENT	SUPERVISOR'S COMMENTS
		(In evaluating an individual's self-concept the nurse determines what the client considers are her strengths and weaknesses and then relates this data to the client's behavior. In this case Ms. V. does not consider herself a good mother, which is indication of a low self-concept. It is now necessary to compare this self-perception with Ms. V.'s behavior with her daughter and analyze the congruence between them.)
NURSE: That's going to be some change—from a working mother to the mother of two *at home.*	I wanted to see how well she had thought out her plans.	You might have said, , "It sounds as though you want to give your children what you missed as a child." The change of focus to a more intellectual level indicates some discomfort on your part in confronting her intense feelings.
MS. V.: Well, Lisa will start nursery school in the fall, so I'll have extra time for the baby. Babies need so much attention and love.		
NURSE: It sounds as though you have thought it through and think you can manage.	Sharing my perceptions. This might enhance her autonomy.	
MS. V.: I thought so, but Mom wants to keep Lisa during the day so that I'll have time for the baby.		
NURSE: (Slight questioning tone.) Your mother-in-law is very attached to Lisa?	Didn't really approach her feelings about this.	Example of the therapeutic communication technique of reflecting.

CASE STUDY: *Fourth Meeting—cont'd*

VERBATIM	STUDENT ASSESSMENT	SUPERVISOR'S COMMENTS
MS. V.: Sometimes I think they are too close. I feel like Lisa belongs to her and visits me. It makes me feel like I'm not such a good mother.	Possible indication of her level of self-esteem and her self-concept. I will pursue this if possible.	
NURSE: You would like to feel closer to Lisa.	Trying to tell her that I care.	Empathic response.
MS. V.: Yes. I don't want Mom to be left out, yet I need more time with my daughter.		
NURSE: Have you discussed this with your mother-in-law?	Trying to explore how client is handling this problem.	
MS. V.: In the beginning I thought she would be hurt and think that I didn't like the way she was taking care of Lisa, but she's getting older now and really doesn't have the energy needed for a toddler. She's really doing us a favor so I can work, but I think she understands how I feel. At least she said she did, and she told Pop, her husband, that taking care of Lisa 10 hours a day was really too much for her. I think everyone will enjoy it better. Lisa will have playmates. I'll feel more like a mother, and Nana will feel like a grandmother.	I thought she was beginning to rationalize here, but it appears that she has objective data and has resolved this conflict. I thought it was interesting that she called her "Nana."	What other behaviors can you identify that she uses to cope with stressors?
NURSE: You call your mother-in-law "Nana."		Good nursing intervention. You seem to have helped client get in touch with her feelings regarding her mother-in-law, increased her sense of autonomy, and helped her think through the problem with her mother-in-law.

VERBATIM	STUDENT ASSESSMENT	SUPERVISOR'S COMMENTS
MS. V.: (Looking away and then down at dominant hand.) Yes. (Smiling.) I guess I'm really fond of her.	Seems to prefer the kinesthetic mode of information processing, looks down at dominant hand and uses verbs such as "feel."	(Neurolinguistic programming helps determine the favored representational system. Body position, verb forms, and breathing patterns are suggestive of the preferred mode. If the nurse uses the same representational system as the client, communication is facilitated.)

At this point Mr. V. and Lisa came in. Lisa ran toward her mother, and they hugged and kissed for a few minutes. Then Ms. V. introduced me to her husband and asked if I would mind if she took Lisa into her bedroom to get her ready for bed. Mr. V. was a tall, slightly obese man (approximately 6 ft, 230 lb). He wore gray slacks and a plaid shirt open at the neck. Lisa was dressed in jeans and a red plaid shirt with tennis shoes and no socks. Ms. V. and Lisa went upstairs. Mr. V. asked me if I wanted something to drink. I said no, then he disappeared into the kitchen. He returned about 5 minutes later with a can of soda and a large bag of potato chips. He offered me some and then turned on the television to the news. We sat watching the news and commenting on it until Ms. V. returned approximately 5 minutes later. She turned off the television, then sat next to her husband on the sofa. I had been feeling uncomfortable and had been glad when he turned on the television. I realized that most of my anxiety about this visit had been connected with meeting Mr. V.

VERBATIM	STUDENT ASSESSMENT	SUPERVISOR'S COMMENTS
MS. V.: Ms. B. came to talk to us, not to watch television.	I felt like an intruder.	Perhaps you could have explained to him your reason for visiting while his wife was gone. You have a contract and a trusting relationship with Ms. V. but not with him. You missed an opportunity to get to know him as an individual. That may be why Ms. V. left you alone with him.
MR. V.: OK. OK. (He closed the top of the potato chip bag.) None for you, Chunky. (He smiled and touched Ms. V.'s hand.)	Their nonverbal communication expressed caring. This put me at ease a little.	
MS. V.: (Smiling.) I haven't been eating my usual snacks. Hopefully I won't be gaining more excess weight like I did last month.	Ms. V. is trying to maintain proper nutrition. She needs positive reinforcement so that she will continue to do so.	You should have given positive reinforcement to both of them.

Continued

CASE STUDY: *Fourth Meeting—cont'd*

VERBATIM	STUDENT ASSESSMENT	SUPERVISOR'S COMMENTS
NURSE:		
(Smiling.) I hope not too. (I reached for the brochure I had brought.) I brought some information on the hospital classes and those of the other childbirth groups I told you about.	Group support from other expectant parents will also help Mr. V. to reassess his beliefs about the father's role.	Do you think he is experiencing role conflict? (Role conflict results when the individual tries to simultaneously conform to different sets of expectations.)
MR. V.:		
Will I be able to see the baby being born? (He seemed to be enthusiastic.)		What nonverbal communication led you to infer that Mr. V. was enthusiastic? What was his metacommunication here?
NURSE:		
(I was shocked. I didn't expect such enthusiasm from him.) Yes, University Hospital allows the husband to be in the delivery room.	Not really sure what happened here—I thought my presence might change his behavior, that he might say he would go just to avoid any conflict, but he seemed to be earnest and truthful.	On what did you base this inference?
MR. V.:		
Good. When do the classes start?		
MS. V.:		
I thought you didn't want to go? (She looked at her husband wide-eyed.)	She seemed as surprised as I was.	
MR. V.:		
You know I like to give you a hard time. (He touched Ms. V.'s hand and looked into her eyes, smiling slightly.) If you really want this, then it's fine with me. You know that you are most important to me. What we decide to do is up to us.	It's the "you and I" communication pattern.	Husband-wife communication in this instance seems to be transactional. (Transactional communication patterns focus on the pattern of relating with minimum emphasis on the actual issue.)
MS. V.:		
(Holding her husband's hand and smiling at him.) Yes, I do want you there for the labor and delivery.	Showed caring between husband and wife.	It also showed open communication. It is efficient in that they are saying what they mean.

VERBATIM	STUDENT ASSESSMENT	SUPERVISOR'S COMMENTS
NURSE: (I began rustling through the papers I had brought. I wanted to leave but didn't know how, so I started talking about the childbirth classes.) The classes at the hospital are held every Wednesday evening from 7 to 10 PM. There is a class starting in 2 weeks and then another in 8 weeks.	I felt like an intruder; they seemed so close. I can't remember everything I said, but it seemed like I talked nonstop for at least 15 minutes. They listened attentively and remained holding hands.	Did the display of affection make you uncomfortable, or was there something else producing this reaction? How would you describe this health teaching? (Feedback is one of the most important aspects of health education. Even in pre-planned structured health teaching, feedback needs to be used for effective health education.)
MR. V.: Well, why don't you leave the application forms here so we can fill them out? (He reached for the papers that I was holding.)		
NURSE: OK. Do you have any questions regarding prepared childbirth classes? Maybe I could . . .	I felt like I was going to start on another speech.	
MR. V.: No, I think you told us enough. We'll find out the rest by going ourselves. (He smiled at me and stood up.)	I felt like I was being dismissed. It's easier in the hospital, where I have more control. The V.'s have so much autonomy at home.	
NURSE: Well, I guess I should be leaving. (I gathered my papers and stood up. Mr. V. shook my hand.)		This ending seems rather abrupt. Several significant events had occurred during the course of the visit. A summary statement would have given a sense of completion to the interaction.
MS. V.: Good-bye, and thank you for coming. Do you want my husband to walk you to your car? It's getting late.	I felt that the client was concerned with my welfare and safety.	

Continued

CASE STUDY: *Fourth Meeting—cont'd*

VERBATIM	STUDENT ASSESSMENT	SUPERVISOR'S COMMENTS
NURSE: No, I'll be OK, but thank you anyway.		
MS. V.: Will I see you next week at the clinic? (She stood up and walked me to the door.)	The client seems to be looking forward to our visits. Perhaps we are finally in the working phase of the relationship.	I agree that you are in the working phase. (The working phase of the relationship is characterized by mutual goal setting and progress toward goal achievement. There is evidence of trust and caring enhanced by an ability to relate empathically.)
NURSE: Yes, I'll be there. Good night.		

NURSING CARE PLAN

Nursing Diagnosis 1:

Altered nutrition: more than body requirements, related to increased food intake during pregnancy, evidenced by excessive weight gain in last pregnancy—priority 3. Client stated that she has been following her diet. No additional health teaching necessary.

Subjective:

Client stated that she has been avoiding snacks.

Objective:

Could not weigh client. Husband did not give her any potato chips during home visit.

Assessment:

Needs are still accurate. Nursing goals and actions are still appropriate and seem to be effective as client verbalizes compliance.

Planned Nursing Actions:

Continue with same.

Nursing Diagnosis 2:

Family Coping: potential for growth, related to marital conflict about natural childbirth, evidenced by client's report of husband's skepticism—priority 1. This was the focus for the home visit. Because client is 25 weeks pregnant, it is necessary for husband and wife to make decision regarding childbirth method and to enroll in prenatal classes.

Subjective:

Couple stated that they want to use prepared childbirth method. Husband stated that he would attend the prenatal classes offered at the hospital with his wife.

Objective:

The V.'s listened attentively to information about prenatal class. They requested and received application forms for University Hospital prenatal classes.

Assessment:

Client needs to feel a sense of self-esteem and autonomy in decision making with husband about method of childbirth.

Expected Outcomes:

Long-Term Goal: Client will use whatever method she desires.

Short-Term Goals: Client will submit application for prenatal classes before next clinic appointment.

• •

Planned Nursing Actions:

1. Ask client at next visit if she has submitted application. If not, discuss with client reasons for not submitting it.
2. Answer any additional questions regarding prepared childbirth.

Evaluation:

Original goal accomplished, because the couple agreed on a childbirth method and to attend University Hospital prepared childbirth classes. Home visit was an efficient and appropriate way to discuss the problem with client and husband. Nursing actions were adequate and effective, because a decision was made. However, my communication while presenting information was not flexible.

Nursing Diagnosis 3:

Situational low self-esteem, related to perception of mothering role, evidenced by client's self-criticism—priority 2. Client spent much time discussing this area. It seemed very important to her.

Subjective:

1. Client stated that she wants to stay home and be a "real mother."
2. Client stated that a "real mother" should stay home with her children and not let other people care for them.
3. Client associates grandmother caring for Lisa with her own past experience with babysitters.
4. Client stated that the new baby will give her a chance to stay home.

Objective:

1. Client is presently working full-time.
2. Daughter was observed running to mother and hugging her when daughter came home.

Assessment:

Client needs increased congruency between self-concept and ideal self in relation to her mothering role.

Expected Outcomes:

Long-Term Goal: Client will have a self-concept congruent with ideal self.

Short-Term Goals: At next visit client will:

1. State her present mothering activities with Lisa.
2. Describe the characteristics of her ideal mother image.
3. State her feelings about how her present behaviors correspond with those of her ideal.
4. State two reasons for working.
5. State her feelings regarding working.
6. State two alternatives to her present work situation.
7. Discuss these alternatives with her husband.

Planned Nursing Actions:

1. Reinforce positive mothering activities identified by client.
2. Share perceptions regarding client's interaction with her daughter.
3. Reinforce those ideal characteristics that client presently demonstrates.
4. Assist client in exploring alternatives to her present work situation.

Supervisor's Comments:

Your goals and actions in dealing with the problem of low self-esteem in relation to her mothering role are concrete and well done. Based on your experiences what changes have you determined in the client's stress state? How has this affected your priorities?

Summary of Fourth Meeting:

In this meeting a change in the context of the relationship adds a new dimension. The hospital environment puts the nurse in charge to a degree, but entering a client's home is a new situation that often results in some temporary role confusion. Just as clients often discuss a feeling of loss of control within the hospital environment, nurses feel the same outside the hospital. Exposure to different environments is encouraged during the learning process, because it allows the student to use new skills within an unfamiliar context. Also, feelings that are common to clients regarding loss of control can be experienced and used as a basis for empathy in future situations.

Not only did the context of the relationship change but also the components. The addition of a new family member, Mr. V., moved the relationship from the dyadic nurse-client relationship previously discussed into a

Continued

CASE STUDY: *Fourth Meeting—cont'd*

larger, group situation. The student needed to be aware of group process and dynamics. The student's preparation for this meeting included a health teaching plan on prepared childbirth. Her inability to be flexible when it was apparent that the couple had decided to enroll in the classes is a common result of increased anxiety in a new situation with a new client.

The development of the student's interpersonal skills is evident in the initial part of this meeting as the student helps the client express her anxieties regarding her role as a mother. During pregnancy a reevaluation of current roles and thoughts concerning future roles is common. With the introduction of a new family member changes are always necessary. These changes produce varying degrees of stress.

The student-supervisor relationship changes throughout the interaction. Initially the supervisor mainly provides positive reinforcement for the student's use of skills. However, when the student becomes anxious as the components of the relationship change, the supervisor takes a more active role, questioning and serving as a role model by offering alternatives.

CASE STUDY: *Fifth Meeting*

I was sick and couldn't make it to the clinic. The evening before her appointment I called Ms. V. to tell her why I would not be there.

The conversation lasted only about 5 minutes. Ms. V. was getting ready to go to a movie with her husband. She said that they had filled out the application the day before and that she had it in her purse to turn in at the clinic the next day. Most of the time she talked of getting ready to see the movie and asked how I was feeling—many people at her workplace were experiencing my symptoms, and Ms. V. was verbal in describing how she protected herself from "their germs."

Supervisor's Comments:

Missed or broken appointments are common in all relationships. By notifying the client before the scheduled appointment the nurse conveys a sense of caring and establishes the importance and legitimacy of the meetings. Often prior notification is not possible, and the effects are more disruptive to the course of the relationship. With or without prior notification, missed appointments must be dealt with in future meetings. Often clients will come late for their next appointment or revert to earlier forms of behavior within the relationship. Missed appointments may bring out feelings of mistrust. Especially in clients who have difficulty trusting, missed appointments can be a major problem; however, dealing with the feelings generated in such circumstances can be a major learning experience.

CASE STUDY: *Sixth Meeting*

Ms. V. arrived late for her clinic appointment. She told the nurse that she had made arrangements to visit a preschool near her home with Lisa immediately after her appointment and then planned to take Lisa shopping and out to dinner. She seemed excited about spending an afternoon with her daughter. Ms. V. told the nurse that she wanted to include Lisa in buying some nursery items for the baby. She had checked out library books for herself and her daughter on the birth of a baby and purchased a special doll for Lisa to feed and bathe while Ms. V. took care of the baby. Ms. V. stated her preference for bottle feeding this child as she had bottle-fed Lisa; she stated convenience and the fact that her husband and in-laws enjoyed feeding the baby as her primary reasons for choosing this method. Ms. V. had gained only 5 lb in the last 4 weeks. She and her husband had attended the first childbirth class and found it both enjoyable and informative.

The topic of termination was introduced at this meeting. Client and nurse agreed to meet 45 minutes before the client's next clinic appointment. No mention was made by either the client or nurse of the previous broken appointment. However, the student expressed feelings of anxiety and guilt to her supervisor about not being able to keep her appointment. In addition, for this appointment the student arrived 30 minutes early, which was seen as a manifestation of these feelings. The client's own lateness for the appointment and making plans that forced this visit to be shortened may have indicated that the client had feelings of anxiety. This possibility was not explored. The supervisor pointed out the behaviors that possibly could have been produced by the stress or uncertainty resulting from the missed appointment. The student's inability to deal with her own feelings prevented any data collection on how the client felt about the situation.

The student's behavior in this situation is a good example of dealing with stress through indirect actions, specifically the use of suppression. The student consciously excluded from the conversation a topic that caused discomfort. By excluding the topic any assessment of how the client dealt with this situation was prevented. Within a therapeutic relationship microsituations like disappointment and loss are played out, and the participants can examine their characteristic modes of responding to similar situations outside the relationship. In this particular instance the student's actions were appropriate. Because she was ill she called the client to notify her. The feelings of guilt and anxiety are not appropriate to this situation; nevertheless, they are present. By identifying the presence of these uncomfortable feelings the student nurse has made a first step. Hopefully at a later time she will be able to express and deal with these feelings. Out of context this incident may be insignificant. However, if it represents the nurse's characteristic way of responding to similar situations, this incident takes on particular significance as a learning experience for this individual at this point in time. Without additional information it is only possible to speculate on the ramifications of the broken appointment for this client at this time.

NURSING CARE PLAN
Nursing Diagnosis 1:

Altered nutrition: more than body requirements, related to increased food intake during pregnancy, evidenced by excessive weight gain during last pregnancy—priority 3. Previous goals being met; therefore nursing actions adequate and effective.

Evaluation:

Client has gained 5 lb in last 4 weeks. Client stated that she is watching her diet and seems pleased with the results. Goals and actions are appropriate and effective; should continue with same.

Nursing Diagnosis 2:

Family coping: potential for growth, related to marital conflict about natural childbirth, evidenced by client's report of husband's skepticism—priority 4. Conflict resolved.

Evaluation:

Couple is attending childbirth classes. Client states that they enjoy the classes.

Nursing Diagnosis 3:

Situational low self-esteem, related to perception of mothering role, evidenced by client's self-criticism—priority 2. Client did not mention this during interaction.

Continued

CASE STUDY: *Sixth Meeting—cont'd*

Evaluation:

No additional data available. At last meeting this seemed to be an important topic to client. Will try to implement nursing actions during next visit.

Nursing Diagnosis 4:

Impaired verbal communication indicating moderate anxiety related to termination, evidenced by avoidance behavior when subject was introduced—priority 1. Not sure if this is the first priority for client, but it is for me. I want this experience to be positive for both client and myself; therefore termination needs to be dealt with directly and thoroughly.

Subjective:

Client stated that she would try to arrive early for our last meeting. She also asked, "Will we have time to talk before I see the doctor?"

Objective:

Client left the room after I mentioned termination. She did not respond directly to my statement about being sad regarding termination.

Assessment:

Client needs a positive experience with termination.

Expected Outcomes:

Short-Term Goals: At next visit nurse and client will:
1. Share feelings about the relationship and termination.
2. Summarize areas of learning.
3. Formulate two goals for the future.

Planned Nursing Actions:

1. Introduce issue of termination early in the interaction.
2. Facilitate open discussion of feelings by sharing own feelings initially.
3. Encourage client to share her feelings.
4. Engage client in summary of events in relationship.
5. Support client in formulating two goals for the future.
6. Give client handmade bootees.

Assessment:

Approach to topic of termination during this interaction was not effective, adequate, or efficient.

CASE STUDY: *Seventh Meeting*

PREINTERACTION

SETTING: Obstetric clinic. There were only two patients waiting. It seemed dark, because the sun was not shining through the windows. It was very quiet. Only the receptionist was there. Most of the staff were attending an afternoon conference.

NURSE: I was feeling very confident. I had just had a good experience in the well-baby clinic that morning and had received a very good evaluation from my advisor. The idea of not seeing Ms. V. again was somewhat depressing, but I think my anxiety regarding termination was gone. Talking about termination in the group last week was helpful. As I looked back on my usual coping response to termination I realized I had never allowed myself to say good-bye to anyone. It was always, "I'll see you someday," or something similar. Only the death of my aunt was a real termination. I began to see the parallels between successful termination of this relationship and coping with past and future losses. I have always felt that this part of the relationship was insignificant and mainly done for the advisor's approval. Two weeks ago I was angry that I had to say good-bye to Ms. V., but now I'm beginning to see the importance and significance of this phase of the relationship. I wish I could go back a few months and begin to prepare both the client and myself adequately.

I arrived at 1:15 and sat in the corner where I had met previously with Ms. V. I wanted to share my feelings with her, allow us to look back over the relationship, and plan for the future.

CLIENT: Ms. V. arrived at 1:40. She was wearing blue pants and a red, white, and blue blouse. She was wearing low-heeled shoes. Her hair was pulled back, and she wore large, round, white earrings. (She looked very pregnant and beautiful, I thought.)

Goals:

Nurse will:
1. Share own feelings regarding this relationship.
2. Summarize areas of learning with the client.
3. Formulate nurse-client goals for the future.
4. Discuss client's present mothering activities and her ideal mother image.
5. Discuss client's reasons for working.
6. Explore possible alternatives to client's present working situation.
7. Discuss Ms. V's diet and weight gain.

Supervisor's Comments:

It seems that your perception of a pregnant woman is changing. A few weeks ago when Ms. V. was talking about her body changes, you stated that you didn't find her new body very attractive. Now you perceive her as "very pregnant and beautiful." Could you explore some reasons for this change? What are the ramifications of this change within the relationship? Also, your preinteraction description shows much growth in self-awareness, observation, and ability to set goals.

Your exploration of your feelings in group supervision seems to have given you some insight into your feelings about termination. Your conclusion that a well-handled termination can be a positive experience is important in your understanding of a therapeutic relationship. This demonstrates the value of a group in assisting the student to explore feelings and receive feedback on planned interventions.

VERBATIM	STUDENT ASSESSMENT	SUPERVISOR'S COMMENTS
NURSE:		
Hello Ms. V. How are you today? (Smiling, I stood up.)		
CLIENT:		
(She sat down next to me as I sat down again.) This is the last time you'll be here, isn't it? (She looked away and sat back in her chair.)	She has introduced the topic of termination. It must be important to her also. She seemed to be physically withdrawing as a coping response.	Assessing the client's pattern organization may show that her characteristic way of responding to loss is by withdrawal.

Continued

CASE STUDY: *Seventh Meeting—cont'd*

VERBATIM	STUDENT ASSESSMENT	SUPERVISOR'S COMMENTS
NURSE: Yes. (I leaned forward to move closer to her. I touched her hand and she placed her other hand over mine.) I feel sad saying good-bye to you. (I looked at the client who was then looking out the windows. There was a silence for about 2 minutes. Ms. V. continued to stare out the window.)	I didn't feel anxious with this silence. During this time I was thinking of all the things I thought would make this a positive experience.	The mutual use of touch indicates that you are both very comfortable with your positive feelings toward each other. (Research has shown a positive correlation between touching and self-disclosure.)[1]
CLIENT: Yes. I'll be rather sad too. I've really enjoyed talking to you. (Direct eye contact.)	I thought it was significant that she used the future tense.	
NURSE: I've learned a lot talking with you. (Smiling.) In fact I almost feel like I'm having a baby too.	I wanted her to know that I appreciated her sharing her thoughts and feelings with me.	Appropriate use of humor can relieve tension and facilitate the relationship.
CLIENT: Yes. (Smiling.) You've really helped me too—my diet, the childbirth classes. I don't think I could have gotten my husband interested without you.		Your careful planning for termination has enabled you to share feelings and summarize areas of learning in a very natural way. You could have been more specific about what you learned from her as she was about what she learned from you.
NURSE: I think that I've helped you think things through and provided information, but you've done all the work.	I wanted her to realize her part in meeting our goals.	Mutuality has characterized your work with this client in the last few meetings.
CLIENT: Saying good-bye is always so very hard for me. (She looked away.)		
NURSE: Yes, I can understand that you feel sad. Saying good-bye is always difficult for me too.	Empathy, focused on feelings of the client.	

VERBATIM	STUDENT ASSESSMENT	SUPERVISOR'S COMMENTS

CLIENT:

| What will you be doing after you leave here? | I felt that sharing of my goals and hopes was appropriate here. She had shared so much of herself with me. | This also helps redefine you as separate people who are becoming more autonomous. This is helpful to the client in remembering you in a positive way. |

I told her about my summer job. She asked about where I lived and my parents. The next 10 minutes or so we discussed my future and her own family in Florida. (Her mother plans to come and stay with her for the first month after the baby is born.) Then Ms. V. was called into the examining room. I weighed her. She had gained only 4 lb. She thanked me for the diet plan, and I gave her positive reinforcement for following her diet. After the examination we returned to the waiting room.

CLIENT:

| Do you have time to talk? I don't have to return to work. (Her eyes searched the waiting room.) | Before I had been feeling slightly disappointed that she hadn't arrived earlier. I was happy that we would have a few more minutes to talk. | This demonstrates the importance of terminating with a feeling of resolution of important issues. She obviously felt a need to discuss more things with you. |

NURSE:

Yes, I do. Would you like to sit down again? (We sat in the same chairs; this time I was facing the windows.)

CLIENT:

| This is my last week at work also. Joe and I decided that I needed more rest now and time to get things ready for the baby. | From this and my home visit I would say that the V.'s use mutual decision making. | This actually parallels the discussion of your future plans. She is reciprocating by telling you what she will be doing. Sharing of future plans is very important in a therapeutic approach to termination. It leaves both people with a sense of continuity beyond the end of the relationship. |

NURSE:

You won't be returning to work?

CLIENT:

Not for a while. It looks like I'm finally going to get that chance to stay home and mother Lisa. (She smiled.)

Continued

CASE STUDY: *Seventh Meeting—cont'd*

VERBATIM	STUDENT ASSESSMENT	SUPERVISOR'S COMMENTS
NURSE: You've mentioned that before. It seems that you believe that a mother needs to be home with her children. (I raised my eyebrows slightly.)	I wanted to further explore and validate her ideal mother image.	
CLIENT: Definitely, but we need the money. . . so I work.		
NURSE: Is there any way that you could work and be home at the same time?		
CLIENT: What do you mean?		
NURSE: Oh, things like babysitting in your home and the like.		
CLIENT: I guess I never thought about that. I used to do typing at home when we were first married. (She gazed across the room.)		
NURSE: You seem to want to be available to your children, and yet you need an added income. That's a real dilemma.	I wanted to verbalize the problem she has implied. This seems to be an approach-approach conflict.	True. The client is pulled toward two goals that are equally attractive, while at the same time mutually exclusive. Such a dilemma of wanting to stay home while simultaneously wanting a career or the income from a job is common for the majority of working women, particularly those with young children who are not in school.

VERBATIM	STUDENT ASSESSMENT	SUPERVISOR'S COMMENTS
CLIENT:		
Yes, sometimes I feel pulled in two opposite directions. Maybe after the baby is born I'll start looking for typing to do at home again. That was fun before because I could do it whenever I felt like it. (She paused and smiled.) Yes, I think I'll talk to Joe about that. It would give us an additional income.	She seemed to be thinking aloud as if I weren't even present. Income is apparently most important from what the client has said about her job. It is probably safe to assume that the client obtains minimal feelings of competency from her present clerical position.	
NURSE:		
And if you do return to work. . .	I wanted her to continue focusing on this area and explore other possibilities.	You are also pointing out the reality of the situation. Financially she may have to work full-time.
CLIENT:		
Well, I don't want to think about that now. (She stood up.) I've kept you long enough. It's after 3 o'clock. I'd better be getting home to Lisa.		However, client doesn't seem ready at this time.
NURSE:		
(Standing up.) I've enjoyed meeting you. (I took her hand.) I'll walk with you to the door. I have a pair of bootees that I made for the baby in my purse at the desk.		In group we discussed the importance of having a sound rationale for gift-giving. I think your idea about the bootees was appropriate and fits in with the recurrent theme of this interaction—positive remembrance of the relationship. It was an especially nice idea to give her something small and handmade. I would like to have seen more of your own reasoning for this action.

We walked to the desk. As I gave Ms. V. the bootees she smiled and thanked me, then kissed me on the cheek.

NURSE:		
I hope you and your family will be very happy. Good-bye. I've really enjoyed knowing you.	I felt sad and yet very pleased. This has been such a positive experience for both of us.	

Continued

CASE STYDY: *Seventh Meeting—cont'd*

VERBATIM	STUDENT ASSESSMENT	SUPERVISOR'S COMMENTS

CLIENT:

Good-bye, and thank you for everything.

The termination was successful in that both you and client were clearly aware that this was the last meeting and confronted this fact together. Feelings were shared, and there was some reminiscence about the course of the relationship. The emphasis on future plans for both of you was very appropriate and helped put the relationship into perspective as a meaningful experience. Goals for the future were not really explicit. This area could have been handled in more depth, particularly in terms of reinforcing the progress the client had made and of encouraging her to continue on in the same way. The extent of your growth in this relationship is well demonstrated by the mature and professional way that you handled the very difficult process of termination.

Summary of Seventh Meeting:

Throughout these interactions the focus has been the student's growth in the use of interpersonal skills, communication, and recording skills. (See Fig. 12-1.) Also, the student's growth in her therapeutic use of the self has been shown, as well as growth in the specific behaviors needed to establish, maintain, and terminate a relationship. In addition to the student nurse's role, the role of the supervisor and the way in which the behaviors of the supervisor change with the needs of the student have been presented.

In this final interaction the student nurse is competent in her use of therapeutic interpersonal skills. In the initial interaction the student constantly changed topics, asked too many direct questions, and had difficulty dealing with silences. By this final meeting silences were used therapeutically and no longer produced anxiety. The student was able to follow the lead of the client regarding content, and her use of therapeutic communication techniques assisted the client in exploring her mothering role and possible alternatives.

Throughout the interactions the student's growing skill in recording nonverbal communication was also evident. Initially the student included minimal nonverbal communication, but by this final interaction nonverbal messages had become an important segment of the process recording.

The student's therapeutic use of self has also been developed throughout the interactions. In initial meetings the student became aware of feelings of anxiety and the like; however, by the final stage of the relationship the student was not only aware of her feelings but of their effect on her behavior and that of the client. Finally she was able to deal with her feelings effectively. A few specific examples will show this progression. After the initial meeting the student retrospectively became aware of her difficulty in meeting strangers and the anxiety associated with such circumstances. In the fifth meeting the student identified feelings of guilt and anxiety produced by a missed appointment. Although aware of these stress-produced behaviors, she was still unable to deal with them. By the final interaction

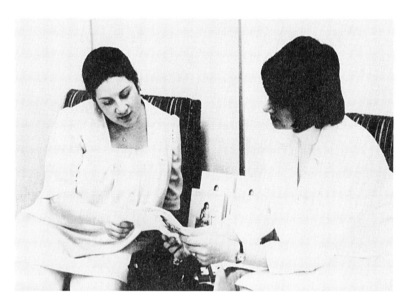

Fig. 12-1 "Caring for the body, disregarding the mind, not caring for the whole man is inhuman, worse than that, dehumanizing." (From Selvini A: An intensive experience in a doctor-patient relationship training group, *Psychother Psychosom* 22:2, 1973.)

the student was aware of her anxiety associated with termination and was also able to deal with her feelings and the feelings of the client regarding termination. In these interactions a progression in learning was depicted. The student moved from retrospective analysis of how feelings *had* affected behavior to a prospective analysis of how emotions *would* affect behavior and the ability to use this analysis within the therapeutic relationship.

The student's skills in the specifics of forming a therapeutic relationship and a concrete example of the progression through the various relationship stages were presented in these interactions. The student's initial difficulty in establishing a relationship can be contrasted with the skills displayed in terminating the relationship, evidencing this development. Also, the student's development of the role identity within the relationship is seen in

her clear sense of purpose, mutual goal formation, and realistic goal accomplishment in the latter interactions.

The role of the supervisor changed throughout the interactions as the skills of the student developed. In this final interaction the supervisor validated the inferences of the student and reinforced her use of therapeutic behaviors. This could be viewed as a somewhat more passive role than that in the initial interactions when the supervisor provided alternatives and used questioning to focus the student on areas of importance. However, throughout the interactions the supervisor served as an objective observer of the relationship. Within this capacity the supervisor was able to explore with the student the rationale for her behavior and the ramifications of her planned nursing actions such as giving a gift at termination.

REFERENCES

1. Cooper C, Bowles D: Physical encounter and self-disclosure, *Psychol Rep* 33:451, 1973.
2. Platt-Koch LM: Clinical supervision for psychiatric nurses, *J Psychosoc Nurs Ment Health Serv* 24:6, 1986.

Suggested Readings

Bodley D: Clinical supervision in psychiatric nursing: using the process record, *Nurse Educ Today* 12(2):148, 1992.

This article explores the need for creative methods of supervision such as the process recording and the role of the supervisory relationship.

Dombeck M, Brody S: Clinical supervision: a three-way mirror, *Arch Psychiatr Nurs* 9(1):3, 1995.

The principles and the process of one model of clinical supervision are described via analysis of two case studies. Peplau's theoretic framework for interpersonal relationships and Bowen's family systems theory are applied.

Farkas-Cameron M: Clinical supervision in psychiatric nursing: a self-actualizing process, *J Psychosoc Nurs Ment Health Serv* 33(2):31, 1995.

This article describes the process of engaging in a potentially supportive and respectful relationship with a colleague to facilitate professional growth and skill development.

Wright L: Live supervision: developing therapeutic competence in family systems nursing, *J Nurs Educ* 33(7):325, 1994.

The importance of supervision to therapeutic competence and nursing education is discussed in this article.

INDEX

A

Acknowledgment techniques, in therapeutic communication, 110, 113t

Acquired immunodeficiency syndrome (AIDS), inducing crisis situations, 296

Adaptations
  in coping with stress, 228-234
  in crisis situations, 291
  model of, *239*
  by nurses to stress, 234-236

Adolescence
  and body image, 58
  developing self concept during, 65
  and peer pressure, 72
  and self-esteem, 67
  theories of development, 45-47

Adrenal glands, responding to stress, 225

Adrenalin, 225

Adrenocorticotropic hormones, in stress response, 224-225

Adulthood
  and body image, 58
  and learning, 253
  and self-awareness, 47-48

Advocacy
  definitions, 263
  ethical and legal considerations of, 272-273
  models of, 263-264
  nursing history of, 263
  referrals and risks, 271-272
  role in nursing, 269-273
  and self-help groups, 264-269

Agency for Health Care Policy And Research, 20

Agendas, 202

Aging; See also old age
  anxiety surrounding, 61
  and midlife crises, 298
  and self-esteem, 67, 73

Alarm reactions, to stress, 226

Anger
  and change, 285
  due to termination phase, 190-191
  versus fear, 183-184

Anger—cont'd
  helping clients deal with, 183-185
  in nurse-client relationships, 176, 178
  over death, 295

Anorexia nervosa, 61

Anticipated life transition crises, 288

Anticipatory planning techniques, in crisis interventions, 291-292

Anxiety
  as a communication barrier, 119
  and crises, 289-290
  versus fear, 182
  in nurse-client relationships, 176, 178
  over body image issues, 61
  over relationship termination, 190-192
  related to fear and stress, 222
  relationship to empathy, 153-154
  relationship to self-esteem, 69
  stress-induced, 222-223

Aphasia, helping clients with, 121

Approach and avoidance conflicts, in coping with stress, 229-231

Arthritis, and stress, 234

Assertiveness
  by clients, 166
  in nurse-client relationships, 184-185

Assessments
  beginning phases of, 178
  of body image, 57-63
  in care plans, 304-306
  of families in crisis, 294
  of groups, *212*
  of health education needs, 252-253
  in the nursing process, 7-10
  of organizational communication, 134-135
  of self-concept, 66
  of self-esteem, 63
  of self-ideals, 63-64
  of senses of humor, 182

Auditory systems; *see also* hearing
  used in communication, 92, 93t

Audits, during evaluation process, 24

Autocratic leadership, 201-202

Autogenic training, 275

Autonomic systems, responding to stress, 224, 226

Page numbers in italics indicate illustrations; *t* indicates tables.

Autonomy
    concept of, 162-166
    correlation with relationship phases, 193t
    definition, 163
    nurses as advocates for, 164-166

B

Behavioral theories, on learning, 250-252
Biofeedback, 274
Blaming patterns, of communication, 98-99
Body image, 57-63
    developmental changes in, 57-58
    differences between genders, 58
    and dressing styles, 60
    effect on self-conceptions, 59-60
    in healthy personality individuals, 75
    ideals of, 60
    nursing assessment of, 60-61
    problems surrounding, 61-63
    readjustments in, 62
Boundaries, setting in relationships, 187
Brain, responding to stress, 224-227
Bulimia nervosa, 61

C

Cancer
    crisis interventions for, 296
    self-examination of breasts, 257
    self-help groups for, 266
    and stress, 234
Care plans
    example of, 305t
    purpose of, 304
Caring
    carative factors of, 158
    concept of, 157-160
    correlation with relationship phases, 193t
    definition, 157-158
    development of, 158-159
    responding to sadness
    and the use of touch, 159-160
Case study, comprehensive, 307-347
Castration anxiety, 42
Changes, basic formula for, 285
Children
    child-proofing homes, 4
    developing language skills, 83
    developing self-concept, 64-65
    developing self-esteem, 67
    development during adolescence, 45-47
    development during early childhood years, 41-43
    development during infancy, 36-39
    development during middle years, 43-45
    development during toddler years, 39-41
    drawing to communicate, 60-61
    forming self-ideals, 63

Children—cont'd
    health education for, 254-255
    interventions with dying, 295-296
    ordinal positions of, 71
    and the process of love, 158
    sexual self-awareness in, 70
    special therapeutic communication needs of, 123-125
Chomsky, on linguistics, 83
Civil disobedience model, of advocacy, 263
Clarification techniques, in therapeutic communication, 111, 113t
Clarifier roles, 207
Client care audits, 24
Clients
    definition within communication process, 129, 135
    versus patients, 263
Clinical pathways, within health care system, 20
Clinical practice guidelines, 20
Code for nurses, 3
Coercive power, 200
Cognitive impairments, and communication, 122
Cognitive reframing, 274
Cognitive theories, on learning, 250-252
Cognitive-field approaches, to coping with stress, 229-231
Coleadership, advantages and disadvantages of, 205t
Communication; *see also* nonverbal and verbal communication; therapeutic communication
    administrative, 129-131
    assertiveness in, 184-185
    assessment of in organizations, 134t, 135
    barriers to, 116-120
    care plans, 304-306
    with children, 123-125
    with community groups, 133
    congruent, 93-94
    cultural considerations, 88-91, 100
    definitions of, 82-83
    descriptive, 98
    dissection and journey styles of, 100
    drawing body images, 60-61
    educator's awareness of, 81
    examination of the process, 94-95
    factors affecting the process, 101-102
    of feelings in nurse-client relationships, 179
    function of, 82
    functional components of the process, 95-96
    games played in, 99-100
    with government, 132-133
    horizontal, 131
    incongruent, 93-94
    and language development, 83-84
    levels of, 83-92
        metacommunication, 92-93
        nonverbal level, 86-92
        verbal level, 83-86

Communication—cont'd
  with media, 133-134
  pattern organization, 82, 101
  patterns of, 97-101
  and process recording, 302
  processes essential to, 96-97
  representational systems, 92, 93t
  and self-disclosure, 180-181
  staff, 131-132
  and time, 102
  time and, 82
  types of speech, 84
  understanding the process, 135-137
  undesirable nursing behaviors, 112-116, 117t
  variances in word meanings, 85-86
Communication process, 81-102
Communication skills
  acquisition of, 135-137
  content considerations, 102
  importance or well-written documentation, 20-22
  nonverbal level, 86-92
  using concise terminology, 14t, 15
  verbal level, 83-86
Compliance, definition in health education, 246-247
Compromiser roles, 208
Computer-assisted instructional (CAI) programs, 257
Computers
  use in health education, 257
  used in documentation, 22
Computing patterns, of communication, 99
Confidentiality, in nurse-client relationships, 177
Conflicts, leading to stress, 222
Confrontations, in nurse-client relationships, 179-180
Confused roles, 207
Congruent communication, 93-94
Consensus taker roles, 207
Consumer education, 4
Consumer intensivity, 268
Context, definition within communication process, 129, 135
Contracts
  components of, 176
  in relationships, 175-176
Controlling speech, 98
Coopersmith, S.
  defining self-esteem for nursing assessments, 67
  studies on children's self-esteem, 67
Coping
  assessing skills of, 294
  with stress, 228-229
  using defense mechanisms, 231-234
Crises; *see also* crisis interventions
  building on stress, 285
  death and dying, 295-296
  definition, 286
  factors involved in, 286-287

Crises—cont'd
  families in, 293
  model of avoidance, *289*
  nursing techniques to prevent, 291-292
  phases of, 287, 291
  situational, 295-297
  types of, 287-288
Crisis interventions
  anticipatory planning techniques, 291-292
  application of techniques, 295
  components of, 290
  family-oriented, 293
  generic models of, 291
  levels of, 290-291
  with life-threatening illnesses, 296-297
  as prevention measure, 263-264, 286
  stages in, 291
  steps in the process, 290
  techniques of, 290-292
  theories on, 288-290
Cultures
  beliefs affecting health education, 246-247
  communication variances between, 88-91, 100
  in group counseling, 203
  and inappropriate humor, 182
  nurse-client language problems, 120-121
  sensitivity to, 88-91
  and stress, 227
  variances in nurse expectations, 272

D

Data collection processes, in nursing assessments, 9-10
Death, and crises, 295-296
Decision making, in groups, 208
Defense mechanisms, characteristics of, 231-234
Defensive patterns, of communication, 98-99
Democratic leadership, 201-202
Demographics, 7
Denial
  of death, 295
  as a defense mechanism, 232, 234t
Depression
  as a communication barrier, 119-120
  in older adults, 61-62
  over change, 285
  over death, 295
  relationship to self-esteem, 69
Descriptive communication, 98
Detachment, in the empathy process, 155-156
Developmental growth
  of body image, 57-63
  of self-concept, 64-66
  of self-esteem, 66-69
  of self-ideals, 63-64
Developmental theories
  comparison of, 50t, 51t
  and dynamics of self, 75-76

Developmental theories—cont'd
    and health values, 276-277
    from infancy to old age, 36-49
    influences on the self, 69-70
    prenatal influences, 70
    and self-esteem, 67
Diagnoses
    classifications of, 12t, 13t
    in the nursing process, 7, 10-13
Dietitians, areas of expertise, 21t
Differentiation phases, of group development, 209t, 210
Diseases
    and crisis interventions, 296-297
    and stress, 234
Displacement, as a defense mechanism, 232, 234t
Dispositional crises, 287
Distracting patterns, of communication, 99
Distress, 219
Documentation; *see also* process recordings
    care plans, 304-306
    computerized systems, 22
    formats for, 20-22
    legalities of, 22
    methods of, 302, 303t, 304t

E

Early adulthood, and body image, 58
Ebbinghaus, language research by, 83
Ectomorphy
    definition, 70
    examples of, *71*
Education; *see also* health education
    health, 125-126, 244-262
    importance in developing child's self-esteem, 72
Egocentric speech, 84
Electra complex, 42
Emergent leadership, 200
Emotions
    associated with stress, 238t
    controlling with clients, 188
    and stress, 224
Empathy, 152-157
    communicating nonverbally, 156
    correlation with relationship phases, 193t
    definition, 152-153
    development of, 154-155
    in everyday life, 153-154
    model of, *155*
    nurse-patient function scale, 157t
    research in, 153
    self-assessment of, 156-157
    steps in the process, 155-156
    versus sympathy, 154
Empowerment
    with advocacy, 165-166
    by mental illness sufferers, 266

Empowerment—cont'd
    models in health education, 249-250
    steps in education process, 249-250
Encounter groups, 203
Encourager roles, 208
Enculturation, 246
Endocrine systems, responding to stress, 224, 238t
Endomorphy
    definition, 70
    examples of, *71*
Epigenetic sequences, 36
Epinephrine, 225
Ergotrophic reactions, to stress, 224
Erikson, Erik, *48*
    on adolescence, 45-47
    biographical information, 35-36
    on development during infancy, 36-39
    on early childhood years, 41-43
    on health values, 276
    on middle age, 48-49
    on middle childhood years, 43-45
    theories on adulthood, 48
    on toddler years, 39-41
Evaluations
    in care plans, 304-306
    of groups, *212*
    of health education programs, 260-261
    in the nursing process, 7, 22-24
    process in communication, 97
Evaluative speech, 98
Exercise, helping with stress, 274
Exhaustion, from stress, 227
Expert power, 200
Explorer roles, 207

F

Faith, and hope, 160
Families, personality development in, 71
Fear
    versus anger, 183-184
    helping clients deal with, 183
Feedback
    activated by stress, 224-228
    in communication, 95
    role of supervisors, 306
"Fight or flight" responses, 224
Fluid retention, due to stress, 225-226
Focusing techniques, in therapeutic communication,
        111-112, 113t
Freud, Sigmund, *41*
    on adolescence, 45-47
    biographical information, 34-35
    on development during infancy, 36-39
    on early childhood years, 41-43
    on middle childhood years, 43-45
    on oedipal stages of development, 41

Freud, Sigmund—cont'd
    on phallic stages of development, 41
    on psychosexual development, 34
    on toddler years, 39-41
Frustration, in stress responses, 221, *230*

G

Gagne, R.M., on stages of learning, 250-252
Gatekeeper roles, 208
General adaptation syndrome, 225-228
Genital phases, of development, 45
Glycocorticoids, responding to stress, 225
Goal setting
    in care plans, 304
    evaluating achievements in, 190
    in groups, 205
    in health education, 251
    in nurse-client contracts, 175-176
    in the nursing process, 15-16
    relationship to self-esteem, 69
Gonadotropic hormones, in stress response, 224
Government, communication with, 132-133
Grief, Kubler-Ross on, 295
Group processes, 206
Group sets, 202
Group therapy, definition, 204
Groups; *see also* self-help groups
    analyzing, *212*
    coleadership in, 204, 205t
    content *versus* process issues, 206
    decision making in, 208
    definition, 199
    goals of therapy, 204
    implications for nurses, 210-211
    phases of development, 208-210
    power in, 200-202
    problems in, 208
    roles in, 207-208
    self-help, 204-205, 264-269
    sets of, 205
    task, 199-205
    therapeutic, 203-205
    types of, 199-205
Growth patterns, in relationships, 178-179
Guerrilla fighter model, of advocacy, 263

H

Habilitation, definition, 5
Harmonizer roles, 208
Health, definition, 243, 245-246
Health belief models, 248, 249t
Health care professionals
    areas of expertise, 21t
    and the team approach, 20
Health care system
    clinical pathways within, 20
    cultural trends in, 7

Health education
    appropriate medium and materials, 255-257, 258t, 259t
    for client empowerment, 249-250
    for communication purposes, 125-126
    cost-effectiveness of, 261
    definitions, 245-246
    establishing programs in, 252-262
    evaluation of programs, 260-261
    goals of, 246-248
    implementation of, 258-261
    importance for nurses, 244-245
    obstacles to, 261-262
    planning goals and objectives, 255
    planning phases of, 253
    for the poor, 253-254
    stages of learning in, 250-252
    theories on, 248-252
Health promotion; *see also* health education
    definition, 243
Health screenings, definition and activities, 19t
Hearing; *see also* auditory systems
    impairments and communication, 121-122
Heart diseases, and stress, 234
Helper-therapy principles, 267
Holistic health care, definition and description, 273
Home health care, 275-276
Homeostasis, 289
Honesty
    in nurse-client relationships, 152
    in old age, 49
Hope
    components and dimensions of, 161
    concept of, 160-162
    correlation with relationship phases, 193t
    definition, 160
    and faith, 160
    and nursing interventions, 161, 162t
Horizontal communication, 131
Hormones, responding to stress, 224-226
Hospitals, communication within, 129-132
Hostility, responding to, 185
Human immunodeficiency virus type 1 (HIV-1), as crisis
        producer, 296
Humor, uses in relationships, 181-182
Hypertension, and stress, 234
Hypothalamus, responding to stress, 224

I

Identification, in the empathy process, 155-156
Identity; *see also* self-concept
    in healthy personality individuals, 76
    importance of sense of, 46
    and intimacy, 48
Illiteracy, 256
Illness prevention
    advocacy and, 264
    health education's role in, 243

Illness prevention—cont'd
 nursing role in, 3-6
 primary, 3-4
 promoting exercise and nutrition, 4-5
 secondary, 4
 tertiary, 5, 264
Imitations, in nonverbal communication, 88
Immediacy, in relationships, 180
Immunizations, 4
Implementation, in the nursing process, 7, 18-22
Imposed leadership, 200
Incongruent communication, 93-94
Incorporation, in the empathy process, 155-156
Infancy
 and body image, 57
 nursing communication techniques, 123
 personal self-development during, 35-39
Information seeker/giver roles, 207
Initiator roles, 207
Intellectualizer roles, 207
Interactional patterns, of communication, 100-101
Interorganizational communication, 129, *130*, 132-134
Interventions
 classification of, 19
 crisis, 288-297
 for empowerment, 165-166
 relating to hope, 161, 162t
Interviews
 communication barriers, 116-120
 conjoint, 306
 between nurse and client, 176-178
 process in assessments, 9-10
 summarizing contracts, 177-178
Intimacy phases, of group development, 209
Intraorganizational communication, 129-131
Introductory phases, of relationships, 174-178
Introjections, as a defense mechanism, 233, 234t
Invisible man/woman roles, 207
Isolation, as a defense mechanism, 233, 234t

J

Johari Windows, *56, 57*

K

Kidneys, responding to stress, 224-227
Kinesthetic systems, used in communication, 92, 93t
Kubler-Ross, on death and dying, 295

L

Laboratory training groups, 203
Laissez-faire leadership, 202
Languages; *see also* communication skills
 development of verbal skills, 83-84
 lack of common, 120-121
 research in, 83
 summary of Piaget's work, 85t

Latency stages, 44
Lead, danger in homes, 4
Leadership
 definitions and behaviors, 200-202
 democratic *versus* autocratic, 201-202
 in group therapy, 204
 model of, 201
 by nurses, 210-211
Learning theories, behavioral *versus* cognitive, 250-252
Legitimate power, 200
Leukocytosis, caused by stress, 225-226
Limbic system, responding to stress, 224
Linguistics
 research by Ebbinghaus, 83
 rules by Chomsky, 83
Listening, importance in therapeutic communication, 107-108
Liver, responding to stress, 224-227
Love; *see* caring

M

Maintenance phases, of nurse-client relationships, 178-189
Maintenance roles, 207-208
Maslow's hierarchy of human needs, 73-75
Maternalism, 163-164
Maturational crises
 and life cycles, 287
 midlife, 298
Maturational/developmental crises, 288
Media, types of, 258t, 259t
Medical diagnosis, *versus* nursing diagnosis, 11
Meditation, for stress reduction, 275
Mental imagery techniques, of stress reduction, 275
Mental ruminations, in stressful situations, 236
Mesomorphy
 definition, 70
 examples of, 71
Metacommunication, definition, 92
Middle age
 and body image, 58
 stage of development, 48-49
Midlife crises, 298
Migraine headaches, and stress, 234
Mineralocorticoids, responding to stress, 225
Monologues, 84
Mutual help groups, 265
Mutuality
 concept of, 162, 166-167
 correlation with relationship phases, 193t
 definition, 163

N

Names, importance of using, 175
Needs; *see also* assessments
 assessing informally and formally, 252-253
Negotiations, 185
Neuroendocrine systems, behaviors related to stress, 238t

Neutrality of speech, 98
Nontherapeutic communication
    problems of commission, 115-116, 117t
    problems of omission, 113-115, 117t
    techniques of, 112-116, 117t
Nonverbal communication
    with actions, 87, *88*
    and cultural sensitivity, 88-91
    definition, 86
    development of, 87-91
    functions of, 85
    gender differences in, 91
    giving meaning to, 91-92
    imitation in, 88
    in nurse-client relationships, 92
    with objects, 87, 89
    with signs, 87
    types of, 87
Noradrenalin, 225
Norepinephrine, 225
North American Nursing Diagnosis Association (NANDA)
    diagnoses classifications, 12t, 13t
    diagnostic statement composition, 11
Nurse-client relationships, 147-167
    behaviors needed in, 148-149
    caring element of, 157-160
    concept of helping in, 147-149
    concept of trust, 151-152
    confidentiality in, 177
    dealing with fear and anger, 183-184
    forming helping, 173-193
    importance of empathy in, 152-157
    importance of supervision, 306
    knowing the client, 148
    maintaining professional boundaries, 187
    nonverbal messages in, 92
    and process recordings, 302, 303t, 304t
    providing hope, 160-162
    questions to help clients, 148-149
    responding to dislike and sadness, 186-187
    responding to hostility, 185
    setting sexual limits, 188-189
    termination phase of, 189-192
    using touch, 159-160
    values clarification in, 149-150
Nursing
    acquisition of communication skills, 135-137
    advocacy role in, 164-166, 269-273
    assessment of body image, 60-61
    clarifying one's value system, 149-150
    code for, 3
    communication barriers, 116-120
    community health, 276
    crisis interventions in, 286
    cultural communication sensitivity, 88
    dealing with families in crisis, 293-294

Nursing—cont'd
    definition and description, 2-3
    education in communication skills, 81
    ethical and legal considerations of advocacy, 272-273
    evaluation of communication skills, 138
    group dynamics in, 210
    health education practices, 244-262
    helping relationships, 147-148
    holistic approaches to, 273-275
    importance of empathy in, 152-157
    importance of interpersonal relationships, 147-149
    importance of supervision, 306
    interventions of hope, 161, 162t
    knowing the client, 148
    preparing care plans, 304, 305t, 306
    prevention measures, 3-6
    primary goals, 243
    process of recording, 302, 303t, 304t
    recognizing stress, 234-236
    roles in client relationships, 176
    and self-awareness, 76-78
    strategies of hope, 161-162
    and stress reactivity, 217
    techniques to prevent crises, 291-292
    therapeutic communication, 107-112, 113t
Nursing diagnosis; *see also* diagnoses
    composition of statements, 11-12
    definition, 11
    versus medical diagnosis, 11
Nursing intervention classification system (NIC), 19
Nursing process, 1-27
    and advocacy, 269-273
    assessment phase, 7-10
    definition, 6
    diagnosis phase, 7, 10-13
    evaluation phase, 7, 22-24
    implementation phase, 7, 18-22
    importance of supervision, 306
    learning dynamics of self, 76
    models of, 9, *25, 26*
    outcome identification phase, 7, 14-16
    phases of, 7-24
    philosophical beliefs of the individual, 1-2
    planning phase, 7, 16-18
    versus problem-solving process, 6t
    recording of, 302, 303t, 304t
Nutrition
    professional areas of expertise, 21t
    and stress, 274

O

Obesity, and body image, 61
Occupational therapists, areas of expertise, 21t
Oedipal phases, of development, 41-42
Oedipus complex, 42

Old age
  and body image, 58
  development during, 49
Oral reports, 126-128
Organizational communication
  assessments of, 134-135
  "intra" *versus* "inter," 129-134
  types of, 129-137
Orientation phases; *see* introductory phases
Outcome audits, 24
Outcome identification
  nursing conditions and behaviors related to, *14*
  in the nursing process, 7, 14-16

P

Pancreas, responding to stress, 224-227
Parents, impact on child's self-esteem, 71
Parent's Creed, 71
Parroting, 114, 117t
Parry, J., on barriers to communication, 117
Passive-aggressive behaviors, 183
Paternalism, 163-164
Pattern organization
  in communication, 82, 101
  influencing nonverbal messages, *90*
Patterns, of communication, 97-101
Peer groups
  in early and middle childhood, 41-45
  in health education, 258
  providing joint supervision, 306
Penis envy, 42
Perception process, in communication, 96
Personal hygiene, 4
Personality; *see also* self
  body image effect on, 57-63
  defining healthy, 73
  and dynamics of self, 75-76
  evolution of, 72
  evolution of theories, *34*
  as a function of environment and heredity, 70
  Maslow's hierarchy of human needs, 73-75
  prenatal influences on, 70
  self-awareness models, 56-57
  and self-concept, 65
Phallic stages, of development, 41
Physical therapists, areas of expertise, 21t
Physicians, areas of expertise, 21t
Piaget, V.
  on imitation, 88
  on stages of language development, 83-84
  summary of work on language development, 85t
Pituitary gland, responding to stress, 224
Placating patterns, of communication, 98
Planning
  in the nursing process, 7, 16-18
  in therapeutic communication, 112, 113t

Play therapists, areas of expertise, 21t
Play therapy
  communication through, 124-125
  educating with, 254-255
Poisonings, 4
Poverty, and health education, 253-254
Power
  and group development, 209
  types of, 200
Preaffiliation phases, 209
Preinteraction phases, of relationships, 174
Prevention; *see* illness prevention
Primary prevention, 3-4
Priority setting, in planning stage, 17-18
Probes, 112
Problem-oriented medical records (POMR), 306
Problem-solving processes, *versus* nursing process, 6-24
Process audits, 24
Process recordings
  care plans, 304-306
  definition, 302
  methods of, 302, 303t, 304t
Projection, as a defense mechanism, 233, 234t
Promotion; *see also* health education and health promotion
  of good health and prevention, 3-4
Psychiatric emergency crises, 288
Psychiatry
  Erikson's influence on, 35-36
  Freud's influence on, 34-35
  Sullivan's influence on, 35
Psychoeducational models, for health education, 248-249
Psychologists, areas of expertise, 21t
Psychology
  and self-esteem, 69
  Sigmund Freud's principles on, 34
  use of group therapy, 204
Psychopathological crises, 288
Psychosexual development, 34-35
Psychosocial moratorium, 46
Psychotherapeutic modalities, 274

Q

Quality control; *see also* quality improvement
  evaluation of, 22-24
Quality improvement, definition and procedures, 23-24

R

Rationalization, as a defense mechanism, 232, 234t
Reaction formation techniques, as a defense mechanism, 232-233, 234t
Record keeper roles, 207
Record keeping; *see* documentation
Records; *see* process recordings
Referent power, 200
Reflecting techniques, in therapeutic communication, 110-111, 113t

Regression, as a defense mechanism, 231, 234t
Rehabilitation, definition, 5
Relating patterns, of communication, 97-98
Relational patterns, of interactional communication, 100
Relationships; *see also* nurse-client relationships
    assertiveness *versus* anger in, 184-185
    assessing within families, 294-295
    beginning assessment process in, 178
    contracts in, 175-176
    correlation with concepts and phases, 193t
    duration of, 177
    helping, 173-193
    immediacy in, 180
    introductory phases of, 174-178
    maintenance phases of, 178-189
    overall purpose of, 176-177
    phases of, 173-192
    preinteraction phase of, 174
    self-disclosure in, 180-181
    use of confrontation in, 179-180
    and use of humor, 181-182
Relaxation responses, to stress, 274
Representational systems, for communication, 92-93
Repression, as a defense mechanism, 232, 234t
Resistance
    patterns in relationships, 178-179
    to stress, 227
Restating technique, in therapeutic communication, 110, 113t
Reverberation, in the empathy process, 155-156
Reward power, 200
Rights to privacy, in nursing code, 3
Rogers, Carl, questions to ask in helping relationships, 148-149
Role ambiguity, 202
Role conflicts, 202
Role differentiation, 202
Role episodes, 202
Role overload, 202
Role sets, 202
Rule of halves, 203
Rule of thirds, 203
Rule of three quarters, 203

S

Satir, V.
    Declaration of Self-Esteem, 68
    on defensive communication, 98, 99t
    definition of communication, 82
Schemas, definition, 118
Schools
    importance in self-esteem development, 72
    nursing role in, 4
    teaching health education skills, 244
Screenings; *see also* health screenings
    for good health, 19t
    and illness prevention, 4
Secondary prevention, description of, 4

Self
    versus concept of self-ideal, 63
    definition, 33
    development during adolescence, 45-47
    development during adulthood, 47-48
    development during early childhood years, 41-43
    development during infancy, 36-39
    development during middle age, 48-49
    development during middle childhood years, 43-45
    development during old age, 49
    development during toddler years, 39-41
    dynamics of, 75-76
    emergence of, 33-51
    therapeutic use of, 55
    variables of, 56
Self-assessment, of communication skills, 136
Self-awareness
    importance for nurses, 33-34
    Johari Windows, 56, *57*
    in nurses, 76-78
    and values, 149
Self-concept
    definition, 64
    developmental changes in, 64
    in healthy personality individuals, 75-76
    nursing assessment of, 66
    personality component of, 65
Self-disclosure, in relationships, 180-181
Self-efficacy, definition, 67
Self-esteem, 35
    assessment of, 63
    and body image, 59
    as a communication barrier, 118
    declaration by Satir, 68
    definition, 66
    developmental changes in, 67-69
    evolution of, 72
    in healthy personality individuals, 76
    importance of, 66
    low, 69
    maintaining, 69
    problems in older adults, 61-62
    versus self-concept and self-ideal, 69
    versus self-ideals, 64
Self-help groups
    as advocates, 264-269
    aprofessional *versus* professional dimensions, 268
    classification of, 266t
    definition, 265
    functions of, 265-266
    interfacing with nursing, 269
    potential problems in, 268-269
    reasons for establishing, 266-267
    referral criteria, 266
    versus task groups, 204-205

Self-ideal, 63-64
    definition of, 63
    effects on personality, 63-64
    in healthy personality individuals, 75
Self-oriented roles, 207
Self-protector roles, 207
Self-worth; *see* self-esteem
Sensitivity, in defining empathy, 153
Sex education
    in schools, 4
    and self-awareness, 70
Sexuality
    between clients and nurses, 188-189
    development of, 41-47
Situational crises, caused by external events, 287
Snob roles, 207
Social engineering, 273
Social Readjustment Rating Scale, 218t
Social workers, areas of expertise, 21t
Speech
    egocentric, 84
    helping clients with impairments, 121
    types of, 98
Speech therapists, areas of expertise, 21t
Spirituality
    and dying clients, 295
    and health promotion, 277
Staff communication, 131-132
Standard setter roles, 208
Stereotypes, 174
Strategic speech, 98
Stress
    adaptation model, *239*
    adaptation to, 228-234
    and anxiety, 222-223
    behaviors related to, 238t
    and conflict, 222
    definitions, 217-219
    and frustration, 221
    holistic approaches to, 274
    in the nursing environment, 2
    physical illnesses caused by, 234, 238t
    psychophysiological responses to, 224-228
    recognizing and dealing with, 234-236
    responses to, 221-223
    self-questioning techniques, 275
    Social Readjustment Rating Scale, 218t
    types of, 220t
    using defense mechanisms, 231-234
Stress states, definition, 219-220
Stressors, definition, 218-219
Strokes, rehabilitation following, 5
Sublimation, as a defense mechanism, 231, 234t
Suicide, relationship to self-esteem, 69
Sullivan, Harry Stack, *45*
    on adolescence, 45-47
    on adulthood, 47-48

Sullivan, Harry Stack—cont'd
    biographical information, 35
    on development during infancy, 36-39
    on early childhood years, 41-43
    on middle age, 48-49
    on middle childhood years, 43-45
    model of infant self-system, *38*
    on toddler year development, 39-41
Summarizer roles, 207
Summarizing, as a therapeutic communication technique, 112, 113t
Supervision
    importance in nursing, 306
    role in evaluation process, 23
Support groups; *see* self-help groups
Support systems, in crisis situations, 294
Supporter roles, 208
Suppression, as a defense mechanism, 232, 234t
Susceptibility, to disease because of stress, 234

T

Task groups, 199-203
Task role behaviors, 207
Teachers
    areas of expertise, 21t
    and communication skills, 136-137
    importance in developing child's self-esteem, 72
Termination phases
    behavioral responses to, 190-192
    of group development, 209t, 210
    in nurse-client relationships, 189-192
Terminology
    hampering communication, 127
    in identifying outcomes, 14t, 15
    variances in word meanings, 85-86
Tertiary prevention
    and advocacy, 264
    description of, 4-5
T-groups, 203
Therapeutic communication, 107-112, 113t
    acknowledgment technique, 110, 113t
    acquiring skills, 136
    asking open-ended questions, 109, 113t
    barriers to, 116-120
    and children, 123-125
    clarification technique, 111, 113t
    definition, 107
    establishing guidelines, 109, 113t
    evaluation of, 138-141
    focusing technique, 111-112, 113t
    helping aphasic clients, 121
    helping sensory-impaired clients, 121-122
    importance of listening, 107-108
    and noncommunicative clients, 122-123
    organizational influences on, 129-135
    problems concerning common languages, 120-121
    reducing distances, 109, 113t

Therapeutic communication—cont'd
    reflecting technique, 110-111, 113t
    restating technique, 110, 113t
    self-assessment of skills, 136
    setting goals, 109, 113t
    skill acquisition handicaps, 137
    structured forms of, 125-129
    in student-teacher relationships, 136-137
    summarizing and planning techniques, 112, 113t
    techniques of, 107-112
    undesirable nursing behaviors in, 112-116, 117t
    use of silence, 108-109, 113t
Therapeutic groups, 203-205
    definition, 203-205
Thought substitution, 185
Threats, stress related, 221-222
Thyroid glands, responding to stress, 224-225
Thyrotropic hormones, in stress response, 224
Time
    and communication, 102
    and stress, 219-220
Toddlers
    and body image, 57
    personal development of, 39-41
Touch, in demonstrating caring, 159-160
Town crier roles, 207
Transmission process, in communication, 97
Traumatic stress crises, 288
Trevarthen, C., on early mother/child communication, 84
Trust
    in beginning phases of relationships, 178
    building, 152
    characteristics of, 152
    correlation with relationship phases, 193t
    definition, 151
    in nurse-client relationships, 151-152

U

Undoing techniques, as a defense mechanism, 233, 234t

V

Values
    clarification of, 149-150
    defining for health promotion, 276
    definition, 149
    in groups, 205
    steps in the clarification process, 150
Vascular dilation, due to stress, 225-226
Vasopressin, secreted due to stress, 224
Venereal diseases, prevention and education, 4
Verbal communication; *see also* communication
    development of, 83-84
    limitations of, 84-86
Vision; *see also* visual systems
    impairments and communication, 121-122
Visual systems; *see also* vision
    used in communication, 92, 93t

W

Watson, J., ten carative factors theory, 158
Weight, problems related to, 61
Wood, B.S., on language development, 83
Work groups; *see* task groups
Working phases; *see* maintenance phases
Written reports, 128-129; *see also* documentation

Y

Yes man roles, 207
Yoga, for stress reduction, 275